D1643629

INTERNATIONAL REVIEW OF
Neurobiology

VOLUME 19

INTERNATIONAL REVIEW OF

Neurobiology

Edited by CARL C. PFEIFFER

Brain Bio Center
1225 State Road
Princeton, New Jersey

JOHN R. SMYTHIES

Department of Psychiatry and the Neurosciences Program
University of Alabama Medical Center
Birmingham, Alabama

VOLUME 19

1976

ACADEMIC PRESS • New York   San Francisco   London
A Subsidiary of Harcourt Brace Jovanovich, Publishers

ACADEMIC PRESS, INC.
111 Fifth Avenue, New York, New York 10003

United Kingdom Edition published by
ACADEMIC PRESS, INC. (LONDON) LTD.
24/28 Oval Road, London NW1

LIBRARY OF CONGRESS CATALOG CARD NUMBER: 59–13822

ISBN 0–12–366819–0

PRINTED IN THE UNITED STATES OF AMERICA

CONTENTS

Octopamine and Some Related Noncatecholic Amines
in Invertebrate Nervous Systems

H. A. ROBERTSON AND A. V. JUORIO

Apomorphine: Chemistry, Pharmacology, Biochemistry

F. C. COLPAERT, W. F. M. VAN BEVER, AND J. E. M. F. LEYSEN

Thymoleptic and Neuroleptic Drug Plasma Levels
in Psychiatry: Current Status

THOMAS B. COOPER, GEORGE M. SIMPSON, AND J. HILLARY LEE

CONTRIBUTORS

Numbers in parentheses indicate the pages on which the authors' contributions begin.

F. C. COLPAERT, *Department of Pharmacology, Janssen Pharmaceutica Research Laboratories, Beerse, Belgium* (225)

THOMAS B. COOPER, *Rockland Research Institute, Orangeburg, New York* (269)

SUSAN D. IVERSEN, *Department of Experimental Psychology, University of Cambridge, Cambridge, England* (1)

A. V. JUORIO, *Psychiatric Research Unit, University Hospital, Saskatoon, Saskatchewan, Canada* (173)

ABRAHAM KARKOWSKY, *Department of Pharmacology, Mount Sinai School of Medicine of the City University of New York, New York, New York* (75)

J. HILLARY LEE, *Rockland Research Institute, Orangeburg, New York* (269)

GIULIO LEVI, *Laboratorio di Biologia Cellulare, Consiglio Nazionale delle Richerche, Roma, Italy* (51)

J. E. M. F. LEYSEN, *Department of Pharmacology, Janssen Pharmaceutica Research Laboratories, Beerse, Belgium* (225)

MARIAN ORLOWSKI, *Department of Pharmacology, Mount Sinai School of Medicine of the City University of New York, New York, New York* (75)

MAURIZIO RAITERI, *Istituto di Farmacologia, Universitá Cattolica, Roma, Italy* (51)

ARUN K. RAWAT, *Departments of Psychiatry and Biochemistry, Medical College of Ohio, Toledo, Ohio* (123)

H. A. ROBERTSON,* *Psychiatric Research Unit, University Hospital, Saskatoon, Saskatchewan, Canada* (173)

GEORGE M. SIMPSON, *Rockland Research Institute, Orangeburg, New York* (269)

W. F. M. VAN BEVER, *Department of Pharmacology, Janssen Pharmaceutica Research Laboratories, Beerse, Belgium* (225)

* Present address: University Laboratory of Physiology, Parks Road, Oxford OX1 3PT, England.

DO HIPPOCAMPAL LESIONS PRODUCE AMNESIA IN ANIMALS?

By Susan D. Iversen

Department of Experimental Psychology
University of Cambridge
Cambridge, England

I. The Effect of Hippocampal and Frontal Lesions on Memory Processes in Humans

A. STUDIES OF NORMAL HUMAN MEMORY

Within the last 10 years few areas in experimental psychology have been as active as that relating to the study of the processes involved in human memory. Not surprisingly, this amount of experimentation has generated a number of competing theories. To grossly oversimplify the situation, these broadly speaking fall into two categories: first, theories proposing that

1

human memory is best described by a two-process model (Broadbent, 1958; Norman, 1969; Atkinson and Shiffrin, 1968), and second, theories proposing that a single-process model can account for the facts (Keppel and Underwood, 1962; Melton, 1963).

In their simplest form two-process models suggest that information is initially processed by short-term or primary memory before being handled by long-term or secondary memory which achieves permanent storage. The storage and retrieval properties of the two memory processes are determined by putting information into the system, extracting it, and studying its condition at various times after entry. While the different properties of the two "boxes" have been described, the relationships between them remain obscure. Much evidence supports the two-process position, which has encouraged casual observers to undermine the importance of the observations of unitary process theorists. Under certain testing conditions (par excellence, verbal paired-associate learning) information appears to be assimilated and handled from then on by a single memory process. The nature of the forgetting shortly after and long after acquisition suggests that the information has been handled by a single process in which interference provides the most important threat to consolidation.

If one adds together all this fact and controversy, it seems possible to preach parsimony. Serial two-process models themselves are already under pressure in that under certain circumstances information appears to reach long-term memory without being processed by short-term memory. Warrington and Shallice (1969) studied a patient with a unilateral lesion in the left parieto-preoccipital region, who has a reduced digit span (considered a prime test for short-term memory) and yet is able to form memories of current events. They therefore propose that under certain circumstances there must be direct input to long-term memory or, in other words, handling by short-term memory is not a prerequisite for long-term storage. Much experimental evidence can be cited which casts doubt on one or another aspect of these three models of memory processing. This cursory view by no means considers all the models with some degree of current favor, and in view of all the evidence, the majority of which appears experimentally valid, one is tempted to ask if it is even reasonable to suppose that any one model of memory will be vindicated. Memory, after all, is a ubiquitous faculty, and it would not be the least surprising to find that it is mediated by a variety of information-handling processes brought into action in a variety of different ways, depending on the nature and amount of information to be memorized and the conditions under which it is assimilated.

A summary of our current synthesis of human memory and the neurological processes underlying it is as follows.

In humans short- and long-term memory processes can be distinguished by their properties. Time is irrelevant in determining whether or not one or another of these processes handles the information. What is relevant is the nature of the information to be stored, its amount, and the conditions under which it is presented.

There are conditions under which short-term memory is not required. If subspan amounts of information are handled and stored, there is no obvious reason why the particular properties of short-term memory should be required or indeed invoked. Long-term memory in such circumstances may well be initiated at the time of reception of the information. Drachman and Arbit (1966) point out that this could well explain why Melton (1963) reports that recall of subspan items decays with the passage of time in the same manner as that of supraspan items. Melton supposes that with subspan items he is studying short-term memory, but in fact short-term memory may not be involved with such items. Sub- and supraspan items are therefore both handled by long-term memory, and it is not surprising to find that forgetting under both conditions can be explained in the same manner. Large amounts of information presented rapidly create the best conditions for guaranteeing that short-term memory is operating and that its operation is a prerequisite for long-term storage to be effective. Language is probably the best natural stimulator of this process. However, because of its nature, language creates an additional source of information to be stored—*order*. Here lies the source of probably one of the greatest pressures on human memory. Language involves the memory of unique sequences of events, i.e., of words or phonemes, which are *not* in themselves unique. Thus interference is maximal.

Memory in humans is not exclusively verbal, but it is clear that language, despite the pressures it creates, provides a highly economical coding process which is favored. In this sense something akin to the classical two-process model of memory may operate for a great deal of the time in the human information processor. A seven-digit telephone number presented in the midst of competing information may depend heavily on the efficiency of short-term processing for its salvation. The same number sequence presented in relative isolation may be handled in quite a different way, perhaps by a process that acquires information and progressively strengthens over time.

The burden of this introduction is not to be viewed as a synthesis of human memory theories, but merely as the puzzled reflections of an animal psychologist who ponders the processes of human memory when attempting to study similar processes in animals. If we could be convinced of the validity of one model rather than another and its peculiarities in relation to the information-processing demands on humans, it would be possible to develop more rational tests of animal memory in a determined effort to define similarities or differences between mnemonic processes in humans and in animals.

B. Memory Disorders Associated with Temporal and Frontal Lobe Lesions in Humans

Turning to the neuropsychological evidence, one may ask if lesions of the brain selectively impair the cardinal facets of memory processing which have been described, notably the ability to retain information and the order of information in supraspan items. Positive results of this kind would greatly strengthen the validity of two-process models of memory.

1. *Memory Deficits Associated with Temporal Lobe Damage in Humans*

In the mid-1950s two series of neurosurgical patients who had sustained radical lesions to the medial temporal lobe became available for psychological study. Quickly it became apparent that severe and global amnesia could result from such a surgical procedure. The amnesia was characterized by intact memory for remote events which had occurred before surgery, unimpaired ability to repeat short lists of numbers immediately after presentation, but a total inability to commit to permanent memory any recent events. One series of patients was operated on at the Montreal Neurological Institute for the relief of epilepsy associated with focal damage in the medial temporal limbic structures of one hemisphere (Penfield and Milner, 1958). In some of these patients it was subsequently discovered that there was abnormal function in the remaining medial temporal region, therefore, functionally speaking, a bilateral lesion. In the other series of patients the surgery was more radical, involving bilateral medial temporal removal; the extent of the removal is illustrated in Fig. 1. This procedure was investigated by Scoville for the treatment of psychosis when all more conservative forms of treatment have failed. However, included in this series was one young epileptic patient, usually referred to in the literature as H.M. and, although Scoville and Milner (1957) found evidence of amnesia in eight of the psychotic patients who sustained similar medial temporal lesions, the amnesic defect in H.M. remains the most severe recorded in the literature. This patient has been assessed regularly, and there has been virtually no improvement in his mnemonic capacity over more than 20 years, despite the fact that the operation produced no decrement in his intelligence quotient. It has gradually become accepted that bilateral damage to the hippocampus is responsible for the global amnesia seen in such patients. In the Scoville surgical series some patients sustained bilateral lesions localized to the amygdala and uncus, and memory deficits were not seen in these patients (Scoville and Milner, 1957). Second, the existence of bilateral damage to the hippocampus was inferred in the Montreal patients, who had originally sustained unilateral lesions, on the basis of abnormal encephalographic activity in the remaining temporal lobe. Recently, one of these patients

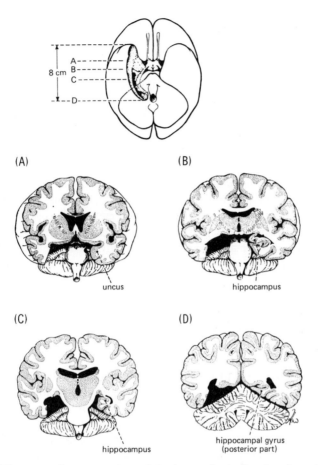

Fɪɢ. 1. Diagrammatic cross sections of the human brain showing the estimated extent of removal in Scoville's medial temporal lobe ablation. All operations were bilateral, single-stage procedures but here, for illustrative purposes, one side has been left intact. (From Milner, 1959.) The letters A–D refer to brain sections from different parts of the temporal lobe; A being the most anterior and D the most posterior as indicated in the ventral brain view at the top.

with a unilateral temporal lobe lesion died, and it was confirmed at post-mortem that the remaining hippocampus was structurally abnormal (Milner, 1970). It is therefore generally agreed that bilateral hippocampal damage severely impedes the ability to form permanent memories.

It should not be supposed that a role for the temporal lobe in memory had not been suspected before the 1950s. In 1900 Bekhterev described a striking memory defect in a patient who at autopsy showed softening of the medial temporal structures. Isolated case reports appeared in the literature over the next 50 years (Terzian, 1958), but it has been the extensive study of H.M. by Milner that has produced the single most conclusive body of evidence on hippocampal involvement in memory. Her observations have reawakened interest in the study of the neurological processes involved in memory storage and in the study of amnesia as a window on the processes of normal memory.

a. Characteristics of Amnesia after Bilateral Medial Temporal Damage. The informal clinical description of H.M. provides as clear a picture as any of the extent and severity of the amnesia associated with bilateral medial temporal damage. His ability to repeat lists of digits is normal, and he can remember a three-figure number or pair of words for many minutes, in fact until he is distracted by another event. He is capable of considerable mental agility, and Milner (1970) describes how on one occasion he was asked to remember the number 584. After sitting quietly for 15 minutes he correctly recalled the number and, when asked how he did it, said, "Its easy. You just remember 8. You see, 5, 8, and 4 add to 17. You remember 8; subtract it from 17 and it leaves 9. Divide 9 in half and you get 5 and 4, and there you are: 584. Easy." Immediately afterward he was quite unable to remember 584, or the train of thought. In a more practical vein his mother reports that he reads the same magazine time and time again without apparent familiarity, and cannot learn where household items are stored despite repeated use. In addition to such informal observations. H.M. has been tested on a wide range of experimental tasks designed to define his mnemonic capacity more precisely. It is now clear that, despite intact perceptual capabilities, H.M. cannot remember verbal or nonverbal stimuli in the auditory, visual, or tactile modality. Information is held for as long as verbal rehearsal allows. However, since under normal conditions rehearsal is prevented or impaired by the normal processes of shifting attention and interference, the severity of H.M.'s deficit can be easily appreciated. The nature of his disability has also been illustrated by Prisko's (1963) study using the delayed paired-comparison task (reviewed in Milner, 1970).

In this procedure, two stimuli in the same sensory modality are presented successively with a short delay. The subject is asked to say whether the stimuli were the same or different. An impression of the first stimulus must be retained in order to compare it with the second one. Task difficulty is varied by increasing the interstimulus delay or by introducing a distraction before the second stimulus. Prisko used five kinds of stimuli: tones, shades of red, nonsense patterns, and rate of presentation of clicks and light flashes. There were at least five stimuli in each category in order to prevent easy verbalization. On this task normal subjects perform virtually perfectly with 60-second delays and distraction. H.M. does the same with zero delay, but his performance deteriorates rapidly toward chance level at 60-second delays. Sidman *et al.* (1968) recently confirmed these findings on H.M., using a matching-to-sample technique. The test required the subject to indicate which of eight ellipses matched a sample ellipse presented immediately or several seconds before. Simultaneous matching was perfect in H.M., again indicating intact perceptual discrimination, but with delays of 5 seconds or more he could no longer match accurately (Fig. 2). Interestingly, however, when verbal stimuli were used (trigrams), his matching performance was excellent at a 40-second delay. Presumably, verbal rehearsal permitted this improvement, as H.M. could be observed mouthing the stimuli during the delays.

It is sometimes suggested that the severity of the amnesia seen in H.M. and other Montreal cases relates to its particular etiology. These were epileptic patients of several years standing at time of surgery, and it has been

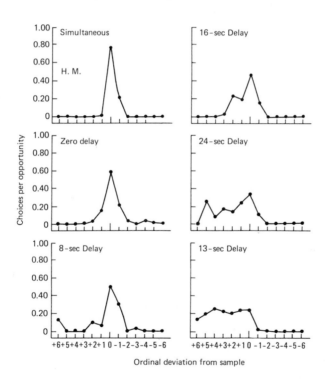

FIG. 2. Gradient of stimulus control in circle-ellipse discrimination in H.M. Responses are plotted against stimulus values which differ progressively from the cue stimulus. Stimulus control is perfect when cue and choice stimuli are presented simultaneously but deteriorates rapidly as the matching delay increases to 32 seconds. (From Sidman *et al.*, 1968.)

suggested that their brains were functionally abnormal, on account of the chronic epilepsy, before surgery was undertaken. However, cases are found in the literature in which acute encephalitis results in a pattern of antero-grade amnesia very similar to that seen in H.M. One such case has been described by Starr and Phillips (1970), in which residual temporal lobe pathology can be inferred on the basis of pneumoencephalographic evidence showing enlargement of the third and lateral ventricles, and disproportion-ate dilation of the temporal horn bilaterally. Several patients of the uni-lateral temporal lobectomy series of Penfield have been assessed on the same tests (Penfield and Milner, 1958), although none has been as extensively tested at H.M. With the more recent use of the sodium amytal test, uni-lateral temporal lobectomy is now less likely to have such irreparable effects. The anesthetic barbiturate sodium amytal is injected into one carotid artery and anesthetizes the ipsilateral cerebral hemisphere. The functional condi-tion of the unaffected hemisphere can then be assessed, and its role in language functions determined. At a subsequent time the other carotid is injected, and the procedure repeated. When the abnormal hemisphere is made temporarily nonfunctional, the ability of the remaining hemisphere to maintain function can be evaluated. With such a procedure, it is possible to detect minimal dysfunction in an apparently normal hemisphere and to avoid the subsequent development of bilateral temporal dysfunction after a unilateral lesion.

b. Characteristics of Amnesia after Unilateral (Left or Right) Temporal Lobe Damage. Milner (1971) reports that the verbal memory defects seen in H.M. are associated with left temporal lobe damage (in normal right-handed patients) and the mnemonic difficulty with nonverbal material with equivalent right temporal lobe damage. Thus left temporal lobectomy, in the hemisphere dominant for speech, selectively impairs verbal memory (Meyer and Yates, 1955; Milner, 1958), regardless of whether the material to be retained is heard or read (Blakemore and Falconer, 1967; Milner, 1967), and regardless of whether retention is tested by recall or recognition (Milner, 1958; Milner and Kimura, 1964; Milner and Teuber, 1968). In contrast, removal of the right, nondominant, temporal lobe similarly im-pairs memory for complex visual and auditory patterns, to which a name cannot be readily given (Kimura, 1963; Prisko, 1963; Milner, 1968; Shank-weiler, 1966; Warrington and James, 1967). Visually (Milner, 1965) or proprioceptively (Corkin, 1965) guided maze learning is also impaired by this lesion. It must be said that this idea of the dissociation of verbal and nonverbal functions to opposite hemispheres is under considerable pressure. This is not because of any doubt that the left hemisphere is concerned with language, but reflects concern that we do not adequately understand the full range of conditions that predispose to verbal coding. A word is a word. But when does a line drawing of a common object cease to be a visual perceptual event and become a word? We are only just beginning to recognize that we know very little about such coding mechanisms. In recent years at the Montreal Neurological Institute, series of patients with right or left temporal lobe lesions, which involve the hippocampus to a varying degree, have become available for study. The role of the hippocampus in producing these more selective amnesias has recently been evaluated by Corsi (reviewed in Milner, 1970, 1971), who has correlated the extent of hippocampal involvement in a series of left and right temporal lobectomy patients with their mnemonic performance on equivalent verbal and nonverbal tests.

In one series of experiments Corsi compared the ability of patients with a left or right temporal lobectomy to recall a group of three consonants or to reproduce the positions of a circle drawn on an 8-inch line, after a short delay occupied with counting. A modified Peterson and Peterson technique was used to vary the duration of the distracting verbal activity interpolated between acquisition and recall. With the verbal task, left temporal lesions produced impairment (Fig. 3), which became more severe when the hippo-

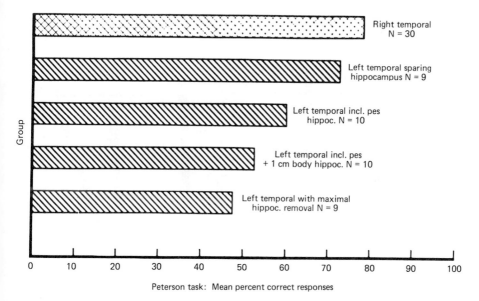

FIG. 3. Verbal memory defect after left temporal lobectomy as related to medial extent of temporal lobe resection. These data for the Peterson task show the progressive reduction in the mean number of consonant trigrams correctly recalled with increasing destruction of the left hippocampus. No impairment is seen after right temporal lobectomy, regardless of whether or not the hippocampus was excised. (From Milner, 1970.)

campus was included in the lesion. With the line position task, a similar correlation with extent of lesion was found after right temporal lobectomy.

Corsi pursued these findings by studying learning situations that extend over several trials in tasks modeled on the recurring digit sequence task described by Hebb in 1961. Strings of unrelated digits, exceeding the subject's immediate memory span by one digit, are presented for immediate recall. Unknown to the subject, the same sequence occurs every third trial. Subjects show cumulative learning of the recurring sequence despite interpolated activity and without any appreciation of the fact that one sequence recurs.

Corsi reports that patients with left temporal lesions involving the hippocampus perform very badly on his task and do not learn the recurring sequence. He constructed a nonverbal analog in which blocks in a spatial array were tapped in a certain order (Fig. 4), the length of the sequence of taps again being one greater than the measured span for the subject. The same spatial array was repeated every third trial, and a relationship found between memory for this sequence and the degree of hippocampal involvement in right temporal lobectomies.

    c. The Nature of Temporal Lobe Amnesia. Not surprisingly, the amnesia seen in H.M. is cited by theorists as evidence for a two-process model. As

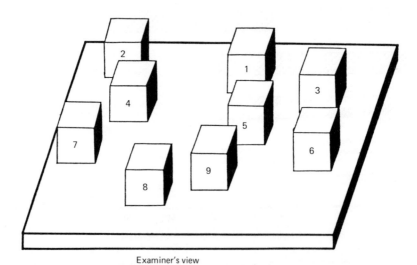

Examiner's view

Fig. 4. Corsi's block-tapping test. Sketch showing the approximate position of the nine black blocks (1¼-inch) on a black board (8 × 10 inches). The blocks are numbered on the examiner's side for ease in recording performance, but the numbers are not visible to the subject.

we have seen, memories of long standing remain relatively intact in this patient, despite an inability to form new permanent memories of recent events. Yet recent events, as they occur, are clearly perceived and held at least temporarily in short-term memory. However, as soon as the load on short-term holding requires transfer of the current information to long-term memory in order to allow assimilation of the next input, the impairment becomes apparent. In patients like H.M. information committed to memory is found to be unobtainable at a subsequent time. Clearly it is difficult to determine at precisely which stage the information was lost, or indeed to know if there is only a single defective node in the memory-processing circuit. For several years, workers had been struck by the power of interfering stimuli to disrupt the ability of H.M. to hold new information. An interpretation of the amnesia was thus proposed in terms of deficient short-to-long transfer due to the need to handle successive interfering signals.

However, Warrington and Weiskrantz (1970) have been impressed with the surprisingly good retention shown by amnesiacs under certain testing conditions. With some ingenious tests they have endeavored to examine the state of the amnesiac's engram at the time of retrieval. Somewhat surprisingly, they found that under some of their testing conditions it could be shown that in amnesiacs information is stored normally in long-term memory but that it is not retrievable when memory is tested with traditional methods, such as recall. If, however, cues are provided at the time of retrieval, retention is much improved. This indicates, it is suggested, that storage in fact occurs in amnesiacs, but that retrieval is impaired. When interference levels are high at the retrieval stage, memory loss is seen but, when reduced as with partial information procedures, retention is improved (Warrington and Weiskrantz, 1972).

2. Characteristics of Amnesia Associated with Frontal Lobe Lesions

Are any other features of memory performance selectively impaired by local brain damage? In humans it seems probable that the frontal lobe has acquired a special role in certain aspects of information processing, although it is not yet clear whether or not these properties relate in any clear way to one or another of the memory components of the two-process models.

Milner (1963) has reported that patients with lesions in the dorsolateral frontal areas are severely impaired on the Wisconsin Card Sorting Test. The test material as it appears to the subject is shown in Fig. 5. Four sample cards are displayed, differing in color, form, and number. The subject is given a pile of 128 response cards which vary along these dimensions. The subject is told to place each card in front of one of the four stimulus cards, wherever he thinks it should go, and is told the examiner will then inform

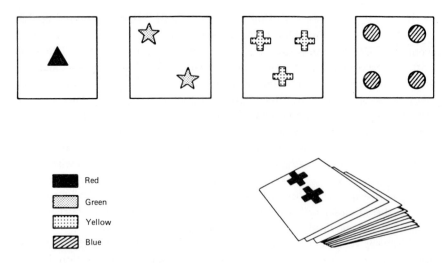

Fig. 5. Wisconsin Card Sorting Test, showing the material as presented to the subject. (From Milner, 1963.)

him whether he is right or wrong. He is told to get as many right as possible. In other words, he has to find out the sorting category required by noting his errors and modifying his strategy accordingly. The sorting categories are arbitrarily arranged as color, form, number, color, form, number. The subject is initially required to sort for color and, when 10 consecutive correct responses have been made, the required sorting shifts to form, and then to number, color, form, and number to complete the six required categories. Patients with posterior cortical lesions achieve almost 5 sorting categories, whereas frontal patients record a mean average of 1.4 categories. Their impairment is characterized by a failure to shift from one sorting category to another. Their apparent perseveration may be a consequence rather than a cause of the impairment and may reflect displacement activity associated with the basic cognitive disorder.

More recently, Corsi (reviewed in Milner, 1971) has described an interesting experimental procedure for evaluating the ability to remember the relative order of preceding events—the so-called recency test. This is prepared with verbal (words) and nonverbal (abstract art pictures) material. In the verbal form of the test the subject is presented with a pile of 184 cards each bearing two words (e.g., cowboy, railroad). He reads the words aloud and then turns to the next card. Periodically a test card appears with a large question mark between the two words, and the subject must indicate which of the words on the test card he has seen most recently. For example, one of them may have been on the card three back and the other on the card eight back. Usually both the words have appeared before, but in the limiting condition one of the words is new. The task then reduces to a simple test of recognition, with the subject merely indicating which of the words he has seen before. Corsi found that patients with left frontal lesions showed excellent recognition memory, although they were significantly impaired when asked to judge "when" they had seen these familiar stimuli. In other words, they remember past experiences but not when they occurred relative to each other. Successful performance on long multichoice mazes also demands an ability to plan a sequence of responses, each of which is determined to some extent by the consequences of previous responses. Frontal patients are severely impaired on visually (Milner, 1965) and tactually (Corkin, 1965) guided maze learning. Further support for the idea that the frontal lobe is important in the coding of sequences comes from the work of Prisko on a delayed paired-comparison task (described in Section I, B, 1, a). Every stimulus must be retained as a unique event, and yet the stimuli themselves are far from unique. They are a small group of easily confused stimuli which occur repeatedly. On any particular trial, success depends on recording the event in relation to those that have gone shortly before, in other words, comparing it with the immediately preceding event and not with the one presented two or three trials earlier. Prisko found frontal patients to be impaired on this task when clicks, flashes, tones, and color stimuli were used. Interestingly enough, when nonsense figures were used, frontal patients performed as well as normal controls. In this subtest a unique pair of stimuli was used on each trial, and it seems likely that with this degree of novelty frontal impairment is overcome. Kimura (1963) presented similar nonsense figures on a recurring figure recognition test and found frontal patients to be as severely impaired as right temporal lobe cases. On this particular test a small number of figures are repeatedly presented intermingled with other stimuli which occur only once. The subject is required to recognize the repeating figures. Thus the repetition of familiar stimuli appears to pose a particular mnemonic problem for the frontal patient.

These are highly selective impairments and suggest that the information in the stimuli and the information about relationships between various of these stimuli are preferentially handled in different parts of the brain. Yet clearly, for efficient memory, these different processing mechanisms must work in harmony. Because these processes of necessity operate together, it is difficult to design tests that will tease apart the various facets of memory processing.

There is a common feature of the tasks described that frontal patients fail. A limited number of stimuli are combined in a variety of ways to provide unique events—but the constituents of these events have no meaning out of context. In other words, identifying a given event is inadequate for

the solution. A particular event achieves a unique identity only by comparison with previous events. It was suggested earlier that the coding of
order seem to be an important corollary of efficient short-term memory.
But it is not at all clear how order is imposed on stream-of-consciousness
experience and coded. Yntema and Trask (1963), for example, have discussed the possibility that time tagging could contribute to this particular
requirement. These impairments need further analysis, but it seems that in
humans the frontal lobe plays a special role in such processes. Patients with
frontal damage are often said to be unable to plan their behavior, to have
difficulty in seeing the relationship between events and the consequences of
responses to these events. Their behavior in more formal testing situations
is consistent with such a hypothesis.

3. *Summary of the Clinical Findings and Their Implications for Animal Studies*

On the basis of the clinical evidence it can be suggested that the medial
temporal structures are crucial to the organization of information required
for successful storage and retrieval. The frontal lobe appears to contribute
to a specialized aspect of this process related to the coding of order.

With reference to neuropsychological studies on animals, the picture is
at first sight by no means as clear. It is generally accepted, and has been for
almost 40 years, that bilateral frontal lesions in the monkey result in difficulty in retaining a brief spatial event, despite an intact ability to remember
difficult discriminations for long periods of time. Jacobsen originally suggested that in some sense this is an immediate memory impairment (see
Iversen, 1972, for review).

However, the search for temporal lobe amnesia in animals has been a
more pessimistic task. Indeed, within the last few years several authorities
have proposed that failure to find such impairments after hippocampal
lesions indicates that the temporal lobe of infrahuman species does not
serve a role in memory processing that can be compared with that observed in humans. In this respect cognitive discontinuity is considered to
exist between monkeys and humans. Many experiments have been performed
on hippocampal lesioned animals, but relatively few of them have been on
monkeys. Theorists have in some cases given only cursory consideration to
the results in this species before concluding that nothing closely resembling
clinical amnesia is seen after hippocampal lesions in animals.

This we feel is an unnecessarily pessimistic view. With the benefit of
more recent electrophysiological, anatomical, and neuropsychological results than were available to the reviewer of the mid-1960s, and with emphasis on the results obtained with monkeys rather than with rats, we plead

for at least a degree of parsimony in hippocampal function. It is clearly that verbal coding has come to dominate human memory function, and it would therefore be foolish not to expect quantitative and qualitative differences in memory performance between the nonverbal animals and humans. The question is whether or not the hippocampus of both animals and humans fulfills a fundamental neurological process common to mnemonic function. The examination of this question has been prefaced by consideration of the processes of normal human memory. Theories pertaining to these processes are derived from experiments on normal human subjects and, if they are valid, disorders of human memory will be identified and clarified within such a framework. Furthermore, the experimental criteria for demonstrating these facets of human memory provide useful guidelines in developing equivalent tests for animals and should be heeded if the search for parsimony is to be attempted.

II. Do Animals Remember and Forget?

Now let us turn to animals, particularly to subhuman primates, to ask:
1. Do they show the same mnemonic processes as humans?
2. Do medial temporal lesions in monkeys produce comparable memory deficits?
3. Do frontal lesions in monkeys produce specific memory deficits?

A. Studies of Memory Processes in Normal Animals

It is clear that the first kind of information is a logical prerequisite for meaningful experiments relating to questions 2 and 3. What is surprising is that in fact very little attention has been given to this basic question. This may explain the currently popular view that there is a basic discontinuity between human and monkey regarding mnemonic processes in general and the role of the hippocampus in such functions in particular. The fact that monkeys with bilateral hippocampal damage are able to learn and remember simultaneous visual discrimination problems is cited as evidence that no memory impairment exists in them. However, until it is clear that visual discrimination learning involves the kind of mnemonic processing we have seen in humans after medial temporal lesions, it is premature to accept the task as a crucial test of memory function in the monkey. What then are the natural demands on the monkey's memory? And when does it appear to use this faculty? The learning commonly studied in laboratory animals is associative learning based on repeated trials or, in other words, habit learning. It is quite apparent from many studies that bilateral medial temporal damage does not impair such learning in the monkey, even when distracting stimuli occupy the intertrial intervals (Orbach *et al.*, 1960).

It is thought that simple associative learning of this kind puts very little pressure on the kind of dynamic information-handling processes envisaged to transfer input from temporary to permanent storage. In everyday human learning there are no strict counterparts of discrimination tasks in which the same piece of information is repeated *ad nauseam*. In humans, motor learning perhaps comes closest to this, and it is widely accepted by human memory theorists that motor memory has properties different from those of verbal memory (Bilodeau *et al.*, 1962; Posner, 1966; Posner and Konick, 1966). It is, for example, not interference-sensitive. Motor learning in humans and discrimination learning in animals may therefore be rather similar.

In this context it is interesting to note that one of the features of H.M's amnesia is his *intact* ability to learn and remember simple motor acts (Corkin, 1968), including short visual and tactual mazes (Milner *et al.*, 1968). More recently, Gaffan (1972) tested one of the amnesiacs from the Warrington and Weiskrantz studies and found, in strict agreement with the results on hippocampal monkeys, that the patient was able to learn visual discrimination tasks presented on repeated trials. A round, white tray had three inverted cups on it. In the middle was a white cup with a black rubber stopper under it. In front of the white cup there were two more cups, one orange and one blue; on successive trials their positions were varied. There was nothing under the orange cup, but under the blue cup there was always a black rubber stopper similar to the one under the white cup. On each trial the tray was placed in front of the subject, the white cup was then displaced to reveal the stopper, and the instructions were, "Under this white cup there is a black stopper; there is another black stopper under one of the other two cups, and I want you to try to tell me which one has the other black stopper under it." On the first day, trials were given at 30-second intervals, which were filled with a distracting task (adding 1 to a number). The discrimination was taught to a criterion of 9 correct out of 10 consecutive responses, which the subject attained in 19 trials. A second pattern discrimination was learned in 2 trials. The day after, the blue-orange task was retested for 5 trials with 10-minute intertrial intervals occupied with distracting tasks. Gaffan reports that the subject said she had never seen the experimenter or the apparatus before and that she did not know where the stopper was hidden. Yet on being asked to choose one of the cups she selected the blue one on all five trials.

If we consider the kinds of tasks on which amnesic patients are impaired it is clear that to find the equivalent in the monkey we must seek tasks in which the animal has to remember sequences of events that are easily confused with each other. When the monkey literature is examined, few tasks of this kind are found and, when they are, one finds that monkeys can be trained on them only with the greatest difficulty. This suggests that monkeys find it difficult to use the particular mnemonic strategies that would interest us. The reasons for this are unclear. Perhaps they do not have the appropriate cognitive ability sufficiently well developed. Maybe they have a very strong tendency to use associative learning processes, which may not be sufficient for certain learning tasks and yet divert the animals from more appropriate mnemonic strategies. There is some evidence for both of these suggestions. When one tests a person's memory, one explains what must be done in the task. For example, in the Konorski paired-comparison test one explains that the significance of the pairs of stimuli to be presented lies in their similarity or dissimilarity. This is the only significance. Their duration, the particular features of the stimuli, and so on, are all irrelevant and must be ignored for successful performance. One is in fact teaching a concept. With a concept nonuniqueness acquires uniqueness or, in other words, an event can be remembered by reference to the rule rather than by its own nature. This is clearly a highly economical cognitive strategy resulting in drastic reductions in the amount of information that must be processed by the nervous system.

There are two studies on chimpanzees which indicate that, even when a concept can be learned to ease the burden of information transmission, it is not. The animal apparently prefers to remember particular responses to particular stimuli.

In 1961 Rholes reported that chimpanzees could be trained on a series of 18 visual oddity problems. They faced three panels with levers below them and were required to press the lever under the odd stimulus of the three. They were originally reinforced for each correct discrimination, but gradually a fixed-ratio requirement was introduced and they were required to make 19 correct responses for each reinforcement. The output of correct oddity responses increased with no loss of accuracy. However, it was noted that the animals often looked away from the panel as they executed the correct sequence of responses. Rholes suggested that they had not bothered to learn on the basis of oddity but had acquired an ordered sequence of 18 responses to the array of levers. They could execute this skilled motor sequence in the absence of stimulus control. Working with chimpanzees and the same apparatus, Farrer (1967) studied matching to sample of forms. After preliminary matching-to-sample training, 24 oddity problems were learned (Fig. 6) successfully. The animals were then retrained on the series without the cue stimulus being presented, i.e., on problem 1 the four matching stimuli were not preceded by the presentation of the X cue. The accuracy

PROBLEM NO.	PICTURES				CORRECT POSITION
	Lever-1	Lever-2	Lever-3	Lever-4	
1	+	ⓖ	|	×	4
2	▲	—	▢	◎	2
3	ⓖ	ⓦ	+	×	3
4	ⓑ	—	ⓡ	▢	1
5	ⓖ	▲	—	×	2
6	+	×	ⓡ	ⓑ	4
7	|	ⓖ	ⓦ	▲	3
8	|	ⓖ	—	◎	1
9	+	◎	ⓞⓡ	×	3
10	▲	▢	|	×	2
11	ⓦ	◎	ⓑ	|	4
12	◎	ⓞⓡ	▢	—	1
13	ⓞⓡ	ⓦ	—	ⓖ	1
14	×	▢	○	ⓡ	2
15	ⓡ	—	+	▢	3
16	▲	ⓖ	|	ⓡ	4
17	×	▢	◎	ⓑ	3
18	ⓑ	|	×	—	4
19	ⓑ	+	▢	—	1
20	+	ⓖ	|	ⓑ	2
21	×	ⓦ	—	ⓑ	2
22	▲	×	ⓖ	ⓡ	1
23	▢	ⓑ	×	|	3
24	▲	—	▢	ⓡ	4

FIG. 6. The 24 problems used in the picture memory test. The position of the stimuli and the correct stimulus are indicated for each problem. (Reprinted with permission of author and publisher from: Farrer, D. N. Picture memory in the chimpanzee. *Perceptual and Motor Skills*, 1967, **25**, 305–315.)

of matching was maintained. The series was also repeated with the four matching stimuli presented in mirror-image positions (i.e., problem 1: +, green disk, 1, X being reversed to X, 1, green disk, +). This did not disrupt the matching performance, indicating that, unlike the animals in Rhole's study, these animals had not learned a series of positioned responses. The only manipulation that disrupted performance was the progressive withdrawal of the negative cues in the problems, which indicated that the animals had learned the problems as constellations of visual forms; accordingly, Farrer entitled his article "Picture Memory in the Chimpanzee."

These results come very close to something like memory for pictures, which is a remarkably well-developed memory faculty in humans (Shepard, 1967). What is unclear is the generality of this picture memory in the chimpanzee. The memory of problem 1 in humans generalizes across methods of retrieval, ways of presenting the stimuli, particularly the nature of the stimuli, and so on. But it seems, from the results obtained when the matching stimuli were reduced in number, that this is not so in the chimpanzee. Memory is very closely tied to that specific stimulus array or, in other words, abstraction did not occur.

In humans verbal mediation plays a large role in memory function when complex information is remembered, regardless of whether the information is essentially verbal or not. Thus the discontinuity between humans and monkeys is likely to show itself dramatically when complex sensory arrays are to be remembered.

Are monkeys closer to humans in any other aspect of their mnemonic performance? There is reason for believing that spatial information is handled in different ways than verbal information. It is therefore possible that, if animals show any mnemonic capacity comparable to that in humans, one should study tasks in which the material to be remembered can be handled in a similar way by both species. This approach has a long and well-established experimental history. When considering the behavior of rats, Tolman (1948) emphasized that the cognitive strategy of choice was concerned with spatial information about events rather than with the events themselves or the responses to them. Rats appear readily to form maps in their heads or spatial memories. This extensive classical literature need not concern us, but recently impressive data of the same kind have been obtained in chimpanzees under virtually natural conditions.

Menzel (1973) describes experiments involving six wild-born chimpanzees now in captivity at the Delta Regional Primate Center in Louisiana. A particular chimpanzee was carried around a field by the experimenter to 18 randomly selected sectors of the field. At each of these sites an accompanying person hid a piece of fruit. The chimpanzee was then returned to the communal cage at the periphery of the field. Ten minutes later, by remote control, all six animals were released into the field, and their movements observed from a tower. Thus five of the animals who had not observed the baiting acted as controls to see if the food could be found by cues other than visual memory. Rarely did these animals find food. However, the test animals usually ran unerringly and in a direct line to the exact clump of grass or leaves, tree stump, or hole in the ground where hidden food lay, grabbed the food, stopped briefly to eat, and then ran directly to the next place, no matter how distant or obscured by visual barriers that place was.

Test animals retrieved the food on a route which proceeded more or less in accordance with a "least distance" principle with no regard for the path along which the experimenter had carried them. Subsequent tests revealed that the chimpanzee also remembered the kind of food hidden at a certain site and which sides of the field contained the greatest number of rewards. The route was altered to take account of this information (preferred site being visited first), but remained ordered and economical. Chimpanzees appeared to perceive directly the relative positions of selected classes of objects and their own position in this selected frame of reference. Menzel wrote, "One is struck again by the parallels between chimpanzee and normal behavior, the necessity for including *representational* processes in any adequate formulation of learning and memory and the apparent evolutionary independence of representational ability and verbal language."

Except possibly in the spatial mode, then, monkeys dislike using concepts and appear to prefer to learn habits. This has been beautifully summed up by Meyer (1971): "Monkeys learn concepts and this affects the way that monkeys learn discrimination habits. Monkeys learn habits, and if they retain them, they fail to make use of their concepts. Thus, a trained monkey is a cognitive machine, but, like human cognitive machines, employs ideas only if a problem it must solve cannot be solved in any other manner." Thus while long-term consolidation processes appear to be utilized by monkeys, there seems to be little demand on short-term processes, either as an information buffer (because information is not handled sufficiently quickly or in sufficient quantity) or as an order processor. Only as far as spatial information goes does the monkey appear to pressure its mnemonic capabilities, and then one can see behavior that apparently demands the coding of a *sequence* of *unique* events—spatial ones. The work of Rholes and Menzel described earlier illustrates this kind of learning. These interesting behaviors have not been studied in rhesus monkeys nor, to the best of our knowledge, are the effects of frontal and temporal lesions on such behavior known.

Possibly, monkeys do have the cognitive abilities required for short-term–long-term memory interactions but, given a choice, prefer not to use them. Weiskrantz (1970) suggests that we have not really designed appropriate tests to answer this question adequately when he says, "The typical human verbal short-term experiment uses material that is highly familiar to the subject and which he has received *ad nauseam* in the past, like digits in various combinations. . . . This general feature of human experiments rarely finds any counterpart in animal experimentation, where we generally teach the animal a novel relationship rather than briefly repeat a particular relationship out of a population of familiar relationships." One must therefore examine the animal literature for tasks that share at least some of these crucial features and which are more readily learned by monkeys. One is therefore looking for tasks in which, at the very least, the animal gives evidence of recognizing more than a single event. If the animal simply responds to a repeated event, we have nothing more than a habit. Immediately we specify more than one event, the natural corollary is interference, which is another cardinal feature of human memory tests.

B. The Effect of Temporal Lobe Lesions on Cognitive Processes in the Monkey

After years of despondency during which experimenters repeatedly demonstrated that bilateral hippocampal lesions in monkeys *do not* impair discrimination habits, reports are beginning to appear that with certain learning and memory tasks such lesions do produce impairments.

1. *Concurrent Visual Learning*

It is quite clear that bilateral hippocampal (Mishkin, 1954) or medial temporal lesions that include the hippocampus and associated white matter and entorhinal cortex (Orbach *et al.*, 1960; Correll and Scoville, 1965a; Drachman and Ommaya, 1964) do not impair simultaneous visual discrimination performance. However, Correll and Scoville (1965a) found that, when monkeys with bilateral medial temporal lesions were required to learn six pattern discriminations concurrently, severe impairment was observed. In the concurrent learning paradigm the animal receives only a single trial on the individual problems at any one time. Learning of the various problems must therefore proceed on the basis of isolated random trials interspersed with interfering trials on the other five problems. The design of this learning task emphasizes interference, making it difficult to learn which of a particular pair of patterns is reinforced.

The more recent study of Correll and Scoville (1970) on concurrent learning after medial temporal lesions takes up the question of interference specifically. The design of the concurrent learning task means, inevitably, that the individual trials on the various problems are separated by a considerable time lag and by interference from the trials on the intervening problems. Do medial temporal animals learn slowly because the memory trace of a trial fades abnormally quickly and is not available for further consolidation when the next trial occurs? Or is trace strength adequate but undermined by abnormal sensitivity to interference? Correll and Scoville (1970) found that monkeys with bilateral medial temporal damage are severely impaired on six-problem concurrent learning tested with 10-second or 45-second intertrial intervals, resulting in about 80–84 seconds or 5 minutes between trials on any given problem. Either rapid fading of the trace or interference could explain such a result but, if trace fading were the most significant factor, one would expect *greater* error scores the *longer* the delay. In fact, at 75-second intertrial intervals medial temporal lesioned animals required more trials and correction trials than at the substantially longer intertrial interval. These investigators comment that the results indicate that the "impairment in serial learning in monkeys with medial temporal lesions is related to interpair interference, rather than to decay of the memory trace." In a similar vein, Douglas *et al.* (1969) have reported that monkeys with bilateral hippocampal damage, while able to learn a simultaneous visual discrimination with two patterns, become increasingly impaired if problems with two, three, or four negative (unreinforced) stimuli, rather than one, are presented. The additional irrelevant negative cues may be increasing interference.

2. Matching to Sample

Correll and Scoville (1965b) and Drachman and Ommaya (1964) found that medial temporal lesions in monkeys impair the postoperative retention of color matching to sample in a two-choice situation. In matching, unlike the situation in simultaneous visual discrimination, there is a changing relationship between the stimuli and the correct response. An independent event (i.e., the sample) determines which of the two match stimuli is correct on a particular trial. Again, in this situation interference between successive trials must be considerable.

3. Delayed Matching to Sample

In both the cited studies *delayed* matching was included and in both cases, although severe impairment was found under delay conditions, it was concluded that the nature of the matching task rather than the delay influenced the deficit. Drachman and Ommaya (1964) found retention loss in 5-second delayed matching and, to dissociate the nature of the task from the delay, they went on to study postoperative learning of matching at a 12-second delay. They found no consistent relationship between the extent of the lesion and the additional training required to perform at the longer delay interval.

4. Delayed Response and Delayed Alternation

In the earliest study of medial temporal lesions, Orbach *et al.* (1960) found both delayed response (DR) and delayed alternation (DA) performance to be impaired. It was clear, however, that DA was more severely affected than DR. In the latter case the monkey must alternately vary its response to left or right, but an external cue is given to direct the behavior. By contrast, in DA, the initiative to respond alternately to left or right is internally generated. As discussed earlier, this is the kind of situation that appears to require mnemonic strategies equivalent to those observed in man in situations in which an interplay between short- and long-term memory occurs.

Correll and Scoville (1967) have reported similar results on DR and DA and have gone on to show again that it is the inherent nature of the task, rather than the delay, that determines the deficit. First, they found that postoperative retention and acquisition of DA was more severely affected than DR. However, when the delay was increased up to 10 seconds in both of these tasks, the performance of the medial temporal group did not deteriorate any faster than that of controls.

It should be noted that the effect of hippocampal damage on DA can be capricious. In a large series of electrolytic hippocampal lesions, Waxler and Rosvold (1970) found that, after two lesions of comparable extent, severe or minimal impairment was observed. They suggest that some animals may adopt spatial orientation strategies in order to solve DA and that this circumvents the need for memory involvement. In other words, having retrieved a reward on the left, the monkey orientates its body or, indeed, moves it to the right-hand position, in readiness for the next trial. With such a strategy, memory is not involved. This observation reinforces the contention that it is difficult to devise a suitable test for monkeys that ensures mnemonic involvement. Even when given the chance to use a highly economical spatial memory strategy, monkeys may prefer to use less cognitive solutions. There is no direct evidence that hippocampal animals which are unimpaired in DA have adopted the nonmnemonic strategy, or indeed whether such changes occur before the operation or are invoked postoperatively, when other strategies are unavailable on account of the brain damage. Certainly in frontal monkeys, we have recently observed the gradual emergence of the spatial orientation strategy after several thousands of unsuccessful trials on DA.

5. Spatial Reversal Tasks

Mahut (1971) has reported that radical hippocampal lesions in the monkey impair performance on a left-right spatial alternation and spatial position reversal test. Similar results were obtained after bilateral section of the fornix in monkeys (Mahut, 1972). These impairments are not thought to be due to difficulty in controlling response tendencies, as the same animals are not impaired in go–no go alternation, which involves a similar degree of response control. This interpretation is further supported by the observation that the lesion does not impair object reversal learning (Mahut, 1971; Jones and Mishkin, 1972). Furthermore, Zola and Mahut (1973) more recently found that acquisition of object reversal is actually facilitated by fornix section.

6. Tasks Requiring Ordering of Responses

Kimble and Pribram (1963) studied sequential responding and reported impairment after bilateral hippocampal resection in the monkey. Preoperatively, the animals were trained with a 16-panel apparatus to discriminate the numerals 6 and 4 under simultaneous discrimination conditions. Post-operatively, they were retrained on this discrimination and were then required to learn a task in which two panels were illuminated with numeral 1 and both had to be pressed to obtain reinforcement. A different two panels were illuminated on each trial and could be pressed in either order. The animal determined the sequence of responses, and this task is said to be "internally ordered." In the next task the numerals 1 and 5 appeared on the panels and had to be pressed in the order 1 and then 5. The reverse order did not bring reinforcement. This task is "externally ordered." Bilateral hippocampectomy impaired acquisition in both of these tasks requiring an ordering of responses.

7. *Elimination of Responses to Unimportant Stimuli*

In all the tasks described so far, the monkey must learn which stimulus is important (i.e., reinforced) under conditions in which the information required to make such a decision is inconsistent either in nature or availability. Douglas and Pribram discussed this problem in 1966 when they proposed that the amygdala and hippocampus worked together in the learning process, the amygdala to register the meaningfulness of events and the hippocampus to strengthen appropriate responses to such stimuli and weaken and eliminate inappropriate ones. It was noted at that time that, in certain discrimination tasks where it was made difficult for the animal to determine which were the important and which the unimportant stimuli, hippocampal lesioned monkeys showed impairment. For example, if in contrast to the usual simultaneous discrimination in which the correct stimulus is rewarded 100% and the incorrect 0%, the positive stimulus is rewarded 70% and the incorrect 30%, learning in the hippocampal animal is retarded. The amygdala codes this information about the reinforcing contingencies, but this information, lacking the vigor or "impellance" of a fully differentiated reinforcement schedule (100%-0%), makes discrimination learning more difficult. In a hippocampal lesioned monkey, the 100%-0% reinforcement coded by the intact amygdala is sufficient information for learning to occur. However, if the reinforcement information is weakened by the 70%-30% contingency, the amygdala information lacks the vigor or impellance to ensure learning in the absence of the hippocampal system. The latter system normally crystallizes responses in favor of one stimulus rather than another. The hippocampal lesioned animal can therefore differentiate its response only under the most favorable conditions. If, for example, a given response is to be made on some occasions and not on others, or if several inappropriate responses are available in a learning situation, the task becomes disproportionately difficult for the hippocampal lesioned animal. All the tasks so far discussed fall within this general framework, but so also do extinction tasks, discrimination reversal tasks, and orientation tasks, all of which have been impaired by hippocampal damage in several species (see Iversen, 1972, for review). The amygdala and hippocampus thus provide a hypothesis-testing mechanism essential to the learning process. A combination lesion to both these structures should render an animal particularly handicapped in situations in which there are changing reinforcement contingencies. Pribram *et al.* (1969) analyzed the impaired reversal performance in monkeys with amygdalohippocampal lesions. These animals learned simultaneous discrimination with ease and were then trained on a 0 versus 5 discrimination to a criterion of 90/100. At this time the 5 rather than the 0 was rewarded. They found that normal monkeys respond for a short time to the previously rewarded stimulus, and then search for a new strategy. Once it is found, the correct performance rises very quickly to criterion. In limbic lesioned animals the learning curve shows the same three segments (wrong strategy, search for new one, and use of new one). The time course is very much the same for both the initial and final segments of the learning curve. It is in the intermediate "strategy-searching" segments that the monkeys with amygdalohippocampal lesions are impaired. They take an inordinate number of trials to find a new appropriate strategy. Once this has been done, it is maintained and learning proceeds rapidly. This indicates that the limbic lesion does not merely dampen all cognitive functioning but selectively impairs a crucial aspect of learning.

Various theories have been proposed to explain the role of the hippocampus in coding learned responses. For many years the emphasis has been on ideas involving response disinhibition. Both Douglas (1967) and Kimble (1968) developed theories which envisaged that the hippocampus plays its role through some direct control of response mechanisms. There can be no doubt that hippocampal deficits are associated with overt emission of inappropriate responses. However, it is not all clear whether this is the cause or the effect of the basic disorder. One is inclined to the latter view. Unlike the inferior convexity of the frontal lobes, the lesioning of which also results in loss of response control, the hippocampus has no obvious connection with motor control centers of the forebrain. It seems more likely that the hippocampus is critically involved in the *fixing of attention* to relevant stimuli, which is a prerequisite of efficient responding. In the rat, Warburton (1972) proposed a sensory role for the hippocampus and, using signal detection methods to analyze the deficits seen in discriminative situations, demonstrated that the apparent lack of response control after hippocampal lesions is due to a change in sensory rather than response bias. Such methods hold great promise for distinguishing among deficits after different brain lesions which superficially appear similar in nature because they result in loss of response control.

C. The Effect of Selective Bilaterial Frontal Lesions on Memory Performance in the Monkey

As regards related questions of frontal memory impairment, the situation is not as clear. It was proposed that the ordering of information in memory is accomplished by the frontal cortex in humans. In the monkey it is clear that only a small segment of the frontal cortex is concerned with memory, and it is presently far from clear whether or not this tissue contributes any unique feature to the memory process. Monkeys with extensive frontal lesions have been tested and found to fail many of the tasks impaired by hippocampal lesions. However, it is now recognized that the frontal lobe includes several dissociable areas concerned with different aspects of behavioral control (see Iversen, 1972, for review). The inferior convexity of the frontal lobe is concerned with response control and, if lesioned, animals fail go–no go discrimination tasks because of their inability to suppress unreinforced responses. As this part of the frontal cortex has been traditionally included in frontal lesions, it is possible that response disinhibition impairment can explain many, if not all, of the defects observed with the specified memory tasks. It can, however, be said that localized lesions to the sulcus principalis of the dorsal convexity do not result in response disinhibition and yet severely impair DA and DR performance. It seems possible that this tissue is the focus of the frontal lobe contribution to memory coding (see Section IV, B, 1), but more partial frontal lesions need to be studied.

In regard to the comparison with clinical data, Corsi's results on the perception of recency provide one of the most novel leads on human frontal function. Equivalent tests have not been made with monkeys. However, performance on the differential reinforcement of low rates of responding (drl) schedule appears to be somewhat related. With such schedules animals are required to organize their responding at a slow rate in order to be reinforced, and must remember when the last response occurred in order to be able to do this. This animal test may involve something akin to time tagging.

It is therefore surprising that Stamm (1969) found drl performance not to be affected by frontal lesions, even extensive ones involving the response control focus in the inferior convexity. Whether or not this is because of the overtraining inherent in the development of efficient drl performance (which is difficult to achieve) remains to be explored.

If one examines the lesion experiments on rats, cats, and monkeys, it is striking that in many instances tests that are sensitive to hippocampal damage are also sensitive to frontal lesions. There is no unique frontal memory test in the monkey and, if these two forebrain areas contribute in different but related ways to memory processing, it has yet to be demonstrated in subhuman species.

III. Anatomical Relationships of the Limbic System

ANATOMICAL SUBSTRATES OF MEMORY PROCESSING

Surprisingly little is clear when one comes to consider the anatomical structures and pathways concerned in memory processing and storage. There are, however, two clear starting points: first, bilateral medial temporal damage such as that in H.M. results in severe amnesia, and second, frontal lesions also produce highly characteristic memory disorders. These facts raise many questions, some of which are beginning to yield interesting answers.

1. The hippocampus is part of Papez's circuit. Are other parts of this circuit of any significance with regard to memory processes?

2. If the frontal cortex is involved in memory processes, is it integrated with the hippocampal system?

3. Where does information make its lasting record in the nervous system?

1. In 1937 Papez described a neural circuit involving the hippocampus, which he suggested may be implicated in emotional behavior (Fig. 7). He pointed out that the connections of the hippocampus are basically efferent and travel via the fornix to the mammillary bodies. The circuit is completed by projections from the mammillary body to the anterior nuclei of the thalamus, from there to the cingulate gyrus, and thence to the entorhinal cortex which gives reentry to the hippocampus. It is now generally accepted, on the basis of animal lesion studies, that different parts of the limbic system are involved in the control and expression of emotional behavior, and it is possible that the connections of the hippocampus noted by Papez play a related role in memory processes.

In humans neurosurgical or spontaneous lesions to all the structures and pathways in the Papez circuit have been reported to produce memory loss (Brion, 1969). Bilateral hippocampal and entorhinal damage such as that in H.M. is fortunately rare, but large groups of patients with unilateral temporal lesions including the hippocampus and entorhinal cortex to varying degrees have been studied at the Montreal Neurological Institute and found to have amnesias (see Corsi's work, Section I,B,1,b).

The most common natural pathology resulting in amnesia is Korsakoff's disease. This condition is a result of thiamine deficiency associated with alcoholism and results in widespread neuron degeneration in the forebrain, in which bilateral degeneration of the mammillary bodies is prominent. Korsakoff patients show a broad range of cognitive deficits, including amnesia. Confabulation accompanies memory impairment, which in any case

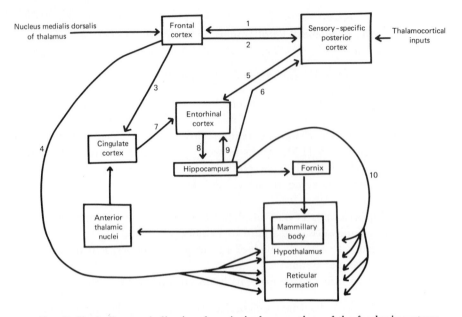

FIG. 7. Block diagram indicating the principal connections of the forebrain systems. The numbers refer to studies that have identified the existence of particular connections. 1 & 2: Pandya and Kuypers (1969); Pandya *et al.* (1971). 3: Pandya *et al.* (1971); Butters and Pandya (1969). 4: Nauta (1964). 5: Van Hoesen *et al.* (1972). 6: Voton (1959, 1960). 7: Pandya and Kuypers, (1969); Van Hoesen *et al.* (1972). 8: Ramón y Cajal (1955), Hjorth-Simonsen and Jeune (1972). 9: Hjorth-Simonsen (1971). 10: Papez (1937); Nauta (1958).

tends to be patchy rather than absolute. Certain isolated events are retained vividly, which together with the tendency to fill the gaps with phantom and misplaced memories produces a somewhat florid amnesia. Korsakoff amnesiacs have many of the features of temporal lobe amnesia. They figure prominently in the patient sample studied by Weiskrantz and Warrington, who showed that memory improved when retrieval mechanisms were aided. However, in addition to retrieval impairment, Korsakoff patients are reported to show abnormal coding strategies when faced with verbal information.

Cermak *et al.* (1973) report that such patients code in verbal memory more by acoustic than by semantic cues, and this lower-order encoding, together with increased sensitivity to interference, subsequently further impairs the storage and/or retrieval of information.

Another interesting feature of the full Korsakoff syndrome is pronounced temporal disorientation. This may be significant in view of the fact that, in addition to hypothalamic pathology, damage also exists in the anterior thalamus and cingulate cortex. It was earlier proposed that temporal information may be important to the frontal lobe with regard to its particular role in memory processing, and that the frontal lobe is anatomically related to the anterior thalamus and cingulate cortex.

In addition to the classical Korsakoff psychosis associated with alcoholism and nutritional deficiency, similar disturbances are seen after a bilateral tumor or vascular damage to Papez's circuit (Brion, 1969).

With reference to other parts of the Papez circuit it is reported that discrete lesions to the anterior thalamic nuclei (Benedak and Juba, 1941), the nucleus medialis dorsalis of the thalamus (Spiegal et al., 1956), or the anterior cingulate gyrus result in amnesia (Whitty and Lewin, 1960), albeit of a somewhat transitory nature. Large groups of such patients have not been available for psychological study, and it is not possible at present to characterize these forms of amnesia and distinguish them from temporal lobe and Korsakoff's amnesia. Damage to these particular sites is often also observed in Korsakoff patients, which encourage clinicians to describe the amnesias associated with their discrete damage as Korsakoff-like. However, as Whitty and Lewin (1960) point out, "Lesions in any of these situations may give rise to memory defects which will have some similarities and also some differences representing the particular 'local sign' of the part affected."

As both the hippocampus and its projection site, the mammillary body, are involved in memory, it is puzzling why fornix lesions that transect the pathway between these sites produce such trivial memory disorders. Perhaps natural pathology to the fornix is rarely sufficiently complete to produce a disorder. In one case reported by Hassler and Rienhart (1957), in which bilateral fornical coagulation was complete, memory disturbance was reported. The presence of direct pathways from the hippocampus to the reticular formation may also be relevant.

Complementing the evidence from lesion material, Bickford et al. (1958) presented evidence of reversible amnesia induced by electrical stimulation of the white fibers in the deep temporal lobe. As such fibers provide crucial links in the Papez circuit, it is not surprising to find that their disruption impairs memory. Indeed, it is almost certainly true that after large temporal lesions that impinge on the hippocampus this white matter is damaged.

Involvement of Papez's circuit in memory processes in the monkey has been suggested but by no means proven. The task is hampered, as we have discussed, both by our incomplete appreciation of the nature of nonhuman memory processes and by the lack of specific tests for such processes. However, the picture looks more hopeful if it accepted that DA and DR tasks come closest to the kind of task that in humans requires dynamic interaction between short- and long-term memory; this type of task is impaired by hippocampal damage (Mahut, 1971), fornix section (Mahut, 1972), and anterior cingulate lesions (Pribram *et al.*, 1962). Lesions to the frontal cortex around the sulcus principalis (Butters and Pandya, 1969), and to the medialis dorsalis of the thalamus (Schulman, 1964) and to the head of the caudate (Rosvold, 1968), sites of reciprocal connections (Akert, 1964; Nauta, 1964; Johnson *et al.*, 1968) with the sulcus principalis, also produced DA or DR impairment.

2. The relationships within Papez's circuit and between it and the frontal cortex are summarized in Fig. 7. The numbers on the lines refer to representative studies which indicate the existence of such connections or refer to the relevant studies.

3. The fact that previously stored memories survive hippocampal damage is usually cited as evidence that memories are not stored in the hippocampus. Where, then, can one look for the permanent record? Lashley's heroic studies demonstrated that there is no unaccounted-for area of the cortex (at least in the rat) acting as a memory repository.

Large areas of the cortex outside the sensory and motor cortices appeared to contribute to the mnemonic capacity of the rat. In humans and monkeys there is localization of sensory modalities within the posterior association cortex (Iversen, 1972). These areas are crucial to perceptual analysis within the modality, and in their absence previously perceived events are no longer recognized. In many ways perception and memory are complementary facets of a single process. In recognition the memory of past events is compared with a present event and, if the match is satisfactory, recognition occurs. The finding that the hippocampus, as well as receiving input from the posterior association cortex, sends projections back to these areas (Whitlock and Nauta, 1956), probably via the entorhinal cortex (Hjorth-Simonsen, 1971), provides the route for such interaction. In addition, many investigators have been impressed by the massive projections from the hippocampus to the hindbrain reticular formation (Nauta, 1958) and see in this area a potential neural substrate for integrating information processed by the hippocampal circuit and by the frontal association cortex which also has strong descending projections to the tegmentum (Kesner, 1973).

IV. Neural Properties of the Hippocampus and Frontal Cortex in Relation to Memory Processing

The evidence reviewed so far suggests that the hippocampus and dorsolateral frontal cortex, together with connecting forebrain circuitry, are essential for the laying down of certain learned experiences. The task is to establish exactly what each of them contributes to such processing, and if these structures have peculiar neural properties which can account for such functions.

A. THE HIPPOCAMPUS

1. *Fine Structure of the Hippocampus*

The general neuronal layout of the hippocampus is illustrated in Fig. 8 together with a stylized diagram of the input and connections. The granule cells of the dentate gyrus (D) give rise to mossy fibers which cross the dendritic fields of the pyramidal fields CA-4 and -3. These pyramidal cells have bifurcating axons, one of which forms an efferent output from the hippocampus; the other, the Schaffer collateral, crosses the dendritic field of the CA-1 pyramidal cells. These cells give rise to another output of the

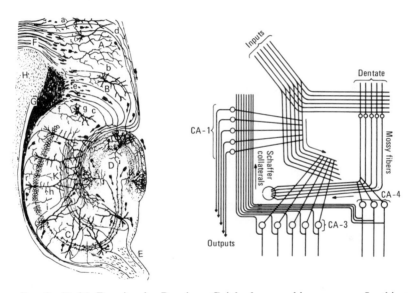

FIG. 8. (Left) Drawing by Ramón y Cajal of mouse hippocampus. In this case the dentate gyrus is just above D; the mossy fibers pass downward through the CA-3 field which is marked C. Each CA-3 neuron gives rise to a bifurcating axon; one part goes off and away at E, but the other part crosses upward to form the pathway marked K. These are the Schaffer collaterals, and they pass through the CA-3 dendrites. These may form the "memory axons," and the CA-1 field may form the motor and emotional outflow aspects of a temporary memory system. (Right) A more complicated schematic drawing of the hippocampus. This shows how the inputs (perforant pathway) sometimes bifurcate to innervate the dentate on one side of the hippocampal cleft and the CA-1 and CA-3 fields on the other side of the cleft. (From Olds, 1970.)

hippocampus. The dentate granule cells and pyramidal cells CA-3 and -4 receive sensory input from subcortical and cortical sites, but these fibers bifurcate also to innervate CA-1 neurons. These neurons also pick up information about activity in CA-3 and -4 neurons by way of the Schaffer collaterals. Olds (1970) sees in this anatomical arrangement the possibility of recording intero- and exteroceptive input together with the responses made to this information, in other words, keeping a running record of outgoing behavior. As we shall see presently, the fact that CA-1 neurons project to the memory circuit and neurons CA-3 and -4 to effector systems may explain how the hippocampus could both initiate and remember responses.

2. *Afferent and Efferent Connections of the Hippocampus*

Introduction of the Nauta silver staining techniques and its various modifications has made it possible for the first time to plot the fine pathways of the forebrain, and with this method unsuspected connections have been revealed. We briefly consider four questions: (1) What are the origins of afferent fibers to the hippocampus? (2) Which areas of the cortex and sub-cortex innervate these areas of "afferent origin"? (3) Where in the hippocampal neurons do the connections terminate? (4) Do the pyramidal fields of the hippocampus project to different areas?

1. The fornix is now known not to be a purely efferent pathway. The septum is the site of neurons projecting to the hippocampus and is the transit site for other fibers innervating the hippocampus (Raisman *et al.*, 1965a). The brainstem tegmentum is the principal source of this input. The amygdala also projects to the hippocampus (Krettek and Price, 1974). The other principal source of hippocampal afferents is the entorhinal cortex, an area that overlies the hippocampus medial to the hippocampal gyrus (Ramón y Cajal, 1955). These inputs are in addition to the "purely limbic" cingulate presubiculum input of Papez's circuit described earlier.

2. The septum receives its input from tegmental areas. It is known to be a site of cholinergic activity, and it has been suggested that one of the cholinergic arousal systems projects to the hippocampus via this route. The amygdala also receives projections from tegmental sites via the medial forebrain bundles. These pathways are thought to be important for coding the meaningfulness of external and internal stimuli, in other words, whether they are reinforcing or punishing to the animal. The medial forebrain bundle and the amygdala are sites that sustain intracranial self-stimulation, which is considered an indication of reinforcement and motivation sites in the brain. It may be significant that the tegmental fibers innervating these sites use norepinephrine or dopamine as their transmitter. Ramón y Cajal was unable to identify the source of afferents to the entorhinal cortex. Re-

cently, this was done in the monkey by Van Hoesen *et al.* (1972). In this species the entorhinal cortex is divisible (on cytoarchitectural grounds) into two distinct segments, 28a and 28b, according to Brodmann's notation. 28a receives its input almost exclusively from the ventral temporal lobe cortex (area TH of von Bonin and Bailey), whereas 28b is innervated by the orbitofrontal cortex (areas 12 and 13 of Walker) and the prepyriform cortex. Van Hoesen *et al.* (1972) go one step further and examine the source of afferents to these three cortical segments. They note that sensory information, once it has reached the primary receiving area in the cortex, is passed to successive sites of association cortex specific for a given modality. The first areas of association cortex have convergent projections to areas in the frontal (around the arcuate sulcus) and parietal lobes. These latter sites project to the cingulate, and thence to the presubiculum and hippocampus. The parietal focus also projects to area TH in the ventral temporal lobe. The first association sites also provide the connections to further modality-specific association areas in the auditory, visual, and somesthetic modes. These second association areas, in contrast to the earlier ones, project to the orbital frontal (areas 12 and 13) and ventral temporal (area TH) cortex. As we have already seen, these are the two sites of input to areas 28a and 28b of the entorhinal cortex. Thus it is clear that there is massive projection of sensory information to the entorhinal cortex, and thence to the hippocampus, from successive sites in the association cortex. The prepyriform cortex is the source of olfactory input to the hippocampus. These observations are summarized in Fig. 9.

3. The projection fields of the various sectors of the entorhinal cortex are proving more difficult to establish, probably because it is technically difficult to produce selective damage to such small areas and fiber tracts. There are three pathways from the entorhinal cortex, the crossed temporoammonic tract, the alvear pathway, and the perforant pathway. Current knowledge indicates that in the rat both medial and lateral areas of the entorhinal cortex contribute to the perforant pathway which innervates both the dentate gyrus and pyramidal fields CA-3 and -4 (Hjorth-Simonsen and Jeune, 1972). There is considerable organization within this pathway, lesions to the medial region resulting in terminal degeneration in the middle layers of the dentate rather than superficially as after lesions to a more lateral area. It also seems that the lateral area innervates the ipsilateral pyramidal fields CA-1, perhaps by the alvear pathway. Certainly the crossed temporoammonic tract innervates this pyramidal field (Raisman *et al.*, 1965a). The picture is broadly similar in the monkey in so far as it has been studied. The lateral entorhinal area (28b) innervates the dentate gyrus and fields CA-3 and -4. However, it appears that the medial sector (28a) selectively innervates the dentate gyrus in this species (Van Hoesen *et al.*, 1972). The afferent input

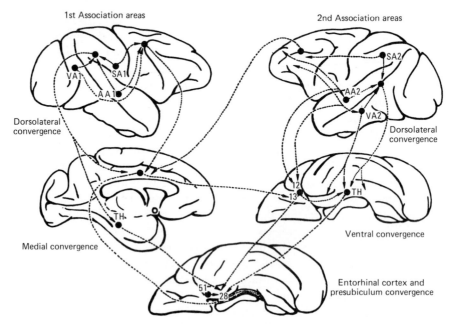

Fig. 9. The probable multisynaptic pathways via which the hippocampus of the limbic system has access to sensory information. These pathways are depicted on dorsolateral, medial, and ventral views of the rhesus monkey brain. Sites of origin (circles) and termination (arrows) refer only to general cytoarchitectonic regions and not to specific points. Primary association areas are labeled VA1, the area for vision; SA1, for somesthesis; and AA1, for audition. Secondary association areas are labeled similarly, except that the digit is changed to 2. TH is the cortical area as designated by von Bonin and Bailey. Orbitofrontal areas 12 and 13 were designated by Walker. Prepyriform cortex (51) and entorhinal cortex (28) were designated by Brodmann. (From Van Hoesen et al., 1972. Copyright 1972 by the American Association for the Advancement of Science.)

from the septal region terminates on the dendrites of dentate granule cells and pyramidal cells CA-3 and -4.

4. Just as the afferent fibers terminate in different areas of the hippocampus, so the efferent fibers innervate different areas. Pyramidal fields CA-3 and -4 distribute fibers to the septofimbrial, medial and lateral septum, diagonal band, and accumbens nuclei. The fields CA-3 and -4 also give rise to fibers which reciprocally innervate the entorhinal cortex. This is a recent and important finding. For many years such connections were inferred on the basis of electrical stimulation studies (Votaw, 1959). Votaw (1960) used the Marchi axon stain in the monkey to demonstrate this connection. Using the Fink-Heimer modification of silver impregnation staining for small unmyelinated axons, Hjorth-Simonsen (1971) has now visualized this projection much more definitively in the rat. In contrast, fields CA-1 and -2 appear to

provide the outputs of the classical Papez circuit, notably to the medial or lateral mammillary nuclei and the anterior thalamic nuclei (Raisman *et al.*, 1965b).

3. *Neuropsychological Theories of Hippocampal Function*

One of the ways of finding out if a certain structure is involved in behavioral control is to damage it and see if and how behavior is disrupted. With appropriate behavioral analysis the nature of the impairment can be identified and if it is found to be specific to this lesion, one is a little closer to understanding the neurological function of the structure. This has been a popular approach in hippocampal studies. But had this approach not been complemented with some of the others discussed, it is doubtful that we would have a very clear picture of the role of the hippocampus. We have proposed that neuronal arrangements in the hippocampus code sensory input and the responses to that input, and hold a record of the correlation between the two. It would not be surprising therefore to find a broad spectrum of learning deficits after hippocampal lesions. This indeed proved to be the case and, while in animals nothing akin to the global amnesia seen in H.M. was found, a variety of other deficits was. Different theorists have chosen to emphasize one deficit rather than another in their efforts to find a unitary theory of hippocampal involvement in behavior. These various results are not mutually exclusive and rather to be expected in view of the complex anatomical relationship we now know to exist in the hippocampus. Warburton (1972) found that synapses in the dorsal hippocampus (dentate gyrus), which employ acetylcholine as their neurotransmitter, are essential for sensory coding functions.

Gray (1970), however, has described a particular form of electrical activity in the hippocampus (the theta rhythm), whose occurrence correlates with the presentation of nonreward.

Vanderwolf (1971), also measuring hippocampal electrical activity, has been impressed with the correlation between certain electrical patterns and voluntary movement.

These theories are only one step from the directly measurable neural properties of the hippocampus. But there are overtly psychological theories. Douglas and Pribram suggested in 1966 that the hippocampus is an essential component of a learning mechanism. The amygdala codes the meaningfulness of events and the hippocampus records the responses made to them and inhibits responses to unimportant events—they suggested that its function is to "error-evaluate." This idea was developed subsequently by Douglas (1967), by Kimble (1968), and by Pribram (1967), who have all elaborated on how the hippocampus achieves its control over response tendencies. The net result of loss of this form of behavioral control would be response disinhibition and, as this impairment had been noted in a large number of rat hippocampal lesion studies, the concept of a hippocampal role in inhibition (by whatever means this is achieved) became widely accepted. Had an equal number of monkey hippocampal lesion studies been viewed, one doubts that the same conclusion would have been reached. The deficits observed in monkeys with medial temporal damage are not characterized in any obvious way by loss of response control. Weiskrantz, in discussing some features of human amnesia, has pointed out that disinhibition of inappropriate responses in memory tasks may account for the retrieval impairment seen repeatedly on recall tasks and the common occurrence of false-positive errors in these cases. This is a form of "cognitive" disinhibition rather than the overtly motor disinhibition observed in rats. However, there is no *a priori* reason why voluntary responses and the memory of such responses should not come under similar forms of neural control. Presumably the same interpretation could be applied to the hippocampal deficits described by Stevens and Cowey (1973). They compared dorsal and ventral hippocampal lesions in the rat in a series of behavioral tests. The lesions do not very clearly conform to any one field of neurons rather than another; however, the dorsal lesion clearly involves the dentate gyrus and the anterior extent of CA-1, whereas the ventral lesion damages CA-3 and -4 in their posterior extent. Dorsal lesions resulted in impaired performance on a task requiring shifting of attention (spontaneous alternation), while ventral lesions resulted in severely impaired performance on a task requiring a changing response strategy (lever-pressing alternation). In the lever alternation task used, a cue was given above the lever that had to be pressed. This clearly contributed to the better-than-control performance observed in the dorsal hippocampal lesioned animals. When it was removed, their performance deteriorated faster than in the controls. This continued attention to an additional external visual cue is seen, Stevens and Cowey suggest, because the normal mechanism of habituation and attention shifting is impaired in these animals. Thus, rather paradoxically, hippocampal lesions can actually *improve* performance on certain tasks.

This dissociation requires further investigation, but the proposal that the dorsal hippocampus mediates input analysis and attention shifts, while the ventral area is concerned with output control, is consistent with some earlier observations of Adey et al. (1962) that electrical activity in area CA-4 is correlated with successful DR performance in the cat.

However, before a response control theory is accepted it should be remembered that, where loss of response control is observed in animals, it is not possible by observation to determine whether the loss is primary or secondary to a loss of sensory control. Only the use of sophisticated methods of behavioral analysis (Warburton, 1972) allows this distinction to be made.

Although Douglas and Kimble both refer to a role for the hippocampus in behavioral inhibition, they believe that this is effected in different ways. Douglas (1972) uses the concept of Pavlovian inhibition, a process by which nonreward induces a state in the nervous system, which prevents one kind of response from occurring and thereby favors another. The hippocampus is central to this switching of attention, and its role is therefore on the sensory side. Kimble, by contrast, has viewed the hippocampus as more overtly concerned with the generation of response strategies. Hippocampal lesioned animals are described as showing impoverished hypothesis behavior, displaying fewer and protracted response strategies (Kimble and Kimble, 1970).

Thus, to date, theorizing has been guided by the desire to find a unitary theory of hippocampal function. Anatomical and neurophysiological findings indicate that this is probably a false aim. The complex anatomy of the hippocampus itself and the afferent and efferent connections of its various segments were discussed earlier. In the context it would be interesting to compare selective lesions to the dentate gyrus, CA-3 and -4, and CA-1. Selective lesions of this kind remain a challenge for the future. It is difficult to damage selectively one neuronal field rather than another. Chemically induced lesions hold some promise; for example, acetylpyridine selectively damages CA-3, and hydrogen sulfide disrupts the zinc-rich cells of CA-2, -3, and -4.

4. Neurophysiological Theories of Hippocampal Function

When forebrain electrical recordings in behaving animals were first made, it quickly became apparent that the hippocampus showed characteristic electrical activity which changed as animals repeatedly experienced learning situations. Grastyan (1954) reported that an electrical response in the hippocampus mirrored orientating behavior and its habituation to repeated stimulation. Adey (1961) studied the temporal coupling of gross brain activity in various structures during discrimination learning in the cat. He found that, early in the acquisition of the task, hippocampal activity preceded that in the entorhinal cortex, but when learning had progressed the reverse was true. Adey believed that the significance of these changes was that at first the input went to the hippocampus and was fed from there to the entorhinal area, where it was stored. Later the information stored in the entorhinal cortex provided a standard against which the input was compared to determine what action should be taken, activity thus being started there before the incoming signal reached the hippocampus. More recent anatomical evidence tends to support such an interpretation. John and Killam (1959) made recordings at many sites in the forebrain during shock avoidance learning in the cat. A cat learned to jump from one compartment of a double-grid box to the other to avoid shock whenever the conditioned stimulus (CS) was presented. The CS was a 10-per-second flashing light (called a tracer CS because it allowed the investigators to trace the path of the signal through the brain by recording the evoked potentials at 10 per second or multiples thereof). A 7-per-second light was not followed by shock. As soon as conditioning started, the *tracer* potentials appeared at all recording sites including sensory cortices, reticular formation, nucleus ventralis anterior (nVA) of the thalamus, fornix, septum, hippocampus, and amygdala. As the cat learned, the tracer potentials disappeared except from the visual cortex, hippocampus, and midbrain reticular formation. When learning was complete, the tracer disappeared from the hippocampus and reappeared in the nVA of the thalamus, a motor nucleus. Again this study implicates the hippocampus only during the initial stages of habit learning. At a later stage successful behavior can occur in the absence of hippocampal activity and of the hippocampus itself as, presumably, in the studies of discrimination behavior cited earlier.

The relatively brief direct involvement of the hippocampus in learning behavior is further emphasized by a study of Uretsky and McCleary (1969) in which they trained cats on a one-way avoidance task. Three hours and 8 days after reaching criterion the hippocampus was isolated from related structures by lesions of the fornix and entorhinal cortex. A retention deficit was found only when the hippocampus was isolated 3 hours after learning, but not 8 days after learning.

As pointed out earlier, the hippocampus does not appear essential for the retention of discrimination habits or indeed their acquisition. Electrophysiological results, however, indicate that at least during the early stages of discrimination learning the hippocampus is active. It is a pity that no recording work has yet been attempted during the acquisition and retention of tasks in which there is persistent pressure on information processing and in which we propose the hippocampus is likely to be permanently involved in successful performance of the task.

Evoked-potential recording techniques will undoubtedly lead to unit recording studies. Hirano *et al.* (1970) have provided some exciting leads in this direction. Rats were reinforced with a food pellet for standing still when one auditory signal rather than another was sounded. Prior to conditioning, blocks of habituation and pseudoconditioning trials had been given. Neuron firing rates were measured during the first 300 msec of the 1-second conditioning stimuli (on response) and during the remaining part of the stimuli (stabilized response).

As conditioning proceeded the midbrain neurons gradually showed a differential increased firing rate in response to the CS+ and CS—. But the difference was not large, developed only in the later stages of conditioning, and was not well maintained in subsequent extinction trials. By contrast, responses in the hippocampal neurons immediately increased as conditioning started, the CS+ inducing a much higher rate than the CS—.

This difference was substantial and remained throughout the extinction periods. Olds (1970) considers that these results are consistent with the proposal that "the hippocampus might function as a temporary memory register participating in the control of operant behavior."

B. THE FRONTAL CORTEX

1. Afferent and Efferent Connections

If the sulcus principalis is involved in memory processes, it too should be examined for appropriate input and output pathways and for possible inter-actions with the hippocampal circuit. No doubt it is true that, if one looks long enough, one can usually convince oneself that convenient connections exist. The traditional counter to this approach was, "Big means important and small means unimportant," and one therefore had to find not just con-nections but substantial ones. However, this safety clause has recently suffered a setback by the demonstration that pathways in the forebrain such as the nigrostriatal pathway, barely visible with fiber-staining techniques, can have immensely important integrative roles in brain organization (Ungerstedt, 1971). Many of our working hypotheses concerning the frontal lobe have had to be revised in the light of evidence that it contains several anatomically and functionally distinct areas (Iversen, 1972). The sulcus principalis con-cerns us in this article, and its isolation as a functionally distinct area suggests that it may have its own particular connections. If one considers the sulcus principalis part of the dorsolateral, as opposed to the orbital frontal cortex, it can indeed be seen to have a unique set of connections. The dorsolateral cortex is reciprocally connected with the specific areas of the posterior association cortex (Pandya and Kuypers, 1969; Pandya et al., 1971). The principal subcortical input arises from the more medial parts (pars parvo-cellularis) of the medialis dorsalis of the thalamus (Akert, 1964), and there are afferent projections to the various elements of the basal ganglia (Johnson et al., 1968) and limbic system (Nauta, 1964).

In each of these cited studies, however, the projections of the total dorsolateral lesions including the sulcus principalis were studied. What we now need to see is a repeat of such studies comparing sulcus principalis, arcuate sulcus, and non-sulcus principalis projections. Butters and Pandya (1969), who have demonstrated that very small lesions within the sulcus principalis produce serve DA impairment, are pursuing the related anatom-ical questions. They have plotted, with the Nauta–Gygax technique, the patterns of degeneration after lesions to the anterior, middle, and caudal third of the sulcus principalis, and to tissue dorsal and ventral to the sulcus. Nonprincipalis lesions result in relatively minor degeneration in other frontal areas, but principalis lesions produce extensive degeneration in other cortical areas or in the juxtallocortex. The caudal third projects to the preoccipito-parietal cortex, whereas the middle and anterior project (1) to the association cortex of the temporal lobe, (2) to the cingulate gyrus, and (3) to the parahippocampal gyrus. These are interesting observations, because both sets of connections ultimately provide access to the hippocampus: connections 1 from the temporal lobe association areas via the entorhinal cortex and connections 2 and 3 in the Papez circuit to the entorhinal cortex, and thence to the hippocampus. Sensory information passes via the modality-specific areas of the association cortex to the dorsal frontal cortex and via area TH and the entorhinal cortex to the hippocampus. Olfactory sensory information travels via the medalis dorsalis to the frontal cortex and via area 28b of the entorhinal cortex to the hippocampus. The amygdala projects to the medialis dorsalis and to the hippocampus, and the tegmentum innervates both areas via the medialis dorsalis and septum, respectively. The inputs, outputs, and relationships between the frontal and hippocampal circuits are summarized in Fig. 10. It may be relevant to think in terms of parallel processing in these

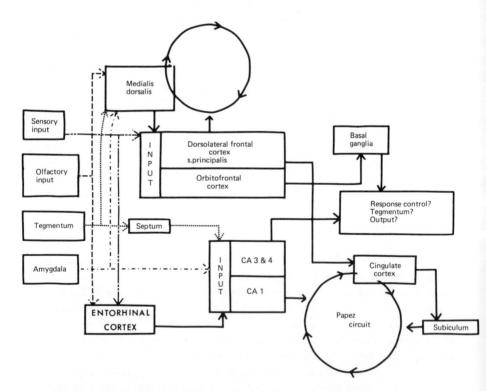

FIG. 10. Block diagram indicating various inputs to the hippocampus and frontal cortex and the relationship between these two areas.

two systems, the task being to identify their unique (yet closely related) contribution to information processing. It has been implied that phylogenetic differences (both of a quantitative and qualitative nature) may be expected to exist with regard to memory processes. In this regard it may be interesting to note von Bonin (1941) stressed that within the primates the temporal lobe cortex has undergone relatively greater expansion than other association cortex. Turning to another part of the proposed memory circuit, Domesick (1969) found in the rat relatively sparse connections from the cingulate cortex to the hippocampus, whereas in the monkey these connections are extensive (Nauta, 1964; Butters and Pandya, 1969).

So far we have emphasized anatomy in relation to the coding of exteroceptive cues. In a recent article, Nauta (1971) has reviewed the anatomy of the frontal cortex, emphasizing the fact that it receives both intero- as well as exteroceptive cues.

Nauta considers what use the frontal cortex might make of this combination of information and suggests:

> It could be suspected—so far on no more than introspective grounds—that the itineraries of anticipated behavior require being registered and "kept on hand" not only in somatic sensorimotor mechanisms but also in structures subserving the organism's affective responsiveness, and thus, that a plan for action cannot be kept in abeyance intact for any length of time unless it is represented in matching somatic and affective registries. If this were indeed the case, it would be readily understandable that loss of the frontal cortex as a major mediator of information exchange between the cerebral cortex and the limbic system is followed not only by an impairment of strategic choice-making, but also by a tendency of projected or current action programs to "fade out" or become over-ridden by interfering influences. . . . In this context it could even be suggested that the "frontal" animal has suffered a memory impairment after all, even though this loss affects the storage of its action plans rather than that of its external-perceptual images.

What is rather surprising is that the hippocampus also has this unique combination of intero- and exteroceptive inputs (Fig. 10). Perhaps the role of the hippocampus is not so much to make the decision as to *what to do* in particular circumstances, as actually to control the basic mechanisms by which one behavior rather than another is generated and to guarantee the memory of the conditions under which this has been done.

2. Electrophysiological Correlates of Frontal Lobe Function

Neuroanatomical studies are clearly making a substantial contribution to our understanding of memory processing. However, we have questions that anatomical methods clearly cannot answer. For example, the hippocampus and frontal cortex are closely related anatomically. We think they may play complementary roles in a memory process, but the details of their afferent and efferent connections do not provide any clue as to what this difference might be. It is at this stage that neurophysiological studies hold promise.

The lesion experiments have, as we have seen, provided clear evidence that the cortex of the sulcus principalis is centrally involved in the mnemonic processes involved in, at least, spatial memory. Electrophysiological techniques provide another way of studying the role of the frontal cortex in information processing, and the kind of information provided by electrophysiology may enable us to determine the role of the frontal cortex and limbic areas in such processes, roles that on the basis of lesion studies alone appear similar (Iversen, 1972).

The approach is yielding interesting results, although interpretation is hindered by a lack of similar studies on the hippocampus.

In 1969 Stamm used electrical stimulation of the frontal cortex as a reversible lesion technique to find out exactly at what point in time the memory of a spatial event was no longer critically dependent on the normal functioning of the dorsolateral frontal cortex. Monkeys were trained on a DR task, and then the frontal cortex was bilaterally incapacitated at various times during DR performance. He found that disruptive electrical stimulation at the time the spatial cue was presented and during the early part of the delay severely impaired performance. Similar stimulation in the later stages of the delay or during the response was largely ineffective (Fig. 11). Stimulation of the ventrolateral caudate nucleus was not disruptive during the cue presentation but was disruptive if given at any time during the delay period.

These results gave the lead to experimenters who could record from single neurons in the frontal cortex in the behaving monkey. Fuster (1973a,b) found that 80% of the neurons in the banks of the sulcus principalis show sustained changes in firing pattern (either excitation or inhibition) during the cue period in the DR task. These changes frequently extended into the delay period. He subsequently studied neurons in the part of the nucleus medialis dorsalis of the thalamus (parvocellularis) that projects to the dorsolateral frontal cortex, and found similar changes in firing related to the presentation of the cue and the early delay period (Fuster and Alexander, 1973). The similarity of the patterns of activity in the neurons of the medialis dorsalis and the sulcus principalis, and the fact that cooling of the frontal cortex impairs DR performance and activity in the thalamic nucleus (Alexander and Fuster, 1973), led Fuster and Alexander (1973) to suggest that reciprocal circuitry between the two sites exists. This could constitute "the substratum for transiently reverberating circuits which contribute to the maintenance of sustained activation in the prefrontal neurones during the delay periods" (Alexander and Fuster, 1973) or, in other words, help the frontal cortex to retain all the external and internal sensory information it

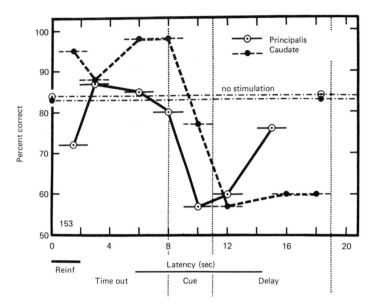

Fig. 11. Performance on 8-second DR by monkey with 2-second stimulation at 3.5 mA applied across principal sulcus and 2.8 mA to head of caudate nucleus. (Horizontal lines indicate periods of stimulus application.) In the principalis group performance was most impaired by stimulation during the cue presentation, whereas in the caudate group stimulation throughout the delay was disruptive. (From Stamm, 1969. Copyright 1969 by the American Psychological Association. Reprinted by permission.)

has received until such time as a response decision is made. Together with Stamm's results, these findings indicate that the sulcus principalis is characteristically active during the coding of spatial events.

Niki and his collaborators were interested in finding neurons that fire in association with the response made after a delay. Monkeys were trained to press alternately two panels with a 5-second delay. A large number of units in the banks of the sulcus principalis were found, which fire during the latter part of the intertrial interval, just before the arm movement to press the panel (Kubota and Niki, 1971). More recently Niki (1974a) found units in the same area, which also fire in conjunction with the response, but in this case the firing pattern differed depending on whether the response was to the left or to the right panel. The DR task has also been investigated, and in a preliminary study neurons were found which fire differentially with left and right responses (Niki, 1974c). In tracking down the parts of the brain involved in this efferent aspect of DA performance, studies have been extended to the caudate nucleus (Niki et al., 1972), a motor structure which receives direct connections from the sulcus principalis and which is known, on the basis of lesion studies, to be involved in DR performance. Neurons found in this structure fire just before the arm movement but not during the preceding delay. Although preliminary in nature these kinds of results indicate the potential value of electrophysiological techniques, and "it remains for further experimentation to clarify these matters and to determine the hierarchical arrangement whereby spatial information is transformed from its arrival in prefrontal cortex into the final mnemonic trace which underlies performance of delayed alternation and delayed response" (Niki, 1974b).

V. Where Now?

The conclusion is therefore that monkeys with medial temporal lesions indeed fail to learn and remember information presented to them under certain conditions. These conditions bear resemblance to those that in the human involve the use of a short-term–long-term memory process. The frontal lobe in humans appears to have acquired a sophisticated corollary of the storage process which adds time marking to the memory process. It is not clear if the frontal lobe of the monkey shares this property, even to a very limited degree. The frontal area with mnemonic function in the monkey appears to share the properties of the hippocampus of that species. The study of these problems in the monkey is difficult, because concept formation seems to be a corollary of high-order mnemonic processes and all the evidence suggests that monkeys are limited either by choice or design in this cognitive area.

It is quite clear that, if the understanding of the neural circuitry concerned in memory processing in the monkey is to advance, much attention must be given to the design of animal memory tests. Neuropsychologists have been all too ready to search on the shelves for some existing task which looks as if it might be a relevant measure for the cognitive process under study. There has also been a tendency to select a task that involves no complicated apparatus or extensive testing. In certain areas of study, for example, the specific visual agnosias associated with temporal cortex lesions, some of the simple tasks have served the science well. But this has not been the case in the study of memory disorders. Hippocampal monkeys have been said not to have memory disorders equivalent to those seen in H.M., because they readily learn visual discrimination tasks when tested for 30 trials per day. In what sense can this test be compared with conditions in humans that involve dynamic activity between short- and long-term memory processes?

Perhaps the next few years will see this remedied, since in several laboratories normal memory function in the monkey is the subject of an increasingly sophisticated body of research. Particularly noteworthy is the use by d'Amato (1973) of delayed matching to sample as a mnemonic test in the monkey, and the efforts of Davis and his collaborators to develop spatial memory tasks for the monkey in which the results can be tested against a predictive model of memory processing. Work of this kind begins to approach the experimentation accepted in the field of human memory.

In the context of what we have said about the dependence of nonhuman primates and other species on spatial memory, the spatial pattern reproduction test of Medin (1969) seems potentially useful. Monkeys faced a panel of 16 square panels (each 4×4 inches) which could be individually illuminated. On any trial one, two, or four lighted panels were exposed for a brief period, and after a delay the monkey was rewarded for pressing those panels that has been lighted. Various factors were uncovered, which determined the accuracy of memory for these patterns with one light; the position within the matrix strongly influenced its ease of reproduction, center panels being the most difficult and corner panels the easiest to remember. With two panels their distance apart (the greater the distance, the easier to remember) and the orientation of the two lights with respect to each other were important. When four panels were lit, the patterns were more easily remembered when the pattern had four sides and least well remembered when separated to form a 16-sided array. Surprisingly, however, symmetry of the patterns was *not* found to influence performance. More recently, Medin (1972) reanalyzed the results from the single-panel task at delays of 0, 1, 2, 5, 10, and 20 seconds. The changing error pattern as the delay increases was tested against predictions derived from one-processor, two-process models of memory. Models assuming a unitary memory trace fading at some constant rate toward zero cannot predict these data accurately, whereas a model assuming both short- and long-term components can account for the results.

In a later study (Borkhuis *et al.*, 1971), two panels were illuminated for 20 seconds, one with white and one with red. After a variable delay the white panel had to be pressed. Two hypotheses were considered which would explain errors in this task: (1) The animals remember which cells were illuminated but forget their color; (2) the animals fail to perceive or encode the red-lighted cells differently from those lighted white. An analysis of the nature of errors at the various delays allows one to distinguish a straightforward loss of discriminative information from confusion in perceptual coding. In the particular experiment performed the errors were best accounted for in terms of perceptual confusion, i.e., interpretation 2.

Experiments of this behavioral and analytical sophistication encourage the view that monkeys indeed have at least to some degree the equivalent of a two-process memory mechanism, and it would be most interesting to study the effects of bilateral medial temporal lesions on such performance. However, it should be noted that the monkeys used in these series of experiments had been trained for *more than 15 years*, and it remains to be seen if the large group of naive monkeys that would be required for a lesion study could master these tasks. It is conceivable that only after extensive training do monkeys give evidence of sophisticated mnemonic performance.

It may also be notable that in the Borkhuis *et al.* experiment the information to be remembered is presented in a spatial framework. Is this a prerequisite for memory? Work on chimpanzees (Farrer, 1967) suggests not. As described earlier, Farrer attempted to train chimpanzees on the concept of form matching. Performance to the match configurations was maintained in the absence of the cue stimulus and when the order of the 24 problems varied, thus eliminating true matching or response sequence learning as the basis of the excellent performance. The animals apparently had learned 24 easily confused, yet unique, stimulus configurations. Here, then, is an example of animal memory that matches the facility of human memory performance. But the animal was a chimpanzee, and many believe that this is the only relevant nonhuman primate to work with if one is seriously comparing the mnemonic capacity of humans and monkeys. Perhaps the chimpanzee does have cognitive properties that closely resemble those of humans, but their study can only be enhanced by comparing it with those of other subhuman primates.

In introducing their symposium volume on animal memory, Honig and James (1971) comment, "After a long period of neglect, experimental and theoretical work in the area of animal memory has recently revived." One may hope that animal neuropsychologists can share and contribute to this resurrection.

REFERENCES

Adey, W. R. (1961). *In* "Brain Mechanisms and Learning" (J. F. Delafresnaye, ed.), pp. 557–588. Blackwell, Oxford.

Adey, W. R., Walter, D. O., and Lindsley, D. F. (1962). *Arch. Neurol. (Chicago)* **6**, 194–207.

Akert, K. (1964). *In* "The Frontal Granular Cortex and Behavior" (J. M. Warren and K. Akert, eds.), pp. 372–394. McGraw-Hill, New York.

Alexander, G. E., and Fuster, J. M. (1973). *Brain Res.* **61**, 93–105.

Atkinson, R. C., and Shiffrin, R. H. (1968). *In* "The Psychology of Learning and Motivation: Advances in Research and Theory" (K. W. Spence and J. T. Spence, eds.), Vol. 2, pp. 89–195. Academic Press, New York.

Bekhterev, V. M. (1900). *Neurol. Zentralbl.* **19**, 990–991.

Benedek, L., and Juba, A. (1941). *Zentralbl. Gesamte Neurol. Psychiatrie* **177**, 282–292.

Bickford, R., Mulder, D. W., Dodge, H. W., Svien, H. J., and Rome, H. P. (1958). *Res. Publ., Assoc. Res. Nerv. Ment. Dis.* **36**, 227–257.

Bilodeau, E. A., Sulzer, J. L., and Levy, C. M. (1962). *Psychol. Monogr.* **76**, No. 20.

Blakemore, C. B., and Falconer, M. A. (1967). *J. Neurol., Neurosurg, Psychiatry* **30**, 364–367.

Borkuis, M. L., Davis, R. T., and Medin, D. L. (1971). *J. Comp. Physiol. Psychol.* **71**, 206–211.

Brion, S. (1969). *In* "The Pathology of Memory" (G. A. Talland and N. C. Waugh, eds.), pp. 29–39. Academic Press, New York.

Broadbent, D. E. (1958). "Perception and Communication." Pergamon, Oxford.

Butters, N., and Pandya, D. N. (1969). *Science* **165**, 1271–1273.

Cermak, L. S., Butters, N., and Gerrein, J. (1973). *Neuropsychologia* **11**, 85–94.

Corkin, S. (1965). *Neuropsychologia* **3**, 339–351.

Corkin, S. (1968). *Neuropsychologia* **6**, 255–266.

Correll, R. E., and Scoville, W. B. (1965a). *J. Comp. Physiol. Psychol.* **60**, 175–181.

Correll, R. E., and Scoville, W. B. (1965b). *J. Comp. Physiol. Psychol.* **60**, 360–367.

Correll, R. E., and Scoville, W. B. (1967). *Exp. Brain Res.* **4**, 85–96.

Correll, R. E, and Scoville, W. B. (1970). *J. Comp. Physiol. Psychol.* **70**, 464–469.

d'Amato, M. R. (1973). *In* "The Psychology of Learning and Motivation: Advances in Research and Theory" (G. H. Bower, ed.), Vol. 7, pp. 227–270. Academic Press, New York.

Domesick, V. B. (1969). *Brain Res.* **12**, 296–320.

Douglas, R. J. (1967). *Psychol. Bull.* **67**, 416–442.

Douglas, R. J. (1972). *In* "Inhibition and Learning" (R. A. Boakes and M. S. Halliday, eds.), pp. 529–553. Academic Press, New York.

Douglas, R. J., and Pribram, K. H. (1966). *Neuropsychologia* **4**, 197–220.

Douglas, R. J., Barrett, T. W., Pribram, K. H., and Cerny, M. C. (1969). *J. Comp. Physiol. Psychol.* **68**, 437–441.

Drachman, D. A., and Arbit, J. (1966). *Arch. Neurol. (Chicago)* **15**, 52–61.

Drachman, D. A., and Ommaya, A. K. (1964). *Arch. Neurol. (Chicago)* **10**, 411–425.

Farrer, D. N. (1967). *Percept. Mot. Skills* **25**, 305–315.

Fuster, J. M. (1973a). *J. Neurophysiol.* **36**, 61–78.

Fuster, J. M. (1973b). *In* "Psychophysiology of the Frontal Lobes" (K. H. Pribram and A. R. Luria, eds.) pp. 157–165. Academic Press, New York.

Fuster, J. M., and Alexander, G. E. (1973). *Brain Res.* **61**, 79–91.

Gaffan, P. (1972). *Neuropsychologia* **10**, 327–341.

Grastyan, E. (1954). *In* "The Central Nervous System and Behaviour (M. A. Brazier, ed.), pp. 119–205. Josiah Macy, Jr. Found., New York.

Gray, J. A. (1970). *Psychol. Bull.* **77**, 465–480.

Hassler, R., and Riechert, T. (1957). *Acta Neurochir.* **5**, 330–340.

Hebb, D. O. (1961). *In* "Brain Mechanisms and Learning" (J. F. Delafresnaye, ed.), pp. 37–46. Blackwell, Oxford.

Hirano, R., Best, P. J., and Olds, J. (1970). *Electroencephalogr. Clin. Neurophysiol.* **28**, 127–135.

Hjorth-Simonsen, A. (1971). *J. Comp. Neurol.* **142**, 417–438.

Hjorth-Simonsen, A. and Jeune, B. (1972). *J. Comp. Neurol.* **144**, 215–232.

Honig, W. K., and James, P. H. R., eds. (1971), "Animal Memory." Academic Press, New York.

Iversen, S. D. (1972). *In* "The Physiological Basis of Memory" (J. A. Deutch, ed.), pp. 305–364. Academic Press, New York.

John, E. R., and Killam, K. F. (1959). *J. Pharmacol. Exp. Ther.* **125**, 252–274.

Johnson, T. N., Rosvold, H. E., and Mishkin, M. (1968). *Exp. Neurol.* **21**, 20–34.

Jones, B., and Mishkin, M. (1972). *Exp. Neurol.* **36**, 362–377.
Keppel, G., and Underwood, B. J. (1962). *J. Verb. Learn. Verb. Behav.* **1**, 153–161.
Kesner, R. (1973). *Psychol. Bull.* **80**, 117–203.
Kimble, D. P. (1968). *Psychol. Bull.* **70**, 285–295.
Kimble, D. P., and Kimble, R. J. (1970). *Physiol. Behav.* **5**, 735–738.
Kimble, D. P., and Pribram, K. H. (1963). *Science* **139**, 824–825.
Kimura, D. (1963). *Arch. Neurol. (Chicago)* **8**, 264–271.
Krettek, J. E., and Price, J. L. (1974). *Brain Res.* **11**, 150–154.
Kubota, K., and Niki, H. (1971). *J. Neurophysiol.* **34**, 337–347.
Mahut, H. (1971). *Neuropsychologia* **9**, 409–424.
Mahut, H. (1972). *Neuropsychologia* **10**, 65–74.
Medin, D. L. (1969). *J. Comp. Physiol. Psychol.* **68**, 412–419.
Medin, D. L. (1972). *Am. J. Psychol.* **85**, 117–119.
Melton, A. W. (1963). *J. Verb. Learn. Verb. Behav.* **2**, 1–21.
Menzel, E. W. (1973). *Science* **182**, 943–945.
Meyer, D. R. (1971). *In* "Cognitive Processes of Nonhuman Primates" (L. E. Jarrard, ed.), pp. 83–102. Academic Press, New York.
Meyer, V., and Yates, A. J. (1955). *J. Neurol. Neurosurg. Psychiatry* **18**, 44–52.
Milner, B. (1958). *Res. Publ., Assoc. Res. Nerv. Ment. Dis.* **36**, 244–257.
Milner, B. (1959). *Psychiatr. Res. Rep.* **11**, 43–52.
Milner, B. (1963). *Arch. Neurol. (Chicago)* **9**, 90–100.
Milner, B. (1965). *Neuropsychologia* **3**, 317–338.
Milner, B. (1967). *In* "Brain Mechanisms Underlying Speech and Language" (F. L. Darlay, ed.), pp. 122–145. Grune & Stratton, New York.
Milner, B. (1968). *Neuropsychologia* **6**, 191–210.
Milner, B. (1970). *In* "Biology of Memory" (K. H. Pribram and D. E. Broadbent, eds.), pp. 29–50. Academic Press, New York.
Milner, B. (1971). *Br. Med. Bull.* **27**, 272–277.
Milner, B., and Kimura, D. (1964). *Pap., 35th Annu. Meet. East. Psychol. Assoc.*
Milner, B., and Teuber, H. L. (1968). *In* "Analysis of Behavioural Change" pp. 268–375. (L. Weiskrantz, ed.), Harper, New York.
Milner, B., Corkin, S., and Teuber, H.-L. (1968). *Neuropsychologia* **6**, 215–234.
Mishkin, M. (1954). *J. Comp. Physiol. Psychol.* **47**, 187–193.
Nauta, W. J. H. (1958). *Brain* **81**, 319–340.
Nauta, W. J. H. (1964). *In* "The Frontal Granular Cortex and Behavior" (J. M. Warren and K. Akert, eds.), pp. 397–409. McGraw-Hill, New York.
Nauta, W. J. H. (1971). *J. Psychiatr. Res.* **8**, 167–187.
Niki, H. (1974a). *Brain Res.* **68**, 185–196.
Niki, H. (1974b). *Brain Res.* **68**, 197–204.
Niki, H. (1974c). *Brain Res.* **70**, 346–349.
Niki, H., Sakai, M., and Kubota, K. (1972). *Brain Res.* **38**, 343–353.
Norman, D. A. (1969). "Memory and Attention: An Introduction to Human Information Processing." Wiley, New York.
Olds, J. (1970). *In* "The Neural Control of Behavior" (R. E. Whalen *et al.*, eds.), pp. 257–293. Academic Press, New York.
Orbach, J., Milner, B., and Rasmussen, T. (1960). *Arch. Neurol. (Chicago)* **3**, 230–251.
Pandya, D. N., and Kuypers, H. G. J. M. (1969). *Brain Res.* **13**, 13–36.
Pandya, D. N., Dye, P., and Butters, N. (1971). *Brain Res.* **31**, 35–46.
Papez, J. W. (1937). *Arch. Neurol. Psychiatry* **38**, 725–743.

Penfield, W., and Milner, B. (1958). *Arch. Neurol. Psychiatry* **79**, 475–497.
Posner, M. I. (1966). *Science* **152**, 1712–1718.
Posner, M. I., and Konick, A. F. (1966). *Org. Behav. Hum. Perform.* **1**, 71–86.
Pribram, K. H. (1967). *Prog. Brain Res.* **27**, 318–336.
Pribram, K. H., Wilson, W. A., Jr., and Connors, J. (1962). *Exp. Neurol.* **6**, 36–47.
Pribram, K. H., Douglas, R. J., and Pribram, B. J. (1969). *J. Comp. Physiol. Psychol.* **69**, 765–772.
Prisko, L. (1963). Unpublished Ph.D. Thesis, McGill University, Montreal.
Raisman, G., Cowan, W. M., and Powell, T. P. S. (1965a). *Brain* **88**, 963–996.
Raisman, G., Cowan, W. M., and Powell, T. P. S. (1965b). *Brain* **89**, 83–108.
Ramón y Cajal, S. (1955). "Studies on the Cerebral Cortex" (L. L. Kraft, transl.). Yearbook, London.
Rholes, F. H. (1961). *J. Exp. Anal. Behav.* **4**, 323–352.
Rosvold, H. E. (1968). *In* "Mind as a Tissue" (C. Rupp, ed.), pp. 21–38. Harper, New York.
Scoville, W. B., and Milner, B. (1957). *J. Neurol., Neurosurg. Psychiatry* **20**, 11–21.
Schulman, S. (1964). *Arch. Neurol. (Chicago)* **11**, 477–499.
Shankweiler, D. (1966). *Pap. 37th Annu. Meet. East. Psychol. Assoc.*
Shepard, R. N. (1967). *J. Verb. Learn. Verb. Behav.* **6**, 156–163.
Sidman, M., Stoddard, L. T., and Mohr. J. P. (1968). *Neuropsychologia* **6**, 245–254.
Spiegel, E. A., Wycis, H. T., Orchinik, C., and Freed, H. (1956). *Am. J. Psychiatry* **113**, 97–105.
Stamm, J. S. (1969). *J. Comp. Physiol. Psychol.* **67**, 535–546.
Starr, A., and Phillips, L. (1970). *Neuropsychologia* **8**, 75–88.
Stevens, R., and Cowey, A. (1973). *Brain Res.* **52**, 203–224.
Terzian, H. (1958). *In* "Temporal Lobe Epilepsy" (M. Baldwin and D. Bailey, eds.), pp. 510–529. Thomas, Springfield, Illinois.
Tolman, E. (1948). *Psychol. Rev.* **55**, 189–208.
Ungerstedt, U. (1971). *Acta Physiol. Scand., Suppl.* **367**, 95–122.
Uretsky, E., and McCleary, R. A. (1969). *J. Comp. Physiol. Psychol.* **68**, 1–8.
Vanderwolf, C. H. (1971). *Psychol. Rev.* **78**, 83–113.
Van Hoesen, G. W., Pandya, D. N., and Butters, N. (1972). *Science* **175**, 1471–1473.
von Bonin, G. (1941). *J. Comp. Neurol.* **75**, 287–314.
Votaw, C. L. (1959). *J. Comp. Neurol.* **112**, 353–382.
Votaw, C. L. (1960). *J. Comp. Neurol.* **114**, 283–293.
Warburton, D. M. (1972). *In* "Inhibition and Learning" (R. A. Boakes and M. S. Halliday, eds.), pp. 431–460. Academic Press, New York.
Warrington, E. K. and James, M. (1967). *Cortex* **3**, 317–326.
Warrington, E. K., and Shallice, T. (1969). *Brain* **92**, 885–896.
Warrington, E. K., and Weiskrantz, L. (1970). *Nature (London)* **228**, 628–630.
Warrington, E. K., and Weiskrantz, L. (1972). *In* "The Physiological Basis of Memory" (J. A. Deutch, ed.), pp. 365–396. Academic Press, New York.
Waxler, M., and Rosvold, H. E. (1970). *Neuropsychologia* **8**, 137–146.
Weiskrantz, L. (1970). *In* "Short and Long-Term Processes in the Nervous System" (R. Hinde and G. Horn, eds.), pp. 63–74. Cambridge Univ. Press, London and New York.
Whitlock, D. G., and Nauta, W. J. H. (1956). *J. Comp. Neurol.* **106**, 183–212.
Whitty, C. W. M., and Lewin, W. (1960). *Brain* **83**, 648–653.
Yntema, D. B., and Trask, F. B. (1963). *J. Verb. Learn. Verb. Behav.* **2**, 65–74.
Zola, S. M., and Mahut, H. (1973). *Neuropsychologia* **11**, 271–284.

SYNAPTOSOMAL TRANSPORT PROCESSES

By Giulio Levi and Maurizio Raiteri

Laboratorio di Biologia Cellulare, Consiglio Nazionale delle Ricerche, Roma, Italy
and
Istituto di Farmacologia, Università Cattolica, Rome, Italy

I. Introduction

In a recent article Osborne and Bradford (1975) stated: "The synaptosome is emerging as a fundamental *in vitro* preparation for studying the dynamic biochemical aspect of neurotransmission and neurosecretion. It qualifies, in many respects, as a functioning presynaptic entity with an impressive range of metabolic and transmission based properties." This statement is justified by numerous studies demonstrating the morphological, metabolic, and functional integrity of synaptosomes (Whittaker, 1973; Abdel-Latif, 1973; De Belleroche and Bradford, 1973a,b; Bradford et al., 1975).

Synaptosomes prepared from whole brain or from grossly dissected brain areas are heterogeneous; in fact, even the purest synaptosomal preparation contains populations of nerve endings synthesizing and utilizing different neurotransmitters. In spite of this heterogeneity, synaptosomes are often preferred to other nervous tissues preparations in studies concerned with properties believed to be specific to presynaptic nerve terminals. This is par-

51

ticularly the case for ion and metabolite transport processes directly or indirectly related to neurotransmission. Since transport phenomena are ubiquitous, and the characteristics of transport of many substrates seem to differ in different structures and cells of the central nervous system, the use of purified synaptosomes offers the advantage of excluding the bulk of the transport due to structures other than nerve endings. Moreover, with synaptosomes it is possible to study the effects of changes in the composition of the suspending medium without the interference of diffusional barriers which may limit or slow down equilibration of the extracellular fluid of more intact preparations, such as brain slices, with the incubation medium.

In this article we discuss some aspects of synaptosomal transport mechanisms, rather than give an extensive survey of the literature on synaptosomal transport studies. Our aim is to emphasize, with some pertinent examples, the multiplicity of interpretations that can be given to many observations made in this field. Several aspects of neurotransmitter transport at nerve endings have been recently reviewed (Snyder *et al.*, 1970, 1973a,b; Bennett *et al.*, 1974; Iverson, 1970, 1971, 1973, Smith, 1973; De Belleroche and Bradford, 1973a; Krnjevic, 1974; De Feudis, 1975).

II. Methodological Aspects of Synaptosomal Transport Studies

Studies on synaptosomal transport processes have been performed under a variety of experimental conditions whose importance in the determination of the results obtained has rarely been evaluated. We give only a few examples of the factors that can lead to quantitatively and qualitatively different results and interpretations.

Whether purified synaptosomes, crude mitochondrial fractions (P_2), or homogenates (1000 g supernatants) are used may be of importance. For example, mitochondria seem to accumulate γ-aminobutyric acid (GABA) and, particularly, glutamate to some extent (Levi *et al.*, 1974), and they avidly accumulate calcium (Lust and Robinson, 1970). Homogenates contain large amounts of free endogenous compounds released during homogenization, which may interfere directly or indirectly with the transport of various substrates. However, purified synaptosomes are less active than cruder preparations in accumulating various compounds. The presence of substrates of endogenous origin in incubation media, which is maximal when homogenates are used, can be significant with washed P_2 fractions or purified synaptosomes also, particularly when fairly high ratios between amount of tissue and volume of medium are used, because of leakage from tissue particles. This may well affect the accumulation of radioactive substrates used at low concentrations (see, for example, Guyenet *et al.*, 1973a).

Localization of the uptake of neurotransmitters and choline into specific nerve endings critically depends on the concentration of substrate used. In fact, it has been demonstrated that, when the concentrations of radioactive amino acid and amine transmitters are increased above a certain level, radioactivity is accumulated by nonspecific synaptosomes also (Iversen, 1970; Snyder et al., 1973a). Obtaining a specific labeling of synaptosomal populations by radioactive neurotransmitters is essential for interpreting data on neurotransmitter release induced by drugs affecting certain systems specifically (Raiteri et al., 1976).

The temperature at which synaptosomes are incubated may affect not only the rates of fluxes measured, but also the affinity constants; it has been shown in other systems that, depending on the substrate studied, a decrease in temperature may bring about an increase or a decrease in the apparent K_m values for transport (Jacquez et al., 1970).

The methods used for collecting synaptosomes after incubation generally include a step in which the transport reaction is stopped by diluting the particles, or by washing them on filters, with medium at a low temperature. As amply discussed elsewhere (Levi and Raiteri, 1973; Raiteri and Levi, 1973a; Levi et al., 1976a), sudden cooling of synaptosomes leads to a differential loss of exogenous as well as endogenous substrates. Depending on the experimental conditions, the loss of amino acids may vary from a small percentage (Simon et al., 1974) to 70–80% (Levi et al., 1976a), whereas that of biogenic amines is minimal even under the most drastic conditions, probably reflecting the different degree of intrasynaptosomal binding of the two classes of compounds (Levi et al., 1976a).

The simultaneous existence of release and reuptake processes at the synaptosomal membrane often makes it difficult to evaluate whether the effect of a given experimental condition (change in the ionic composition of the medium, presence of drugs, etc.) is primarily due to interference with the uptake or with the release process. This difficulty can be circumvented by studying the initial rate of uptake and by monitoring the release under conditions in which reuptake is prevented (Raiteri et al., 1974, 1975a, 1976).

Besides the variations due to nonuniform experimental conditions, different interpretations can be given to identical crude results if they are handled in different ways. For example, in some cases the kinetic analysis of influx revealed the presence of a nonsaturable component of transport, which was subtracted from the overall transport to obtain the saturable components (Lahdesmaki and Oja, 1973). In other instances, however, a "diffusion" component was estimated by measuring the accumulation of the compound under study at 0°C and by subtracting this from the values obtained at higher temperatures. This procedure, utilized for the analysis of choline transport, has led to the conclusion that choline is taken up into synaptosomes only by a high-affinity transport system (Guyenet et al., 1973b), and not by two saturable uptake systems, one of high and one of low affinity (Yamamura and Snyder, 1973; Haga and Noda, 1973). It should be noted that simple diffusion of highly polar solutes across cell membranes is not very likely (Christensen, 1976), and that the characteristics of diffusion at 0°C and at physiological temperatures are probably not superimposable, mainly because of the different physical state of membrane lipids (Oldfield and Chapman, 1972). Moreover, with some substrates, like GABA, a specific saturable and sodium-dependent accumulation is present at 0°C (Weinstein et al., 1965; De Feudis, 1975; Olsen et al., 1975), which makes questionable the correctness of subtracting 0°C "diffusion" rates from transport rates measured at higher temperatures.

III. Uptake Studies

A. CONCENTRATIVE UPTAKE AT THE SYNAPTOSOMAL MEMBRANE

Concentrative synaptosomal uptake has been described for several substrates, including putative neurotransmitters, neurotransmitter precursors, and normal metabolites. The apparent steady-state tissue/medium (T/M) ratios achieved when radioactive substrates are used depend not only on the compound under study (e.g., in cortical synaptosomes: glutamic acid > GABA > dopamine > norepinephrine), but also on the substrate concentration present in the medium (higher T/M radioactivity ratios are achieved at lower concentrations). There is often a relationship between the endogenous concentrations of various substrates and their apparent concentrative accumulation and, for a given substrate, between regional endogenous level and regional accumulation. For example, glutamate synaptosomal concentration and accumulation are higher in telencephalic than in diencephalic areas, and the converse is true for GABA (Levi et al., 1974). Glycine concentration and accumulation are higher in the more caudal areas of the central nervous system (Aprison and McBride, 1973). The highest accumulation of dopamine (DA) is observed in the corpus striatum, where DA levels are the highest (Snyder et al., 1970). This correlation is probably not a general one; for example, no correlation between regional levels and accumulation of taurine was observed (Oja et al., 1976).

It should be noted that, even if the apparent T/M radioactivity ratios corresponded in all cases to a net accumulation of radioactive substrates (but see following paragraph), the experimental values obtained with heterogeneous synaptosomal populations may be misleading. For example, the accumulation of 0.1 μM radioactive GABA is about 10 times higher than that of radioactive norepinephrine (NE) in whole brain synaptosomes, where the average concentration of GABA (about 20 nmoles/mg protein; see Simon *et al.*, 1974; Levi *et al.*, 1974) is about 4000 times higher than that of NE (Blaustein *et al.*, 1972). It thus appears that GABA is concentrated against a much steeper gradient. However, this may not be the case. Let us assume that endogenous GABA is contained and exogenous GABA is accumulated only in "gabergic" synaptosomes, and that the same holds for NE in noradrenergic synaptosomes. Since a high ratio between the number of "gabergic" and of noradrenergic synaptosomes is likely to be present [a ratio of 400 in whole brain may not be too far from the truth, judging from electron microscope autoradiographic studies (Hokfelt, 1970; Iversen and Bloom, 1972)], the difference between the endogenous concentrations of the two neurotransmitters at their specific terminals may not be as large as it appears, and the accumulation of NE in noradrenergic synaptosomes may be even larger than that of GABA at "gabergic" terminals.

In the experimental conditions often encountered in synaptosomal uptake studies (high concentrations of endogenous substrates in the tissue, as compared to low concentrations of radioactive substrates in the incubation medium), false indications of the extent to which the observed accumulation of radioactivity corresponds to an actual net accumulation may derive from at least one of the following situations.

1. The exogenous substrate may exchange with its endogenous counterpart, or with endogenous compounds sharing the same transport system. By this mechanism, which does not lead to changes in the actual concentrations in the medium or in the tissue, a theoretical T/M radioactivity ratio equal to the ratio between the concentration of the substrate in the particles and that in the medium could be reached. Synaptosomes incubated in 0.1 μM radioactive GABA, glutamate, or tryptophan could theoretically reach T/M radioactivity ratios of about 20,000, 100,000, and 1000, respectively, merely by homoexchange (GABA) or by homo- and heteroexchange (glutamate and tryptophan). That exchange processes are present in synaptosomes has been demonstrated for various amino acids (Grahame-Smith and Parfitt, 1970; Levi and Raiteri, 1974; Simon *et al.*, 1974; Raiteri *et al.*, 1975b; Levi *et al.*, 1976b) and for calcium (Swanson *et al.*, 1974; Blaustein and Oborn, 1975).

2. Radioactive substrate that has crossed the membrane can be removed from a free cytoplasmic pool by intracellular metabolic reactions. For example, it is known that a large part of the radioactive choline taken up by synaptosomes incubated in low concentrations of choline is rapidly converted to acetylcholine (Haga, 1971; Yamamura and Snyder, 1973; Haga and Noda, 1973; Guyenet *et al.*, 1973a,b). The described coupling between choline uptake and acetylcholine synthesis is likely to maintain a low concen-

tration of free intrasynaptosomal choline, and it is possible that the uptake of choline is favored by continuous metabolic removal of the substrate; so far it has been impossible to determine the uptake of choline under conditions in which acetylcholine synthesis is specifically inhibited. In this respect, it is noteworthy that a reduction in the activity of cholinergic nerve endings, produced *in vivo*, caused a decreased choline uptake rate in hippocampal synaptosomes (Simon and Kuhar, 1975).

3. The accumulation of a given substrate can also be influenced by other processes causing a decreased cytoplasmic level of free substrate, such as binding or incorporation into subsynaptosomal organelles. These processes may favor the accumulation of extracellular compounds, whether they cross the synaptosomal membrane by an uphill transport mechanism or simply by facilitated diffusion. With many substances, such as amino acids, which, according to the available evidence (Raiteri and Levi, 1973a,b; Levi *et al.*, 1976a), are largely free in the cytoplasm, intracellular binding is not likely to favor accumulation in a significant way. This, however, is not the case for other substrates. Calcium is largely bound intracellularly, and a great part of this element seems to be sequestered in synaptosomal mitochondria (Lust and Robinson, 1970; Swanson *et al.*, 1974). Very little NE seems to exist free in the cytoplasm; [³H]NE in fact is not released from synaptosomes by treatments known to deplete synaptosomal amino acids and potassium (Raiteri and Levi, 1973a,b; White and Archibald, 1974; Levi *et al.*, 1976a), and the cytoplasmic concentration of NE may be so low that the amine may cross the synaptosomal membrane by facilitated diffusion (White and Archibald, 1974). It should be added that overestimation of the net accumulation of radioactive substrates rapidly bound to intracellular sites may derive from a displacement of unlabeled molecules, bound intracellularly, by radioactive molecules, that have recently entered. This possibility is supported by the data of Philippu and Beyer (1973) showing that radioactive DA can displace 90% of the endogenous DA contained in striatal synaptic vesicles.

B. Kinetic Aspects of Synaptosomal Uptake Processes

The accumulation of radioactive substrates in synaptosomes has often been analyzed by Michaelis–Menten kinetics. Synaptosomes seem rather unique, as compared to other nervous tissue preparations or to other tissues, in that they exhibit an apparent high-affinity uptake for a variety of substrates, including glucose (Diamond and Fishman 1973), cyclic AMP (Johnston and Balkar, 1973), non-neurotransmitter and neurotransmitter amino acids (Iversen, 1970; Martin, 1973; Snyder *et al.*, 1973a,b; Peterson and Ragupathy, 1973; Bennett *et al.*, 1974; Belin *et al.*, 1974; Bauman *et al.*, 1974; Levi and Raiteri, 1975; Oja *et al.*, 1976), biogenic amines (Snyder *et* al., 1970; Shore, 1972; Iversen 1973; Bogdanski, 1976), and neurotransmitter precursors such as choline (Haga and Noda, 1973; Yamamura and Snyder, 1973; Guyenet et al., 1973a,b), tyrosine, and tryptophan (Belin et al., 1974; Hamon et al., 1974). Depending on the substrate, tentative roles for the various high-affinity uptake systems have been proposed. So, the high-affinity uptake of glucose may serve to support the high rate of energy production of presynaptic nerve terminals (Diamond and Fishman, 1973); that of neurotransmitters may serve to remove these substances rapidly from the synaptic cleft (Iversen, 1970; Snyder et al., 1973a,b); and that of neurotransmitter precursors may replace the depleted neurotransmitter stores rapidly (Snyder et al., 1973b; Hamon et al., 1974). We are not aware of any proposed role for the high-affinity uptake of non-neurotransmitter amino acids. In addition to high-affinity uptake systems, many of the compounds studied can utilize systems characterized by a lower affinity, generally considered less specific and subserving general metabolic functions, not related to neurotransmission.

The existence of high- and low-affinity transport systems was generally postulated on the basis of the presence of a break in the Lineweaver–Burk plots. However, two-limbed curves in double reciprocal plots may derive not only from the existence of two or more separate transport systems with widely different affinities (Scriver and Mohyuddin, 1968), but also from phenomena of negative allosteric cooperativity, as suggested by Hamon et al. (1974) in the case of tryptophan transport. Moreover, when uptake measurements are based on accumulation of radioactivity, the coexistence of accelerated exchange diffusion and a net uptake process may also simulate the presence of two uptake processes. In the case of GABA, it has been shown that the synaptosomal accumulation of [³H]GABA, in the concentration range of the postulated high-affinity uptake system, can be accounted for by a homoexchange process (Levi and Raiteri, 1974; Raiteri et al., 1975b) having similar kinetic parameters (Simon et al., 1974). An analogous situation may exist with glutamate (Levi et al., 1976b), and possibly with other amino acids.

It should be noted that the calculations of the exchange rates of GABA made by Levi and Raiteri (1974), Raiteri et al. (1975b), and Simon et al. (1974) are based on the assumption that the [³H]GABA used for prelabeling the synaptosomes is homogeneously distributed within the endogenous GABA pool. Although in subsequent studies it has been shown that newly taken up and newly synthesized GABA behave similarly in homoexchange experiments (Levi et al., 1976b), the possibility that the endogenously stored GABA is not as easily exchangeable as the recently entered or formed GABA still remains open. If this is the case, the exchange rates have been overestimated in the studies mentioned above.

The studies on amino acids discussed above raise the question whether or not an exchange process can simulate the presence of a high-affinity net uptake for other classes of neurotransmitters also, such as catecholamines. We decided to determine whether or not unlabeled amines could exchange with radioactive amines preaccumulated by synaptosomes under experimental conditions comparable to those employed with GABA. Figure 1 shows that superfusing synaptosomes, prelabeled with [³H]NE or [³H]DA, with low concentrations of the corresponding unlabeled amine lead to an increase in the release of radioactivity, as observed with GABA. However, even if one assumes that this increased release is due to an exchange pro-

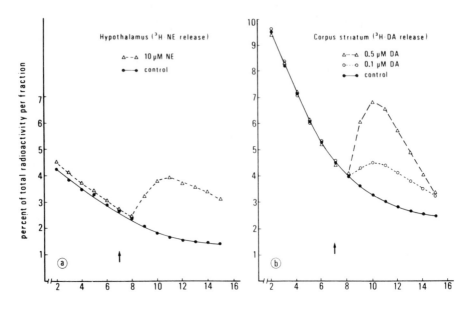

FIG. 1. Stimulation of [³H]NE and [³H]DA release from superfused synaptosomes by unlabeled NE and DA, respectively. Crude synaptosomal preparation from rat hypothalamus (a) or corpus striatum (b), resuspended in 0.32 M glucose and diluted 1:10 in a Krebs–Ringer medium at a protein concentration of 0.8 mg/ml, were equilibrated for 10 minutes at 37°C in a rotary waterbath and then incubated in the presence of 0.1 μM [³H]amine NE in the experiments in (a); DA in those in (b). After 10 minutes, aliquots of the suspension were superfused at 37°C in several parallel superfusion chambers (Raiteri et al., 1974) with a glucose-containing oxygenated medium. After 7 minutes the medium was replaced with new medium containing the unlabeled amine at the concentration indicated in the figure. Incubation and superfusion media contained 12.5 μM nialamide and 1 mM ascorbic acid. The radioactivity released in each 1-minute fraction and that remaining in the tissue at the end of the superfusion were measured by liquid scintillation. Each curve is the average of two duplicate experiments.

cess at the level of the plasma membrane (although other possibilities, such as displacement from intrasynaptosomal binding sites, should probably be favored), a calculation of the NE exchange rates based on the endogenous concentration of the amine would give, for an identical peak of radioactivity, values about 4000 lower than those calculated for GABA. Since the uptake of radioactive NE is only 10 times lower than that of radioactive GABA, it is clear that exchange can account for only a small percentage of the NE accumulated by the synaptosomes.

IV. Sodium Dependence of Synaptosomal Transport Processes

Many studies deal with the ionic requirements of the various synaptosomal transport systems; most of them emphasize the importance of extracellular ions, and only a few reports have drawn attention to the importance of intracellular ionic concentrations (Banay-Schwartz et al., 1976; Bogdanski, 1976), probably because of the technical difficulties inherent in this type of study.

A. EFFECTS OF SODIUM ON INFLUX

The sodium dependence of many synaptosomal uptake processes has been widely analyzed. Extracellular sodium is not required for the transport of some compounds, such as glucose (Diamond and Fishman, 1973) and several non-neurotransmitter amino acids (Grahame-Smith and Parfitt, 1970; Bennett et al., 1974; Bauman et al., 1974). Sometimes sodium has moderate effects, as in the case of the low-affinity uptake systems for putative transmitter amino acids (Bennett et al., 1974; Levi and Raiteri, 1975). In contrast, the high-affinity uptake of putative neurotransmitters and of choline shows an absolute sodium requirement (see recent reviews by Snyder et al., 1973a,b; Bennett et al., 1974; De Feudis, 1975; Bogdanski, 1976). In the case of [³H]GABA (Simon et al., 1974; Raiteri et al., 1975b) and of [¹⁴C]glutamate (Levi et al., 1976b), it has been shown that high-affinity uptake and exchange exhibit an identical sodium dependence, thus supporting the idea that these radioactive substrates are largely accumulated in synaptosomes by a homoexchange rather than by a net uptake process.

There is quite general agreement on the idea that, in sodium-dependent uptake systems, the inward-directed sodium gradient maintained by the sodium pump favors inward transport and intracellular accumulation (Crane, 1965; Weinstein et al., 1965; Bogdanski et al., 1970a,b; Martin, 1973; but see White and Keen, 1971). However, interactions between sodium and the transport system have not been established unequivocally. In a model for GABA transport proposed by Weinstein *et al.* (1965), sodium was considered important for increasing GABA binding to the carrier. Subsequent kinetic studies carried out with various neurotransmitters showed that interaction of sodium with the carrier could lead either to increased affinity for the substrate or to increased mobility of the carrier–substrate complex. For example, Martin (1973) found that an increase in sodium concentration from 19 to 95 mM caused a 10-fold increase in the maximal velocity of GABA uptake and only a 2-fold decrease in the apparent K_m. From kinetic analyses performed in calcium-free media, this investigator concluded that there must be at least three cooperatively interacting sodium sites in the GABA transport system, and noted that this type of stoichiometry greatly favors the concentrative capacity of the particles with respect to GABA.

However, Bennett *et al.* (1973) showed that a decrease in sodium concentration affects synaptosomal glutamate uptake essentially by increasing the apparent K_m, and provided kinetic data suggesting a 1:1 cotransport of sodium and glutamate into the particles. The same investigators showed that the kinetics of the sodium-dependent glycine uptake into medullary and spinal synaptosomes is more complex and may indicate cooperative interaction between sodium and the carrier. In the case of biogenic amines, Bogdanski (1976) supports the idea that sodium increases the affinity between the carrier and NE or 5-hydroxytryptamine (5-HT) and is cotransported at a 1:1 ratio. However, an effect of sodium on the K_m for NE transport was excluded by White and Paton (1972) who proposed two alternative models which, however, still provide for an effect of the sodium electrochemical gradient. According to Holz and Coyle (1974), the K_m for [³H]DA uptake into striatal synaptosomes is not influenced by variations in the sodium concentration, and sodium may be cotransported with the amine across the synaptosomal membrane.

These few examples are sufficient to realize that there is little agreement on the role and the mechanism of action of sodium in synaptosomal sodium-dependent transport processes. Although the uptake of many substrates exhibits apparently similar sodium requirements, it is likely that this ion plays different roles, depending on the compound considered, on its intracellular compartmentation and metabolism, and on the direction (inward or outward) of the flux (see Section II, B).

B. Effects of Sodium on Efflux

The effects of sodium on metabolite efflux from synaptosomes have been studied only sparingly. However, the data available on GABA and NE lend themselves to a discussion that may also be valid for other compounds. Sodium seems to be equally required for the uptake of NE and GABA. However, sodium affects the efflux of these putative transmitters from synaptosomes in a strikingly different way.

Synaptosomes prelabeled with radioactive GABA showed the same retention of radioactivity whether they were subsequently incubated or superfused in the presence or in the absence of sodium (Simon et al., 1974; Raiteri et al., 1975b). It appears therefore that a favorable sodium gradient is not sufficient to trigger an outward transport of the amino acid, in spite of the very steep downhill GABA gradient. In view of this observation, the substantial releasing effect produced by ouabain (Fig. 2) cannot be easily explained by the creation of a sodium gradient more favorable to outward transport, as suggested by Hammerstad and Cutler (1972) on the basis of observations on brain slices. As a matter of fact, the efflux of [³H]GABA

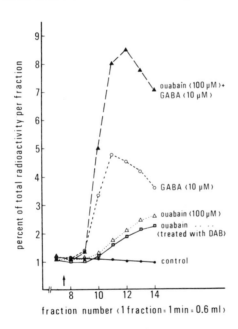

FIG. 2. Effect of ouabain on the release of [³H]GABA from synaptosomes. Purified synaptosomes from rat cerebrum were prelabeled for 10 minutes with 0.5 μM [³H]GABA and superfused as described in the legend for Fig. 1. In a group of experiments, 100 μM L-diaminobutyric acid (DAB) was present in the incubation medium during the prelabeling phase. After 7.5 minutes of superfusion with standard medium, the medium in some of the superfusion chambers was replaced with new medium containing 10 μM ouabain, 10 μM GABA, or both. The incubation and superfusion media contained 10 μM aminooxyacetic acid. Each curve is the average of three experiments run in duplicate.

induced by ouabain does not seem to be mediated by the same agency mediating GABA transport, since the ouabain releasing effect was not decreased in conditions under which the GABA carrier was almost completely blocked by prior incubation of the synaptosomes with L-diaminobutyric acid (Levi et al., in preparation). Ouabain may thus cause a non-carrier-mediated release of [³H]GABA by other mechanisms, such as membrane depolarization and/or increased availability of free intracellular calcium.

In experiments in which unlabeled GABA was added, together with ouabain, to the superfusing fluid, (Levi et al., 1976b,c), the release of [³H]GABA was by and large greater than the sum of the releases induced by either compound alone (Fig. 2). Since double-label experiments (i.e., synaptosomes prelabeled with [³H]GABA and superfused with [¹⁴C]GABA) showed a lower accumulation of [¹⁴C]GABA when ouabain was present, the above results suggest that, if the [³H]GABA released by ouabain and by unlabeled GABA originate from the same intracellular pool, a change in the stoichiometry of GABA homoexchange in the direction of net outward transport may take place under the new ionic intracellular conditions (increased sodium, decreased potassium and, possibly, increased "free" calcium) determined by the drug. It is noteworthy that the potentiating action of ouabain on the GABA-stimulated [³H]GABA release was also present at a GABA concentration (1 mM) giving a maximal stimulation of [³H]GABA release in the absence of the drug. Identical results were obtained by superfusing the synaptosomes with a potassium-free medium (unpublished observations) which, like ouabain, blocks Na⁺-K⁺-ATPase (Schwartz et al., 1972).

In conclusion, if one considers only the sodium gradient as a driving force for GABA fluxes, there seems to be an asymmetry in the requirements for inward and outward carrier-mediated GABA transport at synaptosomal membranes; in fact, the sodium gradient theory is not in accord with the lack of GABA release in the absence of extracellular sodium. The differential effect of a favorable sodium gradient on GABA influx may be a manifestation of the fact that in influx experiments GABA is present on both sides of the membrane, whereas in efflux experiments intracellular GABA must move into a medium free of GABA. A possible consequence of this reasoning is that a carrier-mediated efflux of GABA can be obtained only when GABA (and, obviously, sodium) is present extracellularly, i.e., under conditions in which homoexchange occurs. In this respect, it is interesting that the release of [³H]GABA, triggered by various agents in the absence of extracellular GABA (high potassium; see Fig. 3), ouabain, and spider venom (unpublished), seems to be largely non-carrier-mediated, being scarcely affected by pretreatment of the synaptosomes with L-diaminobutyric acid; this analog strongly inhibits the carrier-mediated homo- and heteroexchange of GABA (Levi et al., 1976b and in preparation).

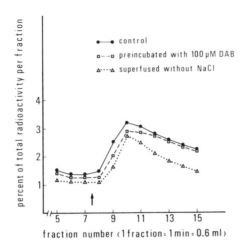

FIG. 3. Effect of 56 mM KCl on the release of [³H]GABA from synaptosomes pretreated with L-diaminobutyric acid or superfused with a sodium-free medium. Experimental conditions were as described in the legend for Fig. 2, except that in one group of experiments the superfusion medium contained 256 mM sucrose instead of 128 mM NaCl. After 7.5 minutes of superfusion, the synaptosomes were exposed to a medium containing 56 mM KCl, replacing an equimolar concentration of NaCl. Each curve is the average of three experiments run in duplicate or in triplicate, except the sodium-free curve which is the average of two experiments (one in duplicate and one in quadruplicate).

A completely different situation seems to exist with NE. In fact, synaptosomes prelabeled with [³H]NE lost much more radioactivity when sodium was not present in the medium (Bogdanski et al., 1968). This increased release of [³H]NE cannot be due only to reuptake inhibition resulting from a lack of sodium, since it was reproduced in our laboratories under superfusion conditions in which reuptake of the released amine was prevented. In the absence of extracellular sodium, a change in the direction of the sodium gradient may allow the outward transport of cytoplasmic NE; the equilibrium between vesicle-bound and free NE would thus be shifted in a direction favoring further detachment of the bound amine. It cannot be excluded that the release of amine from storage sites is facilitated also by a decreased level of high-energy phosphates, a consequence of the lowered sodium concentration.

The release of [³H]NE from synaptosomes was very slightly increased by ouabain (Levi et al., 1976c), under superfusion conditions that excluded any possible effect of the drug on reuptake (Fig. 4). Since ouabain causes a rapid increase in intracellular sodium concentration in synaptosomes (Archibald and White, 1974), the effect of the drug on [³H]NE release could be

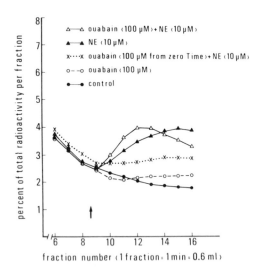

FIG. 4. Effect of ouabain on the release of [³H]NE from synaptosomes. Crude syn-aptosomal fractions from rat cerebrum were prelabeled with 0.1 μM [³H]NE for 10 minutes in the presence of nialamide and ascorbic acid and then superfused as de-scribed in the legend for Fig. 1. After 8.5 minutes the standard superfusion medium was replaced with a new medium containing 100 μM ouabain, 10 μM NE, or both. In one group of experiments ouabain was present in the medium from the beginning of superfusion, and 10 μM NE was added after 8.5 minutes. Each curve is the average of two duplicate experiments. One experiment performed with hypothalamic synaptosomes gave similar results.

explained by the establishment of a more favorable sodium gradient. Other mechanisms may be also involved; e.g., it is likely that sodium hinders the binding of NE to brain synaptic vesicles (Colburn *et al.*, 1968), so that under conditions of abnormally high intracellular sodium more NE may be present in the cytoplasm.

Ouabain, added together with unlabeled NE to the superfusion fluid, had only a brief and modest potentiating effect on the NE-induced [³H]NE re-lease (Fig. 4), which could be explained, as in the case of GABA, by the activation of facilitated exchange diffusion under conditions in which both [³H]NE and sodium are increased in the cytoplasm. After a few minutes, or when unlabeled NE was added to synaptosomes previously superfused with ouabain, the NE-induced [³H]NE release in the presence of the drug was, however, lower than in its absence (Levi *et al.*, 1976c). The latter observa-tion is in keeping with the finding that the glycoside inhibits inward trans-port of NE after a lag period of few minutes (Tissari *et al.*, 1969).

The fact that after a short period of exposure to ouabain the NE-induced [³H]NE release was inhibited suggests that the increased release of [³H]NE elicited by unlabeled NE in control synaptosomes is not due to a simple homoexchange process at the synaptosomal membrane (in this case ouabain would be expected to potentiate the effect of unlabeled NE like it potentiates that of unlabeled GABA) but, rather, to displacement of the [³H]NE from its intracellular binding sites by the unlabeled NE that has recently entered (a process that can be inhibited by ouabain through its inhibitory effect on influx and on the binding of amine that has recently entered).

C. Role of Sodium-Dependent Transport Systems

It has been emphasized (Snyder *et al.*, 1973a,b; Bennett *et al.*, 1974) that only putative neurotransmitters possess a sodium-dependent high-affinity uptake system, and that the presence of such an uptake system represents one of the criteria for considering a given compound a neurotransmitter candidate. Although sodium dependence may be a valuable criterion for discriminating between transport processes of neurotransmitter and non-neurotransmitter amino acids, its physiological significance remains unclear. In fact, under physiological conditions, the extracellular concentration of sodium would favor the high-affinity uptake of neurotransmitter as well as of non-neurotransmitter amino acids. If, under some circumstances (e.g., after the early sodium current following physiological stimulation), the concentration of sodium in the vicinity of the presynaptic membrane decreased in an appreciable way, the sodium-dependent uptake of the neurotransmitters would be depressed. It would be interesting to establish whether or not modulation by sodium of the high-affinity uptake (or exchange) of neurotransmitters has any physiological significance (see also Section VI).

V. Studies on Neurotransmitter Release

A. Spontaneous Release

The process whereby metabolites and neurotransmitters exit from synaptosomes has received much less attention than that of accumulation. Most of the studies concern the modifications induced by drugs and by varied experimental conditions on a basal pattern of release called spontaneous release.

With the present state of knowledge, it is difficult to say whether or not the spontaneous release observed *in vitro* has any correlation with the spontaneous release of transmitters present in the living brain. It is likely that a part, yet undetermined, of the spontaneous release from synaptosomes is accounted for by leakage from damaged particles.

The properties of spontaneous release are in some ascertained cases different from those of stimulated release. For example, the spontaneous release of GABA from synaptosomes is not sodium-dependent (Simon et al., 1974; Raiteri et al., 1975b), is scarcely affected by a decrease in temperature (Simon et al., 1974), and is practically unchanged when the GABA carrier is blocked by prior incubation with L-diaminobutyric acid (Levi et al., in preparation). In contrast, the release of radioactive GABA stimulated by unlabeled GABA or GABA analogs is highly sodium- and temperature-dependent (Simon et al., 1974; Raiteri et al., 1975b) and is strongly inhibited by L-diaminobutyric acid-induced carrier blockage (Levi et al., 1976b). Therefore it seems that the spontaneous release of GABA is largely non-carrier-mediated.

Besides the cases in which spontaneous release is not altered by given experimental conditions, it may be difficult to say whether an increase in the basal rate of release is due to alteration of the spontaneous release process or to activation of a different mechanism of release.

B. Stimulus-Coupled Release

Synaptosomes offer a unique opportunity for studying in vitro the release of neurotransmitters under conditions which, in some ways, mimic the physiological stimulation of nerves. It has been shown that electrical stimulation or high potassium concentrations depolarize synaptosomal membranes and evoke a release of several neurotransmitter amino acids (De Belleroche and Bradford, 1973a; Levy et al., 1974; Raiteri et al., 1975b), of acetylcholine (De Belleroche and Bradford, 1972; Blaustein, 1975), and of NE (Blaustein et al., 1972; Raiteri et al., 1975c). Depolarization of synaptosomes is accompanied by an increased influx of calcium ions (Blaustein et al., 1972; Blaustein, 1975), which is essential for the stimulus-coupled release. Depolarizing drugs, like veratridine, also stimulate calcium uptake and evoke transmitter release (Levy et al., 1974; Blaustein, 1975). The influx of calcium is regulated in a complex manner by the intra- and extra-cellular concentrations of sodium and potassium (Blaustein and Oborn, 1975; Blaustein, 1975), and it is possible that the release of neurotransmitters is indirectly affected by conditions altering the distribution of monovalent cations.

The calcium dependence of neurotransmitter release from synaptosomes is in keeping with the calcium hypothesis (Katz and Miledi, 1967), according to which an increase in the intracellular concentration of free calcium is sufficient to trigger the release of transmitters. Recently, the use of divalent cation ionophores (Foreman et al., 1973), which have been shown to stimulate the release of DA (Holz, 1975), NE (see Fig. 5), GABA, and

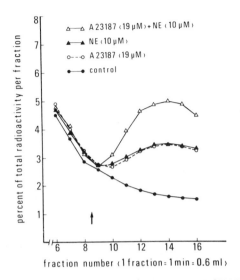

FIG. 5. Effect of the ionophore A23187 on the release of [³H]NE from whole brain synaptosomes. Experimental details were as described in the legend for Fig. 4, except that after 8.5 minutes the standard superfusion medium was replaced with new medium containing 19 μM A23187, 10 μM NE, or both. Each curve is the average of four duplicate experiments. Similar results were obtained in two experiments with hypothalamic synaptosomes.

glutamate (Levi et al., 1976b,c) from synaptosomes in the presence of calcium, has given further support to the calcium hypothesis.

The mechanism by which increased availability of intrasynaptosomal free calcium triggers the release of neurotransmitters is not fully understood. In the case of catecholamines, evidence similar to that obtained in peripheral sympathetic nerves, proving the involvement of an exocytotic mechanism (Douglas, 1968; Weinshilbaum et al., 1971), has not been found in the central nervous system. Some recent observations are not incompatible with the idea that an exocytosis mechanism may be present in central catecholaminergic nerve endings also. For example, it was shown that, under conditions of membrane depolarization, calcium induces a release of unmetabolized [³H]NE from purified synaptosomes (Raiteri et al., 1975c). Moreover, unmetabolized [³H]DA was released from striatal synaptosomes by the calcium ionophore A23187 (Holz, 1975), which was shown to cause an exocytotic release of NE from peripheral adrenergic neurons (Thoa et al., 1974). The simultaneous determination of some ascertained component of synaptosomal vesicles, other than catecholamines, during the stimulus-coupled release would certainly help in elucidating the mechanism of the release process. As an alternative to the exocytotic mechanism, Bogdanski

(1976) favors the idea that calcium mobilizes NE from storage vesicles and that the amine leaves the nerve terminals by carrier-mediated outward transport.

The origin of the neurotransmitter released under stimulation has been the object of investigation also in the case of amino acids (De Belleroche and Bradford, 1973a; Osborne and Bradford, 1975). The data obtained point to release from the main cytoplasmic pool and seem to exclude vesicular origin of the transmitter. In order to exclude vesicular origin of the amino acid released, more concordant data on the amino acid content of synaptic vesicles are necessary. In fact, although very low concentrations of neurotransmitter amino acids were found in synaptic vesicles isolated after osmotic shock (De Belleroche and Bradford, 1973b), recent data obtained with synaptic vesicles isolated in isotonic sucrose by differential centrifugation (Philippu and Matthaei, 1975), indicate that the vesicular concentration of GABA may be at least as high as that present in purified synaptosomes.

The release of neurotransmitter amino acids induced by depolarizing stimuli may or may not be mediated by a carrier mechanism. Studies performed with brain slices have suggested that the release of radioactive GABA and glutamate, induced by electrical stimulation, by ouabain, or by unlabeled exogenous amino acids, is in any case mediated by the same carrier mechanism (Hammerstad and Cutler, 1972). However, with synaptosomes we showed that, when the carrier-mediated transport of GABA was almost completely blocked by preincubation of the particles in the presence of diaminobutyric acid, subsequent potassium stimulation of GABA release was only little affected, suggesting that under these conditions the amino acid can move out of synaptosomes by mechanisms other than membrane transport (Fig. 3). Indirect evidence in favor of this concept comes also from the finding that sodium, which is required for carrier-mediated GABA transport, does not seem to be essential for the potassium-stimulated release of the amino acid (Fig. 3).

Other experiments, however, indicated that, under particular conditions, the release of transmitter amino acids triggered by an elevation of intracellular calcium concentration has a large carrier-mediated component. It has been reported (Martin and Smith, 1972) that the sodium dependence curve of GABA influx into synaptosomes has a sigmoid shape in the absence of extracellular calcium, and that calcium stimulates GABA influx at low but not at high sodium concentrations, abolishing the sigmoid character of the curve (Fig. 6). If the ionic requirements of GABA efflux were similar to those of GABA influx, calcium would stimulate the efflux of GABA under normal conditions of low intracellular sodium. When the calcium concentration of synaptosomes prelabeled with [³H]GABA was increased by superfusing them in the presence of the calcium ionophore A23187, the stimulation of [³H]GABA release observed was modest. However, when the carrier-mediated

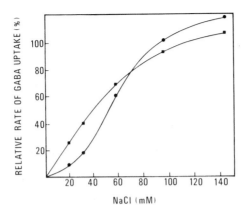

Fig. 6. Dependence of the rate of synaptosomal uptake of [³H]GABA on the sodium concentration, in the absence of calcium (●) or in the presence of 20 m*M* CaCl₂ (■). Uptake was measured over a 3-minute period. NaCl was present as indicated, and osmotic pressure was maintained constant with sucrose (redrawn from Martin and Smith, 1972).

release of [³H]GABA was activated by a small concentration of extracellular GABA, the ionophore had a much more pronounced releasing effect (Fig. 7). This result was qualitatively similar to that previously reported for ouabain (see Fig. 4) and, as in that case, could not be explained on the basis of accelerated homoexchange (in fact, A23187 inhibited GABA influx), but should be interpreted as evidence for a change in the stoichiometry of GABA homoexchange in a direction favoring outward transport (Levi *et al.*, 1976b,c). Thus both ouabain (by increasing intracellular sodium) and the ionophore A23187 (by increasing intracellular calcium) favor the outward carrier-mediated transport of GABA by establishing ionic conditions more favorable than those normally present intracellularly, provided that extracellular GABA is present. Interestingly, the effect of ouabain on GABA-stimulated [³H]GABA release was larger than that of A23187 (cf. Figs. 3 and 4), a finding in keeping with the concept that sodium is more effective than calcium in promoting GABA carrier-mediated transport (Fig. 6).

Since ouabain has been reported to increase the influx of $^{45}Ca^{2+}$ into synaptosomes (Goddard and Robinson, 1975; Swanson *et al.*, 1974), and may also increase intracellular free calcium through other mechanisms (Baker and Crawford, 1975), its effect on GABA release may also be attributed to a raised intracellular concentration of free calcium. However, its effects on GABA release (and uptake) were not calcium-dependent (in contrast to those of the ionophore A23187). Moreover, according to Fig. 6, calcium is not expected to influence GABA transport when the sodium concentration is relatively high, as after ouabain treatment.

As previously mentioned, the increased influx of calcium, determined by

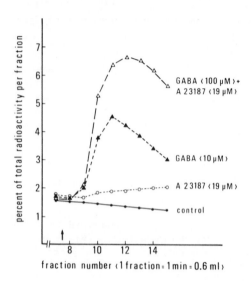

FIG. 7. Effect of the ionophore A23187 on the release of [³H]GABA from synapto-somes. Experimental conditions were as described in the legend for Fig. 2, except that after 7.5 minutes of superfusion the standard medium was replaced with new medium containing 19 μM A23187, 10 μM GABA, or both. Each curve is the average of four duplicate experiments.

the ionophore A23187, causes a substantial release of catecholamines from synaptosomes. In view of the data obtained with GABA, it seemed worthwhile analyzing whether A23187 could potentiate the effect of unlabeled NE on the release of preaccumulated [³H]NE from synaptosomes (Levi et al., 1976c). Figure 5 shows that the releasing effect of A23187 and NE, added together to the superfusion fluid, was approximately equal to the sum of the effects obtained with either compound alone. The lack of a more than additive effect of A23187 and NE agrees with the idea that A23187 causes a direct release of [³H]NE from synaptic vesicles, similar to its effects on DA release (Holz, 1975). In fact, if the ionophore induced release of [³H]NE from the vesicles into the cytoplasm, one would expect an increase in the outward transport of the labeled amine by homoexchange, in the presence of extracellular unlabeled NE, and of a monoamine oxidase inhibitor.

VI. Possible Modulatory Mechanisms of Transmitter Fluxes

During chemical neurotransmission, net entry or net exit of neurotrans-mitters from nerve endings must prevail one over the other, in alternate phases. Therefore the possible existence of regulatory mechanisms modulating neurotransmitter fluxes across the presynaptic membrane should be considered. The experimental approach to the study of this problem must rely essentially on *in vitro* techniques, so that any extrapolation to an *in vivo* situation must be regarded with extreme caution.

From the *in vitro* results discussed in this article, one could suggest that the possibility of obtaining a net inward or a net outward carrier-mediated transport of GABA may be linked to changes in the intracellular concentrations of cations and of GABA itself. Such changes may modulate the stoichiometry of a basic 1:1 homoexchange process. That a carrier-mediated transport system may perform an uphill translocation or a 1:1 homoexchange, depending on even small variations in ionic concentrations, has been proposed for other systems (Schwartz *et al.*, 1972). In the case of GABA, one could envisage the existence of the following situations: (1) a resting phase, in which low extracellular concentrations of GABA are maintained by a 1:1 homoexchange, occurring at normal ionic concentrations; (2) a release phase, in which the ionic changes determined by the stimulation, besides causing release of GABA by themselves, allow modification of the stoichiometry of GABA homoexchange, in the sense of an increased outward/inward flux ratio; (3) a reuptake phase, in which the elevated extracellular concentration of released GABA determines an inversion of the flux ratio. In fact, a net uptake of GABA can be demonstrated by using relatively high concentrations of the amino acid (Iversen and Neal, 1968; Levi and Raiteri, 1974; Simon *et al.*, 1974). Since the uptake at high concentrations of GABA is less sensitive to sodium deprivation than that observed at low amino acid concentrations (Levi and Raiteri, 1975), a decrease in sodium concentration in the vicinity of the presynaptic membrane may favor the establishment of a higher ratio between inward and outward transport.

A scheme of this type, which may be valid for other putative transmitter amino acids, does not seem to hold for biogenic amines. The extremely low intrasynaptosomal concentration of free NE is a condition that does not seem to favor the existence of a prominent exchange process at the synaptic plasma membrane. The net result of membrane inward transport of NE is instead strongly conditioned by the very rapid binding of the amine to its storage sites. Under particular conditions that augment the cytoplasmic content of NE (e.g., reserpine or ouabain, in the presence of monoamine oxidase inhibitors), homo- and heteroexchange processes may become important.

ACKNOWLEDGMENTS

Bibliographic aid was received from the UCLA Brain Information Service, which is part of the Neurological Network of the NINDB. The original work reported was supported in part by Research Grant No. 922 from the North Atlantic Treaty Organization and Grant No. CT 74.00249.04 from the Italian National Research Council. The ionophore A23187 was a kind gift of Eli Lilly & Co.

REFERENCES

Abdel-Latif, A. A. (1973). *Methods Neurochem.* 5, 147–188.
Aprison, M. H., and McBride, W. J. (1973). *Life Sci.* 12, 449–458.
Archibald, J. T., and White, T. D. (1974). *Nature (London)* 252, 595–596.
Baker, P. F., and Crawford, A. C. (1975). *J. Physiol. (London)* 247, 209–226.
Banay-Schwartz, M., Teller, D., and Lajtha, A. (1976). *In* "Transport Phenomena in the Nervous System. Physiological and Pathological Aspects" (G. Levi, L. Battistin, and A. Lajtha, eds.), pp. 349–370. Plenum, New York.
Bauman, A., Bourgoin, S., Benda, P., Glowinski, J., and Hamon, M. (1974). *Brain Res.* 66, 253–263.
Belin, M. F., Chouvet, G., and Pujol, J. F. (1974). *Biochem. Pharmacol.* 23, 587–598.
Bennett, J. P., Jr., Logan, W. J., and Snyder, S. H. (1973). *J. Neurochem.* 21, 1533–1550.
Bennett, J. P., Jr., Mulder, A. H., and Snyder, S. H. (1974). *Life Sci.* 15, 1045–1056.
Blaustein, M. P. (1975). *J. Physiol. (London)* 247, 617–655.
Blaustein, M. P., and Oborn, C. J. (1975). *J. Physiol. (London)* 247, 657–686.
Blaustein, M. P., Johnson, E. M., and Needleman, P. (1972). *Proc. Natl. Acad. Sci. U. S. A.* 69, 2237–2240.
Bogdanski, D. F. (1976). *In* "Transport Phenomena in the Nervous System. Physiological and Pathological Aspects" (G. Levi, L. Battistin and A. Lajtha, eds.), pp. 291–305. Plenum, New York.
Bogdanski, D. F., Tissari, A., and Brodie, B. B. (1968). *Life Sci.* 7, 419–428.
Bogdanski, D. F., Blaszkowski, I. P., and Tissari, A. H. (1970a). *Biochim. Biophys. Acta* 211, 521–532.
Bogdanski, D. F., Tissari, A. H., and Brodie, B. B. (1970b). *Biochim. Biophys. Acta* 219, 189–199.
Bradford, H. F., Jones, D. G., Word, H. K., and Booher, J. (1975). *Brain Res.* 90, 245–259.
Christensen, H. N. (1976). *In* "Transport Phenomena in the Nervous System. Physiological and Pathological Aspects" (G. Levi, L. Battistin, and A. Lajtha, eds.), pp. 3–12. Plenum, New York.
Colburn, R. W., Goodwin, F. K., Murphy, D. L., Bunney, W. E., and Davis, J. M. (1968). *Biochem. Pharmacol.* 17, 957–964.
Crane, R. K. (1965). *Fed. Proc., Fed. Am. Soc. Exp. Biol.* 24, 1000–1006.
De Belleroche, J. S., and Bradford, H. F. (1972). *J. Neurochem.* 19, 1817–1819.
De Belleroche, J. S., and Bradford, H. F. (1973a). *Prog. Neurobiol. (Oxford)* 1, 277–298.
De Belleroche, J. S., and Bradford, H. F. (1973b). *J. Neurochem.* 21, 441–451.
De Feudis, F. V. (1975). *Annu. Rev. Pharmacol.* 15, 105–130.
Diamond, I., and Fishman, R. A. (1973). *J. Neurochem.* 20, 1533–1542.
Douglas, W. W. (1968). *Br. J. Pharmacol.* 34, 451–474.
Foreman, J. C., Mongar, J. L., and Gomperts, B. D. (1973). *Nature (London)* 245, 249–251.
Goddard, G. A., and Robinson, J. D. (1975). *Fed. Proc., Fed. Am. Soc. Exp. Biol.* 34, 715 (abstr.).

Grahame-Smith, D. G., and Parfitt, A. G. (1970). *J. Neurochem.* **17**, 1339–1353.

Guyenet, P., Lefresne, P., Rossier, J., Beaujouan, J. C., and Glowinski, J. (1973a). *Brain Res.* **62**, 523–529.

Guyenet, P., Lefresne, P., Rossier, J., Beaujouan, J. C., and Glowinski, J. (1973b). *Mol. Pharmacol.* **9**, 630–639.

Haga, T. (1971). *J. Neurochem.* **18**, 781–798.

Haga, T., and Noda, H. (1973). *Biochim. Biophys. Acta.* **291**, 564–575.

Hammerstad, J. P., and Cutler, W. P. (1972). *Brain Res.* **47**, 401–413.

Hamon, M., Bourgoin, S., Morot-Gaudry, Y., Héry, F., and Glowinski, J. (1974). *Adv. Biochem. Psychopharmacol.* **11**, 153–162.

Hökfelt, T. (1970). *Brain Res.* **22**, 147–151.

Holz, R. W. (1975). *Biochim. Biophys. Acta* **375**, 138–152.

Holz, R. W., and Coyle, J. T. (1974). *Mol. Pharmacol.* **10**, 746–758.

Iversen, L. L. (1970). *Adv. Biochem. Psychopharmacol.* **2**, 109–132.

Iversen, L. L. (1971). In "Biogenic Amines and Physiological Membranes in Drug Therapy" (J. Biel and L. G. Abood, eds.), Part B, pp. 259–327. Dekker, New York.

Iversen, L. L. (1973). *Br. Med. Bull.* **29**, 130–135.

Iversen, L. L., and Bloom, F. E. (1972). *Brain Res.* **41**, 131–143.

Iversen, L. L., and Neal, M. J. (1968). *J. Neurochem.* **15**, 1141–1149.

Jacquez, J. A., Sherman, J. H., and Terris, J. (1970). *Biochim. Biophys. Acta* **203**, 150–166.

Johnston, G. A. R., and Balkar, W. J. (1973). *Brain Res.* **59**, 451–453.

Katz, B., and Miledi, R. (1967). *Proc. R. Soc. London, Ser. B* **167**, 23–38.

Krnjevic, K. (1974). *Physiol. Rev.* **54**, 419–540.

Lähdesmäki, P., and Oja, S. S. (1973). *J. Neurochem.* **20**, 1411–1417.

Levi, G., and Raiteri, M. (1973). *Brain Res.* **57**, 165–185.

Levi, G., and Raiteri, M. (1974). *Nature (London)* **250**, 735–737.

Levi, G., and Raiteri, M. (1975). *Proc. FEBS Meet., 10th, 1975,* pp. 81–93.

Levi, G., Bertollini, A., Chen, J., and Raiteri, M. (1974). *J. Pharmacol. Exp. Ther.* **188**, 429–438.

Levi, G., Coletti, A., Poce, U., and Raiteri, M. (1976a). *Brain Res.* **103**, 103–116.

Levi, G., Poce, U., and Raiteri, M. (1976b). In "Transport Phenomena in the Nervous System. Physiological and Pathological Aspects" (G. Levi, L. Battistin, and A. Lajtha, eds.), pp. 273–289. Plenum, New York.

Levi, G., Roberts, P. J., and Raiteri, M. (1976c). *Neurochem. Res.* (in press).

Levy, W. B., Haycock, J. W., and Cotman, C. W. (1974). *Mol. Pharmacol.* **16**, 438–449.

Lust, W. D., and Robinson, J. D. (1970). *J. Neurobiol.* **1**, 303–316.

Martin, D. L. (1973). *J. Neurochem.* **21**, 345–356.

Martin, D. L., and Smith, A. A., III. (1972). *J. Neurochem.* **19**, 841–855.

Oja, S. S., Kontro, P., and Lähdesmäki, P. (1976). In "Transport Phenomena in the Nervous System. Physiological and Pathological Aspects" (G. Levi, L. Battistin, and A. Lajtha, eds.), pp. 237–252. Plenum, New York.

Oldfield, E., and Chapman, D. (1972). *FEBS Lett.* **23**, 285–297.

Olsen, R. W., Bayless, J. D., and Ban, M. (1975). *Mol. Pharmacol.* **11**, 558–565.

Osborne, R. H., and Bradford, H. F. (1975). *J. Neurochem.* **25**, 35–41.

Peterson, N. A., and Raghupathy, E. (1973). *J. Neurochem.* **21**, 97–110.

Philippu, A., and Beyer, J. (1973). *Naunyn-Schmiedeberg's Arch. Pharmacol.* **278**, 387–402.

Philippu, A., and Matthaei, H. (1975). *Naunyn-Schmiedeberg's Arch. Pharmacol.* **287**, 191–204.

Raiteri, M., and Levi, G. (1973a). *Nature (London) New Biol.* **243**, 180–183.

Raiteri, M., and Levi, G. (1973b). *Nature (London) New Biol.* **245**, 89–91.

Raiteri, M., Angelini, F., and Levi, G. (1974). *Eur. J. Pharmacol.* **25**, 411–414.

Raiteri, M., Bertollini, A., Angelini, F., and Levi, G. (1975a). *Eur. J. Pharmacol.* **34**, 189–195.

Raiteri, M., Federico, R., Coletti, A., and Levi, G. (1975b). *J. Neurochem.* **24**, 1243–1250.

Raiteri, M., Levi, G., and Federico, R. (1975c). *Pharmacol. Res. Commun.* **7**, 181–187.

Raiteri M., Bertollini, A., del Carmine, R., and Levi, G. (1976). *In* "Transport Phenomena in the Nervous System: Physiological and Pathological Aspects" (G. Levi, L. Battistin, and A. Lajtha, eds.), pp. 319–335. Plenum, New York.

Schwartz, A., Lindenmayer, G. E., and Allen, J. C. (1972). *Curr. Top. Membr. Transp.* **3**, 1–82.

Scriver, C. R., and Mohyuddin, F. (1968). *J. Biol. Chem.* **243**, 3207–3213.

Shore, P. A. (1972). *Annu. Rev. Pharmacol.* **12**, 209–226.

Simon, J. R., and Kuhar, M. J. (1975). *Nature (London)* **255**, 162–163.

Simon, J. R., Martin, D. L., and Kroll, M. (1974). *J. Neurochem.* **23**, 981–991.

Smith, A. D. (1973). *Br. Med. Bull.* **29**, 123–129.

Snyder, S. H., Kuhar, M. J., Green, A. I., Coyle, J. T., and Shaskan, E. G. (1970). *Int. Rev. Neurobiol.* **13**, 127–157.

Snyder, S. H., Young, A. B., Bennett, J. P., and Mulder, A. H. (1973a). *Fed. Proc., Fed. Am. Soc. Exp. Biol.* **32**, 2039–2047.

Snyder, S. H., Yamamura, H. I., Pert, C. B., Logan, W. J., and Bennett, J. P. (1973b). *In* "New Concepts in Neurotransmitter Regulation" (A. J. Mandel, ed.), pp. 195–222. Plenum, New York.

Swanson, P. D., Anderson, L., and Stahl, W. L. (1974). *Biochim. Biophys. Acta* **356**, 174–183.

Thoa, N. B., Costa, J. L., Moss, J., and Kopin, I. J. (1974). *Life Sci.* **14**, 1705–1719.

Tissari, A. H., Schonhofer, P. S., Bogdanski, D. F., and Brodie, B. B. (1969). *Mol. Pharmacol.* **5**, 593–604.

Weinshilbaum, R. M., Thoa, N. B., Johnson, D. G., Kopin, I. J., and Axelrod, J. (1971). *Science* **174**, 1349–1351.

Weinstein, H., Varon, S., Muhleman, D. R., and Roberts, E. (1965). *Biochem. Pharmacol.* **14**, 273–288.

White, T. D., and Archibald, J. T. (1974). *Brain Res.* **82**, 360–364.

White, T. D., and Keen, P. (1971). *Mol. Pharmacol.* **7**, 40–45.

White, T. D., and Paton, D. M. (1972). *Biochim. Biophys. Acta* **266**, 116–127.

Whittaker, V. P. (1973). *Naturwissenschaften* **60**, 281–289.

Yamamura, H. I., and Snyder, S. H. (1973). *J. Neurochem.* **21**, 1355–1374.

GLUTATHIONE METABOLISM AND SOME POSSIBLE FUNCTIONS OF GLUTATHIONE IN THE NERVOUS SYSTEM[1]

By Marian Orlowski and Abraham Karkowsky

Department of Pharmacology
Mount Sinai School of Medicine of the City University of New York
New York, New York

[1] This work was supported in part by grants from the National Institute of Neurological Diseases and Stroke, and the National Institute of Arthritis, Metabolism and Digestive Diseases.

I. History and Introduction

Glutathione was first discovered in yeast cells by de Rey-Pailhade (1888a,b), who named it philothion. It was isolated in crystalline form by Hopkins (1921). Glutathione is probably the most ubiquitous peptide found in living cells. The biosynthesis of the peptide bonds of glutathione was studied by Bloch and his co-workers (1949–1955) in the hope that it would lead to an understanding of the mechanism of protein synthesis. Its degradation by γ-glutamyl transpeptidase was studied by Hanes and co-workers (1950, 1952), who were inspired by the same expectations. Although none of these hopes have been fulfilled, studies of the biochemistry and metabolism of glutathione continue to attract the interest of researchers from diverse fields. New information acquired about the significance of the sulfhydryl group and the γ-glutamyl linkage of glutathione, and the recognition of clinical disorders associated with defects in its biosynthesis justify this interest. The sulfhydryl group of glutathione is credited with an important role in maintaining the sulfhydryl groups of proteins and enzymes in a reduced state, in protecting cell membranes against oxidative stress, and in detoxifying a great number of foreign compounds. Glutathione also plays an important role as a coenzyme in several enzymic reactions. The enzymic reactions of the synthesis and degradation of glutathione have recently been linked in a cyclic process called the γ-glutamyl cycle (Orlowski and Meister, 1970a). It was proposed that the cycle functions in amino acid transport. Pyrrolidone carboxylate,[2] formed by cyclization of the γ-glutamyl moiety of γ-glutamyl amino acids in a reaction of the γ-glutamyl cycle, is now accepted as a normal intermediate of mammalian metabolism.

Of the reviews covering aspects of glutathione biochemistry the most informative are those by Knox (1960) and by Waley (1966), a recent review on glutathione biosynthesis by Meister (1974a), and a monograph by Jocelyn (1972). Other information on the biochemistry of glutathione can be found in proceedings of symposia held in 1953 (Colowick et al., 1954), 1959 (Crook, 1959), and most recently in 1973 (Flohe et al., 1974). This article summarizes newer information on glutathione metabolism and emphasizes aspects related to its metabolism and function in the central nervous system (CNS). The detection of neurological disorders in patients with inherited deficiencies in glutathione synthesis indicates the importance of this tripeptide in brain function.

---

[2] Synonyms of pyrrolidone carboxylate are 5-oxoproline, pyroglutamic acid, 5-oxopyrrolidine-2-carboxylic acid, and 2-pyrrolidone-5-carboxylic acid.

II. Biochemistry of Glutathione

A. CHEMICAL PROPERTIES

Glutathione is a tripeptide, γ-glutamylcysteinylglycine:

$$
\begin{array}{l}
\text{CH}_2\text{—SH} \\
\quad | \\
\text{CO—NH—CH} \\
| \qquad\quad | \\
\text{CH}_2 \qquad \text{CO—NH—CH}_2\text{—COOH} \\
| \\
\text{CH}_2 \\
| \\
\text{HCNH}_2 \\
| \\
\text{COOH}
\end{array}
$$

Glutathione has two structural features responsible for much of its biochemistry. These two features are its sulfhydryl group (due to cysteine) and the γ-glutamyl bond (the bond linking cysteine to glutamate). The sulfhydryl group is responsible for most of the catalytic and reactive properties of glutathione. It confers on glutathione the ability to participate both in oxidation-reduction reactions and nucleophilic displacement reactions. Because of its tendency to participate in oxidation-reduction processes, glutathione occurs both in reduced (GSH) and oxidized (disulfide, GSSG) forms. The nucleophilic properties of the sulfhydryl group are such that it readily participates both as an incoming and exiting nucleophile.

The γ-glutamyl bond of glutathione makes it resistant to the actions of most peptidases. In addition, the presence of this bond makes glutathione the most abundant naturally occurring substrate for γ-glutamyl transpeptidase.

B. OCCURRENCE OF GLUTATHIONE IN THE NERVOUS SYSTEM

High concentrations of glutathione are found in the brain (Martin and McIlwain, 1959). Glutathione has been reported to comprise 97% of the acid-soluble thiols in the cerebral cortex (Martin and McIlwain, 1959), and approximately 80% of the total soluble thiol groups in the cerebral cortex, which react rapidly with 5,5'-dithiobis(2-nitrobenzoic acid) (DTNB) (Boyne and Ellman, 1972). In whole brain, the concentration of total glutathione, consisting of both its oxidized and reduced forms, is 0.5–3.4 μmoles/gm tissue (Table I). A similar range of concentrations has been found in various regions of the brain. The large range of GSH concentrations reported by various investigators is probably due in part to differences in methodology.

TABLE I

CONCENTRATION OF GLUTATHIONE IN RAT BRAIN AS
DETERMINED BY VARIOUS METHODS

Concentration[a]	Method of determination	Reference
3.44	Glyoxalase	Martin and McIlwain (1959)
3.43	Glyoxalase	Martin and McIlwain (1959)
2.01	Glyoxalase	Davidson and Hird (1964)
2.03	Glutathione reductase	Davidson and Hird (1964)
3.16	Iodometric	Varma et al. (1968)
1.10	Ion exchange	Reichelt and Fonnum (1969)
1.40	Ion exchange	O'Neal and Koeppe (1966)
0.95[b]	Ion exchange	Minard and Mushahwar (1966)
0.266[c]	Ion exchange	Agrawal et al. (1966)
0.358[d]	Ion exchange	Agrawal et al. (1966)

[a] Mean concentrations in micromoles per gram of tissue are given.

[b] This value was obtained by adding twice the value found for glutathione disulfide to that obtained for reduced glutathione.

[c] Adult.

[d] Newborn.

In general, it seems that enzymic methods for the determination of GSH yield higher values than those obtained after separation on ion-exchange columns using amino acid analyzers. In addition to total brain levels, the subcellular localization of glutathione in rat brain has been studied. These studies have shown that glutathione is located primarily in the soluble supernatant fraction (62%) and partially in the crude mitochondrial fraction (34%). When the crude mitochondrial fraction was further fractionated, 41% of the glutathione was recovered in the mitochondrial fraction, 35% in the synaptosomal fraction, and 24% in the myelin fraction (Reichelt and Fonnum, 1969).

In the brain, glutathione occurs primarily (97%) in its reduced form. It is partially oxidized postmortem. Though the proportion of oxidized and reduced glutathione changes with time after the death of the animal, the magnitude of this change is a matter of some controversy (Martin and McIlwain, 1959; Hais et al., 1965). Glutathione levels in the brain change during development. Glutathione concentrations, on a wet weight basis, in neonate cat neocortex are about 80% of adult levels. Glutathione levels markedly increase during the postnatal period and reach adult levels by the end of the second week. The time course of this glutathione increase parallels the morphological development of neocortical elements in the cat (Berl and Purpura, 1963). During this period, glutathione levels also increase in the hippocampus, brainstem, cerebellum, and mesodiencephelon, though the last-mentioned attains its maximal glutathione levels later in development (Berl and Purpura, 1966). Glutathione concentrations have been reported to decrease in some stressful situations (Varma et al., 1968; Purpura et al., 1960; Berl et al., 1959; Sanders et al., 1969), and to remain normal in others (De Ropp and Snedeker, 1961; Tews et al., 1963). Hallucinogenic drugs such as mescaline and LSD also decrease brain glutathione concentrations (Varma et al., 1968).

C. Glutathione Analogs and γ-Glutamyl Peptides

   In addition to glutathione, other naturally occurring γ-glutamyl peptides have been found (for reviews, see Waley, 1966; Pisano, 1969; Sano, 1970). Aside from pteroylglutamic acids, the first γ-glutamyl peptides discovered in mammalian tissues were ophthalmic acid (γ-L-glutamyl-L-α-amino-n-butyrylglycine) (Waley, 1956) and norophthalmic acid (γ-L-glutamyl-L-alanylglycine) (Waley, 1957) isolated from calf lens. γ-Glutamyl derivatives of leucine, isoleucine, and valine have been isolated from human urine (Buchanan et al., 1962). γ-Glutamylglutamate and γ-glutamylglutamine were the first γ-glutamyl peptides isolated from mammalian (bovine) brain (Kakimoto et al., 1964). Six additional γ-glutamyl peptides, γ-glutamylglycine (Kanazawa et al., 1965a), γ-glutamyl-L-β-aminoisobutyric acid (Kakimoto et al., 1965), γ-glutamylserine, γ-glutamylalanine, γ-glutamylvaline, and S-methylglutathione, were also isolated from bovine brain (Kanazawa et al., 1965b). In addition, a substance containing glutamyl, α-aminobutyryl, and glycyl residues, suggestive of ophthalmic acid, was also isolated (Sano, 1970). γ-Glutamyl peptides have also been isolated from monkey brain, including two peptides, γ-glutamylisoleucine and norophthalmic acid, not reported in bovine brain (Reichelt, 1970). The concentration of these peptides in bovine brain ranges from approximately 30 nmoles/gm wet tissue for γ-glutamylglutamine and γ-glutamylglutamate to about 0.5 nmoles for γ-glutamylvaline and S-methylglutathione (Sano et al., 1966). Relatively high concentrations of γ-glutamylglutamine were found in the intestine, kidney, liver, and brain of several species (Kanazawa and Sano, 1967). Two pathways for the origin of these γ-glutamyl peptides have been suggested. The peptides may be formed by transpeptidation, catalyzed by γ-glutamyl transpeptidase, between glutathione and amino acids. Some of the peptides may, however, be synthesized directly by γ-glutamylcysteine synthetase from the free amino acid and glutamate (Sano, 1970).

III. Enzymology of Glutathione, Glutathione Analogs, and γ-Glutamyl Amino Acids

A. Biosynthesis

The biosynthesis of glutathione was first studied by Braunstein and his co-workers (1948) in liver slices. Its complete synthesis in cell-free preparations from the component amino acids was first accomplished by Bloch (1949) and his co-workers. The overall reaction proceeds in two steps (Snoke and Bloch, 1952) catalyzed in sequence by γ-glutamylcysteine synthetase [reaction (1)] and glutathione synthetase [reaction (2)].

$$\text{L-Glutamate} + \text{L-cysteine} + \text{ATP} \xrightarrow{\text{Mg}^{2+}} \text{L-}\gamma\text{-glutamyl-L-cysteine} + \text{ADP} + \text{P}_i \quad (1)$$

$$\text{L-}\gamma\text{-Glutamyl-L-cysteine} + \text{ATP} \xrightarrow{\text{Mg}^{2+}} \text{L-}\gamma\text{-glutamyl-L-cysteinylglycine} + \text{ADP} + \text{P}_i \quad (2)$$

The same two enzymes also catalyze the synthesis of ophthalmic acid in calf lens and rabbit liver (Cliffe and Waley, 1958, 1961).

1. γ-Glutamylcysteine Synthetase (EC 6.3.2.2)

Partially purified preparations of this enzyme have been obtained from hog liver (Mandeles and Bloch, 1955; Strumeyer, 1959), bovine lens (Rathbun, 1967), human erythrocytes (Majerus et al., 1971), and sheep brain (Richman, 1975). The isolation of an apparently homogeneous preparation of γ-glutamylcysteine synthetase from rat kidney was described by Orlowski and Meister (1971a,b). It was calculated that the enzyme constitutes 2–3% of the soluble protein fraction of rat kidney homogenates. The enzyme isolated from rat kidney has a sedimentation coefficient of 5.6 S and a molecular weight of approximately 92,000 (Orlowski and Meister, 1971c). The rate of reaction in the presence of Mg^{2+} is similar for L-α-aminobutyrate and L-cysteine, however, the K_m for the latter (0.35 mM) is much lower than for the former (1.25 mM). Significant activity is obtained with several cysteine-related amino acids. Among protein amino acids L-threonine, L-alanine, glycine, and L-serine show some activity (Table II); other amino acids have little or no activity. γ-Glutamylcysteine synthetase is apparently a "sulfhydryl" enzyme. Strong inhibition is obtained with relatively low concentrations of thiol-blocking agents, such as p-chloromercuribenzoate, p-chloromercuribenzenesulfonate and iodoacetamide.

L-Methionine-S-sulfoximine is an effective inhibitor of γ-glutamylcysteine synthetase (Orlowski and Meister, 1971c; Richman et al., 1973). This methionine analog has long been known as a convulsive agent which provokes recurrent bouts of seizures (Mellanby, 1946; Moran, 1947; Bentley et al.,

TABLE II
SPECIFICITY OF γ-GLUTAMYLCYSTEINE SYNTHETASE
FROM RAT KIDNEY IN THE PRESENCE OF Mg^{2+}

Amino acid	Relative activity[a]
L-α-Aminobutyrate	100
L-Cysteine	96
S-Methyl-L-cysteine	85
DL-C-allyglycine	74
β-Chloro-L-alanine	59
L-Norvaline	48
L-Threonine	20
L-Alanine	10
Glycine	3.7
L-Serine	3.1

[a] The specific activity of the enzyme was 520 μmoles of L-γ-glutamyl-L-α-aminobutyrate synthesized per milligram of protein per hour. (Taken from Orlowski and Meister, 1971c.)

1950). It is also an irreversible inhibitor of glutamine synthetase (Pace and McDermott, 1952; Lamar and Sellinger, 1965; Ronzio et al., 1969). The mechanism of inhibition of both enzymes involves phosphorylation of the inhibitor to methionine sulfoximine phosphate (Richman et al., 1973; Ronzio and Meister, 1968). Several studies have attempted to correlate the convulsive action of methionine sulfoximine with its inhibition of brain glutamine synthetase, thereby affecting the metabolism of glutamine, glutamate, and γ-aminobutyrate (Kolousek et al., 1959; De Robertis et al., 1967). In view of the postulated excitatory and inhibitory neurotransmitter function of glutamate and γ-aminobutyrate (Roberts, 1960; Curtis and Watkins, 1965), such an effect would be expected to have profound physiological significance. Other studies, however, have questioned the existence of any causal relationship between the inhibition of glutamine synthetase and the occurrence of seizures (Peters and Tower, 1959; Folbergova, 1963).

Recent studies (Orlowski and Wilk, 1975a) have shown that in vivo methionine sulfoximine inhibits the activity of γ-glutamylcysteine synthetase in the brain, liver, and kidney after administration to mice. It also affects the concentration of glutathione and pyrrolidone carboxylate in several tissues. The data are consistent with the interpretation that methionine sulfoximine affects the in vivo metabolism of glutathione and that this action may contribute to the convulsive properties of this drug. γ-Glutamylcysteine synthetase is widely distributed in animal tissues and is found associated with the soluble protein fraction of tissue homogenates. The highest activity was found in rat kidney. The activity of the enzyme in mouse and rabbit kidney, and in rat and mouse liver, is approximately 20 times lower (Orlowski and Wilk, 1975b) than in rat kidney. γ-Glutamylcysteine synthetase activity was found in the CNS of several animals. The activity, although somewhat lower, is of an order of magnitude similar to that of activity in the liver of the same species (Table III). The activity of the enzyme in the choroid plexus is in general higher than in the cerebral cortex and in other regions of the brain (Tate et al., 1973). The available data indicate that the activity of γ-glutamylcysteine synthetase in the CNS is sufficient to account for the synthesis of brain glutathione, and for maintaining a glutathione turnover in excess of that actually observed. It seems that the activity of γ-glutamylcysteine synthetase together with glutathione synthetase can account for the finding of small amounts of glutathione analogs in the CNS, such as S-methylglutathione and ophthalmic acid (Kanazawa et al., 1965a; Sano, 1970).

2. Glutathione Synthetase (EC 6.3.2.3)

The synthesis of glutathione from γ-glutamylcysteine and glycine by an enzyme present in extracts from acetone-dried pigeon livers was first demonstrated by Snoke and Bloch (1952). Highly purified preparations of the enzyme were obtained from yeast (Mooz and Meister, 1967), human red blood cells (Majerus et al., 1971), and bovine red blood cells (Wendel et al., 1972). The enzyme also catalyzes the synthesis of ophthalmic acid from L-γ-glutamyl-L-α-aminobutyrate and glycine (Cliffe and Waley, 1958), and norophthalmic acid from L-γ-glutamyl-L-α-alanine and glycine (Waley, 1956, 1958). The molecular weight of the enzyme from yeast was estimated

TABLE III

Activity of γ-Glutamylcysteine Synthetase in the CNS
of Several Animals

Tissue	Specific activity, mean[a]	Reference
Rat brain	0.15	Orlowski and Meister (1971a)
Mouse brain	0.19	Orlowski and Wilk (1975b)
Bovine cerebral cortex	0.16	Okonkwo et al. (1974)
Rabbit cerebral cortex	0.17	Okonkwo et al. (1974)
Bovine choroid plexus	0.24	Okonkwo et al. (1974)
Rabbit choroid plexus	0.25	Okonkwo et al. (1974)

[a] Specific activity is expressed in terms of μmoles of L-γ-glutamyl-L-amino-butyrate synthesized per milligram of protein per hour in the coupled enzyme assay (Orlowski and Meister, 1971a).

as 123,000 (Mooz and Meister, 1971). A similar molecular weight was reported for the enzyme isolated from bovine erythrocytes. Polyacrylamide gel electrophoresis in a sodium dodecyl sulfate-containing buffer system yielded a protein band with a molecular weight of 61,000 (Wendel et al., 1972). It was suggested that the native enzyme is a dimer composed of two subunits.

Glutathione synthetase shows an absolute requirement for Mg^{2+} ions and has a pH optimum close to 8.0. The enzyme catalyzes an exchange of free glycine with glycine in glutathione or ophthalmic acid, in the presence of ADP or ATP and arsenate or inorganic phosphate (Snoke and Bloch, 1955). Aminomethanesulfonic acid and hydroxylamine can substitute for glycine in the synthetic reaction (Snoke, 1955). The rate of glutathione synthesis by the enzyme from bovine erythrocytes is approximately twice as high as the rate of synthesis of ophthalmic acid (Wendel et al., 1972). The enzyme has been found in mouse brain (Orlowski and Wilk, 1975b). Its mean activity was 43 nmoles of ophthalmic acid synthesized per milligram of protein per hour. This activity is considerably less than the activity of brain γ-glutamylcysteine synthetase. It is of interest that the activity of glutathione synthetase is also lower than the activity of γ-glutamylcysteine synthetase in mouse liver and kidney (Orlowski and Wilk, 1975b), in rat kidney (Orlowski and Meister, 1970a), and in human erythrocytes (Minnich et al., 1971; Sass, 1968). The capacity of the enzyme to synthesize glutathione nevertheless exceeds the rate of turnover of the tripeptide in all these tissues.

Little is known about the in vivo control of glutathione synthesis. Although the activity of glutathione synthetase in most tissues seems to be lower than that of γ-glutamylcysteine synthetase, the availability of γ-glutamylcysteine may actually limit the rate of GSH synthesis. The concentration of this intermediate in tissues it not yet known, except for human red blood cells, where its level was determined as 20 μM (Wendel et al., 1975a). Such low levels, if present in other tissues, would limit the rate of tripeptide synthesis. It seems unlikely that the concentration of glutamate, which is rather high in most cells, is the rate-limiting factor. It is more likely that the low concentration of cysteine in tissues limits the availability of this amino acid for tripeptide synthesis. An additional controlling factor may be feedback inhibition of γ-glutamylcysteine synthetase by physiological concentrations of glutathione (Jackson, 1969; Richman, 1975; Richman and Meister, 1975).

Efficient utilization of γ-glutamylcysteine in glutathione synthesis requires a mechanism for protection of this dipeptide against degradation by γ-glutamyl cyclotransferase. This cytoplasmic enzyme converts γ-glutamylcysteine into pyrrolidone carboxylate and free cysteine. Such protection could be achieved by a tight coupling or compartmentalization of the two reactions in glutathione synthesis. As a result, γ-glutamylcysteine would not be released into the cytoplasm as a free intermediate. Indications for the existence of such a coupling came from experiments with mice in which the influence of cysteine and related amino acids on the concentration of pyrrolidone carboxylate was determined in the brain, liver, and kidney (Orlowski and Wilk, 1975b). The administration of L-α-aminobutyrate and S-methyl-L-cysteine led to the formation *in vivo* of the corresponding γ-glutamyl derivatives and to an increase in pyrrolidone carboxylate in all three tissues. No such increase was observed after administration of L-cysteine, indicating that the L-γ-glutamyl-L-cysteine formed is protected from attack by γ-glutamyl cyclotransferase. This protection is apparently not completely effective in the *in vivo* synthesis of ophthalmic acid and S-methylglutathione. The γ-glutamyl dipeptide precursors of these glutathione analogs are accessible to attack by γ-glutamyl cyclotransferase and are partially degraded, leading to an accumulation of pyrrolidone carboxylate.

B. DEGRADATION

1. γ-Glutamyl Transpeptidase (EC 2.3.2.2)

It has long been known that extracts from kidney and other tissues are capable of degrading glutathione. This activity has been variously referred to as antiglyoxylase (in view of the coenzyme function of GSH in the glyoxlase reaction) (Dakin and Dudley, 1913b; Woodward et al., 1935; Schroeder et al., 1935) or glutathionase (Binkley, 1961). The discovery that the degradation of glutathione by γ-glutamyl transpeptidase is amino acid-dependent is credited to Hanes and co-workers (1950, 1952). The enzyme catalyzes transfer of the γ-glutamyl group of glutathione to amino acids according to the following reaction.

Glutathione + amino acid (or peptide) →
$$\gamma\text{-glutamyl amino acid (or peptide)} + \text{cysteinylglycine} \quad (3)$$

All the natural amino acids (with the exception of proline), and a large number of peptides, can serve as acceptors of the γ-glutamyl group. In addition to the transfer reaction [reaction (3)] the enzyme is also capable of hydrolyzing the γ-glutamyl bond of glutathione [reaction (4)] and catalyzing an autotranspeptidation in which the substrate itself serves as an acceptor [reaction (5)].

$$\text{Glutathione} + H_2O \rightarrow \text{glutamic acid} + \text{cysteinylglycine} \quad (4)$$

$$\text{Glutathione} + \text{glutathione} \rightarrow \gamma\text{-glutamylglutathione} + \text{cysteinylglycine} \quad (5)$$

γ-Glutamyl transpeptidase is associated with particulate fractions of tissue homogenates. Solubilization of the enzyme can be achieved by treatment of the particles with detergents, such as deoxycholate, and also by treatment with 1-butanol (Fodor *et al.*, 1953; Szewczuk and Baranowski, 1963; Orlowski and Meister, 1965; Szewczuk and Connell, 1965; Taniguchi, 1974).

γ-Glutamyl transpeptidase is a glycoprotein containing up to 36% carbohydrate as hexose, hexosamine, and sialic acid (Szewczuk and Baranowski, 1963; Orlowski and Meister, 1965; Taniguchi, 1974). The enzyme from various sources is greatly resistant to digestion by trypsin and other proteolytic enzymes. The large amount of carbohydrate apparently renders the sensitive peptide bonds inaccessible to attack. Advantage has been taken of this property to obtain purified preparations of the enzyme from hog (Leibach and Binkley, 1968), human (Richter, 1969), rat (Tate and Meister, 1975), and sheep kidneys (Zelazo and Orlowski, 1975). The isolated enzyme from sheep kidney has a molecular weight of approximately 90,000. It is composed of two polypeptide chains, one with a molecular weight of 27,000, and the other with a molecular weight of 65,000. The activity of the enzyme toward glutathione and the activating effect of metal ions and various acceptors are shown in Table IV. The release of cysteinylglycine is strongly activated by Na^+ and K^+, and even more so by the divalent cations Ca^{2+} and Mg^{2+}. The activating effect of metal ions (Orlowski *et al.*, 1973) was shown to result entirely from acceleration of the transfer reaction (Zelazo and Orlowski, 1975). Among the L-amino acids the greatest acceleration of the reaction is obtained with methionine and glutamine. A similar specificity was reported for enzymes isolated from other sources. γ-Glutamyl transpeptidase from hog kidney (Orlowski and Meister, 1965) shows significant activity with the γ-methyl, γ-ethyl, and γ-benzyl esters of glutamate. In the presence of hydroxylamine the enzyme catalyzes the formation of γ-glutamyl hydroxamate from several γ-glutamyl derivatives.

γ-Glutamyl transpeptidases from various sources are inhibited by sulfhydryl-blocking agents such as iodoacetic acid, iodoacetamide, *N*-ethylmaleimide, *p*-chloromercuribenzoate, and dithionitrobenzoic acid. The degree of inhibition varies greatly with different enzymes and different inhibitors (Orlowski, 1963; Szewczuk and Connell, 1965; Richter, 1969). Some enzyme preparations are little affected by these inhibitors (Taniguchi, 1974). It seems therefore rather unlikely that a sulfhydryl group is directly involved in the catalytic process. An interesting observation is that γ-glutamyl transpeptidase is inhibited in a competitive manner by a mixture of borate and serine (Revel and Ball, 1959). Other known inhibitors of γ-glutamyl transpeptidase include Bromsulphalein, bromcresol green, several other phthaleins (Binkley, 1961), and γ-glutamyl hydrazones of several α-keto acids (Tate and Meister, 1974a).

Studies of the enzyme have been facilitated by the introduction of syn-

TABLE IV
ACTIVATION OF γ-GLUTAMYL TRANSPEPTIDASE BY METAL IONS AND
SEVERAL ACCEPTOR AMINO ACIDS[a]

Addition	Activity	
	Specific	Relative
None	20	100
Na^+ (150 mM)	44	220
K^+ (150 mM)	46	230
Ca^{2+} (10 mM)	150	750
Mg^{2+} (10 mM)	140	700
Mg^{2+} (10 mM) plus Na^+ (150 mM)	80	400
Glycylglycine (20 mM)	660	3300
Glycylglycine (20 mM) plus Mg^{2+} (10 mM)	840	4200
Glycine	253	1300
L-Leucine	242	1200
L-Phenylalanine	253	1300
L-Aspartate	104	520
L-Asparagine	412	2100
L-Glutamate	205	1000
L-Glutamine	709	3500
L-Methionine	784	3900
L-Arginine	429	2100
L-Lysine	366	1800

[a] The reaction mixtures contained glutathione (0.005 M), tris–HCl buffer (0.08 M, pH 8.8), dithiothreitol (0.005 M), enzyme, and additions indicated in the table in a final volume of 0.5 ml. Activity is expressed in terms of micromoles of cysteinylglycine released per milligram of enzyme per minute. Relative activities are expressed relative to those obtained in the absence of activators. The concentration of all amino acids was 20 mM. The activity in the presence of amino acids was measured in the presence of 10 mM Mg^{2+}.

thetic substrates (Szewczuk and Orlowski, 1960; Goldbarg et al., 1960; Orlowski and Szewczuk, 1961, 1962; Orlowski and Meister, 1963, 1965). The γ-glutamyl derivatives of 1- and 2-naphthylamine were successfully employed for histochemical localization of the enzyme (Albert et al., 1961; Glenner and Folk, 1961; Orlowski, 1963). L-γ-Glutamyl-p-nitroanilide is the substrate presently most frequently used for determination of the enzyme activity in both biochemical and clinical studies. γ-Glutamyl transpeptidase is widely distributed in animal tissues, being most prominent in the kidney. Histochemical studies have shown that the enzyme is highly concentrated in the brush border of the cells of the proximal tubules of the kidney (Albert et *al.*, 1961, 1964; Glenner *et al.*, 1962; Rutenburg *et al.*, 1969), in the apical portion of the cells of the intestinal epithelium (Kokot *et al.*, 1965; Gibinski *et al.*, 1967; Greenberg *et al.*, 1967), in several glandular epithelia, in the epithelium of the cells of the cilliary body, and in the capsule of the lens (Reddy and Unakar, 1973; Ross *et al.*, 1973).

Studies on the localization of γ-glutamyl transpeptidase in the CNS (Albert *et al.*, 1966) have shown that the enzyme is concentrated in the brush border of the epithelium that covers the choroid plexus, and in the endothelium of capillaries in the cerebrum, cerebellum, and medulla. In addition, activity is localized in ependymal cells and in cells lining the central canal of the spinal cord. It is of interest that distinct γ-glutamyl transpeptidase activity was found in some groups of neurons in the diencephalon. Later studies have confirmed the association of γ-glutamyl transpeptidase with brain capillaries. When this enzyme was used as a marker, a fraction rich in capillaries was isolated by differential and density gradient centrifugation of homogenates of bovine brain (Orlowski *et al.*, 1974). It is notable that the activity of the enzyme in the endothelium of larger vessels is much less prominent than in the capillaries. This difference is especially visible in places where a larger vessel gives off capillary branches.

Biochemical studies have shown the presence of γ-glutamyl transpeptidase in the brain of several animal species (Albert *et al.*, 1966) and have confirmed the finding of high enzyme activity in the choroid plexus (Orlowski *et al.*, 1973; Tate *et al.*, 1973; Okonkwo *et al.*, 1974). The activity of γ-glutamyl transpeptidase in rabbit choroid plexus is of the same order of magnitude as that in the kidney. A somewhat lower activity was found in bovine choroid plexus. The determination of serum γ-glutamyl transpeptidase is one of the most sensitive indicators of liver disease (Orlowski, 1963). Two recent reviews of the subject have been published (Kokot and Sledzinski, 1974; Rosalki, 1975). Elevated serum γ-glutamyl transpeptidase activity was reported in patients with epilepsy (Ewen and Griffiths, 1971). It is not clear whether this change is due to the disease itself or to the treatment of patients wih drugs inducing hepatic synthesis of the enzyme (Rosalki *et al.*, 1971). Only traces of enzyme activity are found in the cerebrospinal fluid (Swinnen, 1967), no elevation being observed in patients with epilepsy. The activity of the enzyme in patients with tumors of the CNS is generally normal, however, increased activity was observed 3–5 days following surgical removal of the tumor, the highest elevation being attained during the second week (Ewen and Griffiths, 1973). Increased serum enzyme activity was also reported in patients with vascular brain lesions. It is of interest that γ-glutamyl transpeptidase activity increased in the brain of rats after halothane and diethyl ether anesthesia, indicating the possibility of induction of the enzyme in the brain (Lawinski *et al.*, 1969). Recently, increased serum γ-glutamyl transpeptidase activity was reported in 12 patients with myotonic dystrophy (Alevizos et al., 1975).

2. γ-Glutamyl Cyclotransferase (γ-Glutamyl Lactamase) (EC 2.3.2.4)

This enzyme catalyzes the conversion of γ-glutamyl amino acids to pyrrolidone carboxylate and free amino acid as follows.

$$\gamma\text{-Glutamyl amino acid} \rightarrow \text{pyrrolidone carboxylate} + \text{amino acid} \qquad (6)$$

Pyrrolidone carboxylate and glutamate were observed as products of glutathione metabolism in kidney extracts by Woodward and Reinhart (1942). That the formation of pyrrolidone carboxylate is due to an enzyme different from γ-glutamyl transpeptidase was first shown by Connell and Hanes (1956). Later studies showed that γ-glutamyl cyclotransferase is inactive toward reduced and oxidized glutathione, and that the formation of pyrrolidone carboxylate in kidney extracts occurs in two separate reactions catalyzed in sequence by γ-glutamyl transpeptidase and γ-glutamyl cyclotransferase (Orlowski et al., 1969; Orlowski and Meister, 1971d) :

$$2GSH \xrightarrow[\text{transpeptidase}]{\gamma\text{-glutamyl}} \gamma\text{-glutamylglutathione} + \text{cysteinylglycine} \qquad (7)$$

$$\gamma\text{-Glutamylglutathione} \xrightarrow[\text{cyclotransferase}]{\gamma\text{-glutamyl}} \text{pyrrolidone carboxylate} + \text{glutathione} \qquad (8)$$

Glutamate is not formed in the cyclotransferase reaction, and attempts to demonstrate the reversibility of the reaction were unsuccessful (Connell and Hanes, 1956).

Highly purified preparations of γ-glutamyl cyclotransferase have been obtained from human brain (Orlowski et al., 1969; Orlowski and Meister, 1970b), pig liver (Adamson et al., 1971), and rat liver (Orlowski and Meister, 1973). The enzyme is associated with the soluble protein fraction of tissue homogenates. Two forms (isozymes A and B) of the enzyme differing in isoelectric point were found in human brain, pig liver, and all tissues of the rat. The molecular weight of the enzyme from pig liver was estimated by sedimentation equilibrium as approximately 22,000 (Adamson et al., 1971) for both forms. The amino acid composition of both isozymes was quite similar, and the N-terminal amino acid was glycine. The two isozymes isolated from rat liver also had identical molecular weights of approximately 27,000, as determined by gel filtration. The specificity of both isozymes toward various γ-glutamyl amino acids was identical.

γ-Glutamyl cyclotransferase is widely distributed in animal tissues, high activities being found in the kidney, liver, testes, and brain. The specificity of the enzyme is similar in all tissues of the rat. However, marked differences

GLUTATHIONE IN THE NERVOUS SYSTEM

89

in specificity are found among enzymes from different animal species. γ-Glutamyl cyclotransferase is significantly active with the γ-glutamyl derivatives of L-α-aminobutyrate, L-methionine, L-glutamine, glycine, and L-glutamate. Little activity is obtained with γ-glutamyl derivatives of L-leucine and L-phenylalanine (Table V). Similarly, low activities were found with γ-glutamyltyrosine and γ-glutamylvaline tested with purified human and sheep brain enzyme. These studies indicate that γ-glutamyl derivatives of aromatic and branched-chain amino acids are poor substrates for mammalian γ-glutamyl cyclotransferases. It seems that a free carboxyl group in the amino acid attached directly to the γ-glutamyl group is required for activity. The results shown in Table V indicate that considerable activity of γ-glutamyl cyclotransferase is present in mammalian brains. The activity of the enzyme in the choroid plexus was found to be higher than in the cerebral cortex or in other parts of the brain (Tate et al., 1973; Okonkwo et al., 1974).

3. Cysteinylglycine Dipeptidase (EC 3.4.3.5)

Extracts of kidney and other tissues contain one or more peptidases capable of hydrolyzing cysteinylglycine, the dipeptide released from gluta-

TABLE V

SPECIFICITY OF γ-GLUTAMYLCYCLOTRANSFERASE IN MOUSE, RAT, AND HUMAN BRAIN[a,b]

Substrate	Mouse[c]	Rat[c]	Human[d]
L-γ-Glutamyl-L-γ-glutamyl-p-nitroanilide	100	100	100
L-γ-Glutamyl-L-2-aminobutyrate	132 (2970)	538 (834)	11
L-γ-Glutamyl-L-methionine	264	1040	10
L-γ-Glutamyl-L-glutamine	402	1920	43
α-N-(L-γ-glutamyl)-L-lysine	11	188	—
L-γ-Glutamylglycine	8	76	14
L-γ-Glutamyl-L-glutamate	8	126	—
L-γ-Glutamyl-L-leucine	3	0	0.9
L-γ-Glutamyl-L-phenylalanine	3	—	0.5

[a] From Orlowski and Wilk (1975a), Orlowski and Meister (1973), and Orlowski et al. (1969).

[b] The activity is expressed relative to that found with L-γ-glutamyl-L-γ-glutamyl-p-nitroanilide arbitrarily set at 100. Values in parentheses represent specific activity (nanomoles of product per milligram of protein per hour) determined with L-γ-glutamyl-L-2-aminobutyrate.

[c] Homogenates.

[d] Purified enzyme.

thione by the action of γ-glutamyl transpeptidase (Binkley and Nakamura, 1948; Semenza, 1957; Marks, 1970). The reaction proceeds as follows.

$$\text{L-Cysteinylglycine} + H_2O \rightarrow \text{L-cysteine} + \text{glycine}$$

The enzyme or enzymes that catalyze this reaction require further characterization.

C. ATP-Dependent Pyrrolidone Carboxylate Hydrolase

When [^{14}C]L-pyrrolidone carboxylate is administered to mice, $^{14}CO_2$ rapidly appears in the exhaled air. Analysis of tissues has shown that most of the label is converted into glutamate and glutamine (Orlowski and Meister, 1970a; Ramakrisha et al., 1970). Rush and Starr (1970) observed that a soluble rat liver preparation converted [^{14}C]pyrrolidone carboxylate into [^{14}C]glutamate in the presence of ATP, and that this conversion was a necessary step in the incorporation of pyrrolidone carboxylate into tRNA. Subsequent studies have shown that rat tissues contain an enzyme that converts L-pyrrolidone carboxylate into L-glutamate in an ATP-requiring reaction (Van Der Werf et al., 1971) as follows.

$$\text{L-Pyrrolidone carboxylate} + \text{ATP} + 2H_2O \xrightarrow{\text{enzyme}} \text{L-glutamate} + \text{ADP} + P_i$$

The enzyme requires for activity both a divalent (Mg^{2+} or Mn^{2+}) and a monovalent (K^+ or NH_4 but not Na^+) cation in addition to ATP. The enzyme is widely distributed in animal tissues. Significant activities were found in the kidney, liver, spleen, lungs, and brain. The enzyme is strongly inhibited by sulfhydryl-blocking reagents like iodoacetamide, p-chloromercuribenzoate, and N-ethylmaleimide. A recently obtained preparation from rat kidney was reported to have a molecular weight of 460,000 and to be composed of four subunits each with a molecular weight of 115,000 (Wendel et al., 1975b). L-2-Imidozolidone-4-carboxylate was found to be a competitive inhibitor of the enzyme (Van Der Werf et al., 1973). Pyrrolidone carboxylate hydrolase activity was found in rat, mouse, and rabbit brain (Tate et al., 1973; Okonkwo et al., 1974; Orlowski and Wilk, 1975b). The activity of the enzyme in the choroid plexus is significantly higher than in the brain.

D. Enzymic Reactions Involving the Sulfhydryl Group of Glutathione

In addition to the reactions that affect the net concentration of glutathione, there are also enzymic reactions of physiological interest, which utilize the oxidation and reduction properties of glutathione. These reactions are reviewed in this section.

1. Glutathione Peroxidase (EC 1.11.1.9)

Glutathione peroxidase was first isolated by Mills (1957) as a glutathione-utilizing enzyme which protects hemoglobin from oxidation. Its activity has been separated from that of catalase (Mills, 1959). Glutathione peroxidase catalyzes the following reaction.

$$2GSH + ROOH \xrightarrow[\text{peroxidase}]{\text{glutathione}} GSSG + ROH$$

In this reaction glutathione reduces hydrogen peroxide to water, or a hydroperoxide to an alcohol, and is itself oxidized in the process. The specificity requirements for both the reducing agent and the hydroperoxide have been investigated. Of the possible reducing agents tested, glutathione is the most effective (Mills, 1959). With other sulfhydryl compounds, the rate of the reaction is increased with the degree of sulfhydryl ionization. An amino group near the sulfhydryl group inhibits this reaction (Flohe et al., 1971b). The enzyme, however, shows little preference in the nature of the hydroperoxide to be reduced. The hydroperoxide can be hydrogen peroxide ($R = H$), an organic hydroperoxide (e.g., R = t-butyl), or a fatty acid hydroperoxide (e.g., R = linoleic acid) (Holmberg, 1968; Little and O'Brien, 1968). The enzyme, however, is not reactive with dialkyl peroxides (Tappel, 1974).

Glutathione peroxidase has been partially purified from bovine lens (Holmberg, 1968) and obtained as a homogeneous protein from bovine blood (Flohe et al., 1971a), rat liver (Nakamura et al., 1974), and ovine erythrocytes (Oh et al., 1974).

Glutathione peroxidase prepared from bovine blood has been reported to have a molecular weight of 83,000 and is composed of four subunits, each with a molecular weight of 21,000 (Flohe et al., 1971a). The enzyme contains 4 gm-atoms of selenium per mole, presumably 1 gm-atom per subunit (Flohe et al., 1973). Analogous physical characteristics were observed with the purified enzymes from rat liver (Nakamura et al., 1974) and ovine erythrocytes (Oh et al., 1974). Since glutathione peroxidase contains no heme or flavin (Flohe et al., 1971c), it is supposed that its catalytic activity resides in changes in the oxidation state of selenium (Flohe et al., 1973). An oxidation state change has been demonstrated by X-ray photoelectron spectroscopy (Wendel et al., 1975c).

The tissue distribution of glutathione peroxidase in rat has been determined. High glutathione peroxidase activity was found in the blood and liver, intermediate activity in the heart, kidney, and lungs, and low activity in the intestine and muscles (Mills, 1960). Similar tissue distributions of glutathione peroxidase activity were found by De Marchena et al. (1974). These workers, however, found little glutathione peroxidase activity in brain

homogenates from the seven animal species studied. The activity of glutathione peroxidase in the brain of a given species was about 10% (2–25%)
of that found in the liver. Low glutathione peroxidase levels in rat brain were
also found by Lawrence et al. (1974). The markedly low levels of glutathione
peroxidase in brain, coupled with the low levels of other enzymes involved in
disposing of peroxides (e.g., catalase), suggests that brain possesses a unique
mechanism for dealing with peroxidative stress (De Marchena et al., 1974).
Studies on the subcellular distribution of glutathione peroxidase in rat brain
showed low activity in all subcellular fractions (De Marchena et al., 1974).
Glutathione peroxidase plays a major role in the protection of living cells
and biological membranes against oxidative damage. This protective role
may result from its ability to degrade the low levels of hydrogen peroxide
normally generated in living cells (Cohen and Hochstein, 1963), or its
ability to degrade lipid peroxides formed through environmental oxidation of
cellular fatty acids (Neubert et al., 1962; Christophersen, 1966). Selenium is
an essential trace element. This nutritional role of selenium is dependent on
its being required for the synthesis of glutathione peroxidase.

2. Glutathione Reductase (EC 1.6.4.2)

The enzyme responsible for maintaining cellular glutathione in the reduced state is glutathione reductase. The early work concerning glutathione
reductase has been reviewed by Vennesland and Conn (Colowick et al., 1954,
p. 105). Glutathione reductase catalyzes the following reaction:

$$\text{GSSG} + \text{NADPH} + \text{H}^+ \xrightarrow{\text{glutathione}\atop\text{reductase}} 2\text{GSH} + \text{NADP}^+$$

The substrate specificity of this reaction in red blood cells has been investigated and has been recently reviewed (Beutler, in Flohe et al., 1974, p. 109).
In enzyme preparations, NADH can substitute for NADPH as the reducing
agent. Reductase activity with either cofactor, however, resides with a single
enzyme (Kaplan, 1968; Beutler and Yeh, 1963), and in intact erythrocytes
NADH seems to be ineffective (Beutler and Yeh, 1963). Disulfide specificity
has also been investigated. The reductase reaction is relatively specific for
oxidized glutathione, though other disulfides such as dihydrolipoic acid and
di-γ-glutamylcysteine can also be utilized as substrates (Smith, 1971; Scott
et al., 1963). These disulfides, however, have lower affinities for the enzyme
and react at rates markedly lower than that of GSSG. Mixed disulfides of
proteins and glutathione, such as hemoglobin-glutathione (Srivastava and
Beutler, 1970) and lens crystalline-glutathione (Srivastava, 1971), are substrates for glutathione reductase.

Glutathione reductase has been isolated from several sources (Hosoda
and Nakamura, 1970; Ray and Prescott, 1975; Scott et al., 1963; Icen, 1967;

Staal *et al.*, 1969, Worthington and Rosemeyer, 1974; Mize and Langdon, 1962). Glutathione reductase activity has, in addition, been found in all rat tissues studied (Rall and Lehninger, 1952; Wendell, 1968). In guinea pig brain, glutathione reductase activity is dependent on the method of tissue preparation. Under optimal conditions (acetone-dried extract, EDTA) the brain can reduce 250–300 μmoles of glutathione per gram of fresh tissue per hour. The significance of this high glutathione reductase activity is still unclear. It seems to be an important enzymic pathway for the utilization of NADPH in the brain. Reduction of NADPH by cytochromes, and transhydrogenation of NADPH to NAD^+, are probably lesser pathways for its utilization (McIlwain and Tresize, 1957; McIlwain, in Crook, 1959, p. 66). Studies of the subcellular distribution of glutathione reductase activity have shown that it is primarily localized in the soluble supernatant fraction (Rall and Lehninger, 1952; Hosoda and Nakumura, 1970). Glutathione reductase, depending on its origin, has been found to occur either as a monomer with a molecular weight ranging between 44,000 and 60,000 (Ray and Prescott, 1975) or as a dimer with a molecular weight ranging between 102,000 and 124,000 (Ichio and Sakai, 1974). Glutathione reductase is a flavoprotein containing one FAD molecule per subunit. FAD can be dissociated from the intact enzyme by acid treatment in the presence of ammonium sulfate, resulting in the loss of reductase activity. The enzyme can be reactivated by the addition of FAD. FMN or riboflavin, however, was ineffective in restoring activity (Mapson, in Crook, 1959, p. 28).

The NADPH needed for reducing glutathione can be produced either by the oxidation of glucose via the hexose monophosphate shunt, or by the oxidation of malate by malic enzyme. In red blood cells, only the glucose oxidation pathway is operative, and NADPH can therefore be produced only by the hexose monophosphate shunt. In rat liver, where both oxidative pathways operate, it has been suggested that malate can also supply NADPH for glutathione reduction (Stark *et al.*, 1975). In red blood cells and leukocytes, the amount of glucose oxidized by the hexose monophosphate shunt is stimulated by oxidative stress. The process linking oxidative stress to increased glucose oxidation occurs as follows. Oxidative stress results in higher GSSG levels. The GSSG is subsequently reduced to GSH, by glutathione reductase, with a concomitant elevation of $NADP^+$ levels. These elevated $NADP^+$ levels are believed to be the primary stimulus for oxidative stress enhancement of hexose monophosphate shunt activity (Jacob and Jandl, 1966; Reed, 1969; Beck, 1958; Metz *et al.*, 1974). The hexose monophosphate shunt also operates in the brain to maintain glutathione in its reduced form (Hotta, 1962). CNS-active drugs, such as chlorpromazine, quinacrine, and Amytal, were shown to affect both the ability of subcellular preparations of guinea pig brain to reduce glutathione, and the activity of the hexose monophosphate shunt, in these preparations. It has been suggested that these changes are a reflection of the drugs' pharmacological action, possibly through their alteration of the oxidation state of certain key sulfhydryl groups (Hotta, 1966, 1967; 1970; Hotta and Seventko, 1968; Tarantino and Hotta, 1974). By maintaining cellular sulfhydryl groups in the reduced state glutathione reductase prevents cellular damage by oxidative stress. This antioxidant activity of glutathione reductase results from two distinct actions of this enzyme. First, glutathione reductase can directly reduce certain disulfides formed during oxidative stress, such as the mixed disulfides hemoglobin-glutathione and lens crystalline-glutathione. Second, glutathione reductase can also reduce GSSG to GSH, thereby maintaining a sufficient supply of the reduced substrate for the glutathione peroxidase reaction. Since glutathione peroxidase functions to eliminate cellular hydrogen peroxides (or hydroperoxide), the coupling of glutathione peroxidase and glutathione reductase results in the net reduction of hydrogen peroxide (or hydroperoxides) and the net oxidation of NADPH, with no net change in the oxidation state of glutathione.

3. Transhydrogenases

Other disulfide compounds aside from oxidized glutathione occur naturally (Jocelyn, 1972; Mannervik and Eriksson, in Flohe et al., 1974, p. 120). There are two known enzymic pathways for the reduction of these disulfides (Tietze, 1970a). The first pathway, as represented in reaction (9), is the direct reduction of the disulfide by a reduced nucleotide.

$$R^1SSR^2 + H^+ + NAD(P)H \rightarrow R^1SH + R^2SH + NAD(P) \quad (9)$$

This reaction is analogous to the reaction catalyzed by glutathione reductase. An alternate pathway for disulfide reduction is represented by reactions (10) through (12):

$$
\begin{aligned}
R^1SSR^2 + GSH &\rightarrow R^1SSG + R^2SH & (10)\\
R^1SSG + GSH &\rightarrow GSSG + R^1SH & (11)\\
GSSG + H^+ + NAD(P)H &\rightarrow 2GSH + NAD(P) & (12)
\end{aligned}
$$

$$\text{Sum } R^1SSR^2 + H^+ + NAD(P)H \rightarrow R^1SH + R^2SH + NAD(P)$$

In this case each half of the disulfide bond is sequentially replaced by reduced glutathione [reactions (10) and (11)], resulting in oxidized glutathione and two free thiol groups. The oxidized glutathione is subsequently reduced by glutathione reductase. The sum of these three reactions is equivalent to reaction (9).

The enzymes that catalyze the sequential replacement of disulfide bonds by glutathione are called transhydrogenases (Racker, 1955) or thiol transferases (Askelof et al., 1974). The term transhydrogenase is used here, since this is the term more frequently cited in past literature. Nucleotide-linked reducing systems that are nonspecific for disulfides, such as the thioredoxin system, are capable of reducing disulfide bonds as shown in reaction (9) (Tietze, 1970b). Reductases specific for homocystine (Racker, 1955), cystine (Romano and Nickerson, 1954), and glutathione-CoA disulfide (CoASSG) (Ondarza and Martinez, 1966; Ondarza *et al.*, 1974) have also been described. It has been suggested, however, that these substrate-specific reductase activities may be artifacts attributable either to direct reduction by glutathione reductase, an enzyme not totally specific for glutathione, or to coupled transhydrogenation and reduction, as shown in reactions (10) through (12) (Black, 1963; Mannervik and Eriksson, in Flohe *et al.*, 1974, p. 120; Eriksson *et al.*, 1974).

The transhydrogenase activity described by reactions (10) and (11) was first demonstrated by Racker (1953). Transhydrogenase activity is widely distributed in animal tissues (Tietze *et al.*, 1972; States and Segal, 1969; Katzen and Stetten, 1962; Wendell, 1968; Kohno *et al.*, 1969; Chandler and Varandani, 1972; Varandani and Nafz, 1974). It is possible to divide transhydrogenases on the basis of their disulfide specificity. It should, however, be stated at the outset that such a classification is by no means rigorous. One group of transhydrogenases has marked specificity for small disulfides such as cystine and CoASSG. An enzyme with this specificity has been purified from bovine kidney (Chang and Wilken, 1966). This enzyme is capable of reacting with small disulfides but is relatively inactive with proteins such as insulin and RNase. It is a small protein, having a molecular weight of approximately 12,000. There are, however, enzymes such as glutathione insulin transhydrogenase and RNase-reactivating enzyme that preferentially react with proteins and peptides. Glutathione-insulin transhydrogenase reacts readily with insulin, oxytocin, and vasopressin, but has little activity with cystine (Katzen and Stetten, 1962). Glutathione-insulin transhydrogenase from various sources has a molecular weight of about 60,000 (Varandani, 1973). RNase-reactivating enzyme has a molecular weight of about 42,000 (De Lorenzo *et al.*, 1966). RNase-reactivating enzyme catalyzed the reactivation of proteins such as RNase, egg-white lysosome, and soybean trypsin inhibitor, by thiol disulfide exchange (transhydrogenation) (Fuchs *et al.*, 1967).

The physiological function of these transhydrogenases can probably be related to their specificity. Thus enzymes with specificity toward small disulfides probably maintain these disulfides in their reduced form (Chang and Wilken, 1966). There is probably more than one enzyme capable of reducing small disulfides, as judged by differences in specificity and tissue distribution. The physiological function of transhydrogenases, which preferentially utilize proteins or peptides, is probably to either activate or terminate protein or peptide activity (De Lorenzo *et al.*, 1966; Tomizawa, 1962; Katzen and Stetten, 1962; Varandani and Nafz, 1974). It is not yet known whether the activities of glutathione-insulin transhydrogenase and RNase-reactivating enzyme are functions of the same or different enzymes (Katzen and Tietze, 1966; Ansorage *et al.*, 1973). There are similarities and differences between these enzymes (Varandani and Nafz, 1974; Varandani, 1973). It should be noted that the enzyme capable of degrading oxytocin, a peptide, has little activity with insulin. It does, however, have activity with small disulfides (e.g., cystine and homocystine) and some proteins (e.g., bovine albumin) (Small and Watkins, 1974).

The specificity of the thiol needed for transhydrogenation has been investigated for glutathione-insulin transhydrogenase. It has been found that protein sulfhydryl groups, as well as GSH, can act as the thiol cosubstrate to effect insulin degradation. Proteins are effective in concentrations much lower than that required for GSH. This effectiveness suggests that protein sulfhydryl groups may also function as cosubstrates in the physiological process of insulin degradation (Chandler and Varandani, 1973). The importance of transhydrogenase reactions in brain function is difficult to evaluate. There has been one report that high transhydrogenase activity is found in the brain (rat) (Chang and Wilken, 1966) when CoASSG is used as the disulfide substrate. Other transhydrogenase activity utilizing thiamine disulfide derivatives (Kohno *et al.*, 1969), insulin (Chandler and Varandani, 1972), or partially reoxidized RNase (De Lorenzo and Molea, 1967) as the disulfide substrate have only slow to moderate activity in the brain.

IV. Turnover of Glutathione in the CNS

Glutathione is synthesized rapidly in the brain. Brain glutathione is labeled within minutes after intravenous administration of [^{14}C]glutamate to rats and mice (Lajtha *et al.*, 1959). Intracisternal administration of [^{14}C]glutamate to cats rapidly labels glutathione in the brainstem, cerebellum, mesodiencephalon, and hippocampus (Berl and Purpura, 1966). In addition to these *in vivo* studies, *in vitro* experiments have shown incorporation of [2-^{14}C]glycine and DL-[1-^{14}C]glutamic acid into glutathione (Takahasi and Akabane, 1961). The first-order rate constants for glutathione synthesis in the brain have been calculated as 0.17×10^3 min^{-1}. This value is higher than that calculated for human erythrocytes (0.12×10^3 min^{-1}) and rabbit muscle (0.11×10^3 min^{-1}), though it is much lower than that calculated for liver (2.9–5.8×10^3 min^{-1}) and kidney (24×10^3 min^{-1}). These calculations assume a homogeneous pool of both precursors and products (Sekura and Meister, 1974). Glutamate metabolism in the brain is believed to occur in at least two compartments or pools. It was found that glutamine is more readily converted to glutathione in the brain than glutamate (Berl *et al.*, 1961), as was similarly found in the lens (Kern and Ho, 1973). A computer simulation of the dynamics of glutamate metabolism in the brain was, in general, in accord with experimental data when the simulation was modeled assuming two glutamate pools. The data also suggested a model in which glutathione occurs in two pools, one of which has a rapid turnover time (Garfinkel, 1962, 1966).

The half-life of glutathione in rat brain after intracisternal injection of labeled glycine was 71 hours (Douglas and Mortensen, 1956). Though the half-life of glutathione in the brain is longer than that reported in mouse kidney (0.5 hour) and in mouse, rabbit, and rat liver (2–4 hours) (Sekura and Meister, 1974; Waelsch and Rittenberg, 1942), it is shorter than that reported for human erythrocytes (96 hours) (Dimant *et al.*, 1955) and rabbit muscle (103 hours) (Henriques *et al.*, 1955). It should be noted that turnover does not include glutathione utilization by processes such as oxidation, reduction, and transhydrogenation. These processes, in general, yield no net synthesis or degradation of glutathione, and would not be expected to affect glutathione turnover. In addition, a small pool with a rapid turnover, performing an important metabolic function, could account for most of the observed glutathione turnover. Such a pool could be associated with the choroid plexus and could function in amino acid transport.

V. Possible Functions of Glutathione

A. DETOXIFICATION

Glutathione is able to conjugate with certain substances and thereby prepare these substances for eventual excretion (for recent reviews, see Boyland and Chasseaud, 1969; Wood, 1970; Boyland, 1971; Chasseaud, 1973, and in Flohe *et al.*, 1974). The conjugates formed with glutathione are either excreted unchanged into the bile or are further metabolized to mercapturic acids. Mercapturic acids are N-acetyl-S-substituted derivatives of cysteine. They are generally water-soluble and can be excreted in the urine. Conjugation with glutathione limits the lifetime and toxicity of exogenous substances in the body. The reaction of the nucleophilic thiol group of glutathione with the electrophilic substance prevents other cellular nucleophilic sites from reacting with the electrophile. Conjugation with glutathione generally occurs enzymically, but can also occur nonenzymically. Enzymic conjugation with glutathione is catalyzed by a series of enzymes called glutathione S-transferases (Combes and Stakelum, 1961; Booth *et al.* 1961).

The formation of mercapturic acid from the initial glutathione conjugate involves enzymic removal of the γ-glutamyl and glycine moieties of the conjugate, followed by enzymic acetylation. The γ-glutamyl moiety of the conjugate is removed by the action of γ-glutamyl transpeptidase. It is of interest that several S-substituted derivatives of glutathione are more active substrates for γ-glutamyl transpeptidase than glutathione (Tate and Meister, 1974a). Several glutathione S-transferase activities have been found. These activities are characterized by the nature of the substrate conjugated to glutathione. They include glutathione S-aryltransferase (Booth et al., 1960; Combes and Stakelum, 1961; Al-Kasseb et al., 1963), glutathione S-alkyltransferase (Johnson, 1966a), glutathione S-aralkyltransferase (Suga et al., 1967), glutathione S-epoxide transferase (Boyland and Williams, 1965; Booth et al., 1961), glutathione S-alkenyltransferase (Boyland and Chasseaud, 1967, 1968), and glutathione S-estrogen transferase (Jellinck et al., 1967; Kuss, 1967). Five enzymes containing glutathione S-transferase activity have been identified in rat liver. These enzymes have been designated glutathione S-transferase A to E. Four of these enzymes, glutathione S-transferase A (Pabst et al., 1974), B, C (Habig et al., 1974a), and E (Fjellstedt et al., 1973) have been purified to homogeneity. Each of these purified enzyme preparations has, to a greater or lesser extent, activity with aryl, alkyl, aralkyl, epoxide, and alkenyl substrates.

In addition to glutathione S-transferase activities, there are degradative activities that are glutathione-dependent but do not form glutathione conjugates. These activities include that of DDT dehydrochlorinase (Sternburg et al., 1954; Lipke and Kearns, 1959a), organic thiocyanate-degrading enzyme (Ohkawa and Casida, 1971), and nitrate ester reductase (Heppel and Hilmoe, 1950), and thiosulfate ester reduction (Mannervik et al., 1974). Detoxification of compounds by their conjugation with glutathione seems to occur primarily in the kidney and liver. Little detoxification seems to take place in the brain. Rat brain contains little glutathione S-alkyltransferase activity (Johnson, 1966b). Similarly, rat cerebrum, cerebellum, and brainstem contain little glutathione S-arene oxide (epoxide) transferase activity (Hayakawa et al., 1974). In addition, ligandin, or Y protein (Litwack et al., 1971), a protein capable of binding organic anions (Levi et al., 1969), has been shown to be associated with glutathione S-transferase activity (Kaplowitz et al., 1973). It has in fact been shown to be identical with glutathione S-transferase B (Habig et al., 1974b). Little ligandin (Levi et al., 1969), hence little glutathione S-transferase B activity, has been demonstrated in the brain.

B. Coenzyme Functions of Glutathione

Glutathione can function as a coenzyme in the catalysis of several reactions. These reactions include hydration, dehydrogenation, isomerization, and dehydrochlorination (Jocelyn, 1972).

1. Hydration

Glutathione functions as a coenzyme in the hydration and rearrangement of methylglyoxal (pyruvic aldehyde) to lactic acid in a reaction catalyzed by glyoxalase. Glyoxalase (Neuberg, 1913; Dakin and Dudley, 1913a) is composed of two enzymes, glyoxalase I and glyoxalase II. Both enzymes are necessary to catalyze this reaction sequentially (Crook and Law, 1950; Racker, 1951). Glyoxalase I catalyzes the conversion of methylglyoxal in the presence of glutathione to S-lactoylglutathione. Glyoxalase I from several sources has been purified to apparent homogeneity (Vander Jagt and Han, 1973; Kester and Norton, 1975; Uotila and Koivusalo, 1975). The molecular weight of the enzyme from mammalian sources ranges from 43,000 to 52,000 (Uotila and Koivusalo, 1975; Mannervik et al., 1972). A subunit molecular weight of 21,000 was found for the sheep liver enzyme (Uotila and Koivusalo, 1975). The specificity of glyoxalase I toward other keto aldehydes seems to be similar to the specificity observed for the complete glyoxalase system (Knox, 1960; Vander Jagt et al., 1972; Uotila and Koivusalo, 1975).

Glyoxalase II, which catalyzes the hydrolysis of S-lactoylglutathione to D-lactic acid and glutathione was first separated from glyoxalase I by Racker (1951). This enzyme has been extensively purified from human liver (Uotila, 1975). Glyoxalase II isolated from human liver seems to be specific for thiol esters of glutathione but relatively nonspecific for the structure of the acyl group. The distribution of the total glyoxalase system has been investigated. Glyoxalase activity is widely distributed in plants and animals (Dakin and Dudley, 1913b). It has a relatively high activity in the brain (Geiger, 1935; McIlwain, in Crook, 1959; Jowett and Quastel, 1934).

The physiological function of the glyoxalase system is not known. Numerous attempts have been made to associate this system with glycolysis. However, methylglyoxal is not an intermediate in the glycolytic pathway. It has been suggested that the function of glyoxalase is to utilize other naturally occurring keto aldehydes as substrates (Green and Elliott, 1964; Jerzykowski et al., 1973). Glyoxalase may be a promoter (promine) of cell growth, reacting with keto aldehydes that show growth-retarding abilities (retine) (Szent-Györgyi et al., 1967).

2. Dehydrogenation

Formaldehyde dehydrogenase (EC 1.2.1.1) is one of several enzymes that catalyze the dehydrogenation of formaldehyde. This enzyme, first isolated from beef and chicken liver, is a NAD-dependent enzyme distinct from acetaldehyde dehydrogenase (Strittmatter and Ball, 1955). This enzyme reversibly catalyzes the dehydrogenation of formaldehyde, in the presence of

NAD$^+$, to S-formylglutathione. S-Formylglutathione is subsequently hydro-lyzed by a second enzyme, S-formylglutathione hydrolase, to formic acid and glutathione as a cofactor, which cannot be satisfied by other sulfhydryl groups

Formaldehyde dehydrogenase has a specific requirement for reduced glutathione as a cofactor, which cannot be satisfied by other sulfhydryl groups (Strittmatter and Ball, 1955). This enzyme is not totally specific for NAD$^+$, and at lower pH values can also utilize NADP$^+$ as the oxidizing agent. Other aldehydes, including methylglyoxal and glyoxal, can act as substrates in place of formaldehyde (Uotila and Koivusalo, 1974b).

The molecular weight of the enzyme from human liver has been esti-mated as 89,000 (Goodman and Tephly, 1971) and 81,400 (Uotila and Koivusalo, 1974b). The enzyme was found to have a subunit molecular weight of 39,500 (Uotila and Koivusalo, 1974a). Formaldehyde dehydro-genase activity has been found in every tissue examined, including: rat brain, kidney, heart muscle, and skeletal muscle; bovine brain and adrenal gland; sheep liver; mouse ascites tumor cells; and human brain. The enzyme is associated with the soluble fraction of homogenates (Uotila and Koivusalo, 1974b).

3. Dehydrochlorination

GSH is a necessary cofactor in the dehydrochlorination of dichlorodi-phenyltrichloroethane (DDT) to dichloro-2,2-bis(p-chlorophenyl)ethylene (DDE) catalyzed by DDT dehydrochlorinase (EC 4.5.1.1) (Sternburg et al., 1954). Other thiol compounds, with the exception of cysteinylglycine, are ineffective in effecting DDT dehydrochlorination. Cysteinylglycine can serve as a cofactor but is only 60% as effective as GSH (Lipke and Kearns, 1959b). DDT dehydrochlorinase activity in flies has been correlated with the degree of their resistance to DDT (Sternburg et al., 1954). The enzyme was purified from DDT-resistant flies. It has a monomeric molecular weight of 30,000–36,000 (DiNamarca et al., 1969; Lipke and Kearns, 1959a). Aggregation of monomeric DDT dehydrochlorinase is stimulated by DDT. Glutathione stabilizes the aggregated enzyme. DDT dehydrochlorinase tetramers are 10 times more active than the corresponding trimers; dimeric and monomeric DDT dehydrochlorinases are without activity (DiNamarca et al., 1969, 1971).

4. Isomerization

Glutathione serves as coenzyme for the cis-trans isomerization of maleyl-acetoacetate to fumarylacetoacetate as catalyzed by maleylacetoacetate iso-merase (Edwards and Knox, 1956). It also serves as a coenzyme in the isomerization of maleylpyruvate to fumarylpyruvate as catalyzed by maleyl-pyruvyl isomerase (Lack, 1961). Maleylacetoacetate and maleylpyruvate are degradation products of homogentisic acid and gentisic acid, respectively. The isomerizing enzymes require GSH for activity; other thiol compounds cannot substitute for GSH (Seltzer, 1972).

C. MAINTENANCE OF CELLULAR THIOL GROUPS

Glutathione also acts to maintain the thiol-disulfide status of cells. The thiol-disulfide status of a given cell is defined as the total pattern of thiols and disulfides within that cell (Kosower et al., 1972). This maintenance function is similar to that described by the euphoristic theory of glutathione action. Glutathione is euphoristic in the sense that it keeps enzymes "happy" by preventing their oxidation and protecting them from reacting with heavy metals (Racker, in Colowick et al., 1954). There are many agents that have the potential to introduce changes in the cellular thiol-disulfide status. These agents include peroxides, radiation exposure, hyperbaric oxygen, airborne oxidants such as ozone and nitrogen dioxide, and drugs such as primaquine and nitrofurantoin. Such changes are transitory as long as sufficient glutathione reductase and NADPH are available. Glutathione peroxidase and the glutathione-dependent transhydrogenases can also play an important role in mitigating the effects of oxidation stress. Glutathione peroxidase can divert the oxidation stress from key sulfhydryl groups, while the glutathione-dependent transhydrogenases are capable of regenerating these key sulfhydryl groups. Both these processes occur at the expense of reduced glutathione. The resulting oxidized glutathione is subsequently reduced by glutathione reductase.

The pathological consequences of altered thiol-disulfide status include cataracts and anemia. In addition, convulsions of central origin are the primary manifestations of oxygen toxicity, presumably also due to alteration in the cellular thiol-disulfide status. The possible cellular thiols affected include enzymes, coenzymes (e.g., dihydrolipoic acid and CoASH), flavoproteins, and glutathione. Sulfhydryl compounds, such as glutathione, which can compensate for aberrations in the thiol-disulfide status, have been found to moderate oxygen toxicity (Haugaard, 1968; Williams and Haugaard, 1970; Sanders et al., 1969). The importance of the reduced-oxidized glutathione status in cellular function can be determined by alteration of this status. Rapid and stoichiometric oxidation of glutathione can be accomplished by the addition of diamide, or other similar thiol-oxidizing agents (Kosower and Kosower, 1969). Among the various cellular sulfhydryl groups diamide preferentially reacts with glutathione (Kosower et al., 1972).

The consequences of altering the thiol-disulfide status of glutathione include inhibition of thiol-dependent steps in protein synthesis, insect feeding behavior, muscle contraction, ionic transport in rabbit lens, growth of

Escherichia coli, development of sea urchin eggs, the feeding response of *Hydra* (Kosower *et al.,* 1972, and references cited therein), and amino acid transport (Hewitt *et al.,* 1974). Diamide treatment also produces changes in the neurophysiological characteristics of frog nerve-muscle preparations. These changes include an increase both in frequency of miniature end-plate potentials and height of neurally evoked end-plate potentials (Werman *et al.,* 1971). The physiological changes induced by diamide are probably mediated by changes in the thiol-sulfide status of enzymes secondary to direct oxidation of glutathione.

D. The γ-Glutamyl Cycle

The reactions of the amino acid-dependent degradation of glutathione, and the reactions leading to its resynthesis, have been linked in a cyclic process called the γ-glutamyl cycle (Fig. 1) (Orlowski and Meister, 1970a). It was proposed that the γ-glutamyl cycle functions in amino acid transport. Evidence in favor of this proposal has been reviewed (Orlowski and Meister, 1970a; Meister, 1973, 1974b,c). Here we summarize the current status of research in this field, with special emphasis on aspects related to the function of the γ-glutamyl cycle in the CNS.

The hypothesis linking the γ-glutamyl cycle to amino acid transport is based on the assumption that membrane-bound γ-glutamyl transpeptidase functions in the translocation of amino acids across cellular membranes. The

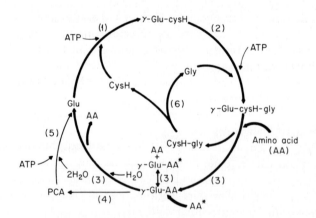

Fig. 1. The γ-glutamyl cycle. (1) γ-Glutamylcysteine synthetase, (2) glutathione synthetase, (3) γ-glutamyl transpeptidase, (4) γ-glutamyl cyclotransferase, (5) pyrrolidone carboxylate hydrolase, (6) cysteinylglycine dipeptidase. AA, Amino acid; PCA, pyrrolidone carboxylate.

possibility that the enzyme may be involved in amino acid transport was mentioned by several investigators (Hird, 1950; Binkley, 1951; Ball *et al.*, 1953).

The hypothesis that γ-glutamyl transpeptidase functions in amino acid transport has its limitations. Many cells have little if any γ-glutamyl transpeptidase and yet are capable of transporting amino acids. It therefore seems unlikely that the enzyme is part of a general amino acid transport system in all tissues. Its function is probably limited to sites where it is highly concentrated (Orlowski, 1963). The affinity of amino acids *in vivo* for γ-glutamyl transpeptidase is not known. Although γ-glutamyl transpeptidase has a broad specificity when tested with optimal concentrations of amino acids *in vitro*, the reaction may be restricted *in vivo* to a limited number of amino acids. The concentration of the amino acid in plasma and its affinity for the enzyme, or for a binding site (recognition site) from which it can interact with the enzyme, may be the causes of such a restriction. The enzyme can also interact with peptides as acceptors, including γ-glutamyl peptides which can act as both donors and acceptors of the γ-glutamyl residue. It remains to be established which of these substrates is preferentially handled by the enzyme.

Several distinct transport systems specific for certain groups of amino acids have been described. At the present time no single system can account for all transport phenomena of all amino acids described in experiments *in vivo* and *in vitro*. The well-documented transport of nonmetabolizable amino acids (Christensen *et al.*, 1956), e.g., α-aminoisobutyric acid or cycloleucine, probably cannot be explained by the function of the γ-glutamyl cycle, since these amino acids are not substrates for γ-glutamyl transpeptidase.

The hypothesis that γ-glutamyl transpeptidase is active in amino acid transport assumes that the enzyme interacts at the cell membrane with glutathione and amino acids to form the corresponding γ-glutamyl derivatives of amino acids. The free amino acid can be then released from its γ-glutamyl linkage and brought into the cell by one of three possible mechanisms. First, since γ-glutamyl amino acids are substrates for γ-glutamyl transpeptidase, the amino acid can be released from its γ-glutamyl linkage in a reaction with a new incoming amino acid. Repetition of this process would allow reutilization of the γ-glutamyl moiety of GSH in several transfer reactions. Functioning of this mechanism *in vivo* would require coupling of the reaction to an energy-yielding process in the cell membrane, allowing a conformational change in the enzyme and permitting translocation of the amino acid into the cell. Second, the hydrolytic function of γ-glutamyl transpeptidase, although slow under experimental conditions, may be of significance in release of the amino acid from γ-glutamyl linkage *in vivo*. The significance of this function of the enzyme increases with a decrease in pH. Third, those γ-glutamyl amino acids that escape into the cytoplasm would be converted to pyrrolidone carboxylate and free amino acid by the action of γ-glutamyl cyclotransferase.

The high concentration of the enzymes of the γ-glutamyl cycle at sites where high transport activity is expected is consistent with its function in transport. Thus γ-glutamyl transpeptidase is concentrated in the brush border of the proximal tubules of the kidney and at other sites with high transport activity. The localization of γ-glutamyl transpeptidase in the endothelium of brain capillaries, in ependymal cells, and in the brush border of cells covering the choroid plexus (Albert et al., 1966), and the much higher activity of the enzymes of the γ-glutamyl cycle in the choroid plexus than in other brain regions (Tate et al., 1973; Okonkwo et al., 1974), suggest that the enzyme functions in brain amino acid transport.

The concentration of a wide variety of substances, including glucose and amino acids, is lower in cerebrospinal fluid than in plasma. Active transport of glucose from the ventricles into the blood by the choroid plexus has been shown to be a factor responsible for the low level of glucose in the cerebrospinal fluid (Csaky and Rigor, 1968), and a similar mechanism is implied for amino acids (Lorenzo and Cutler, 1969). Several studies indicate that there is a continuous exchange of amino acids between blood and brain (Lajtha, 1956, 1968) and that this movement of amino acids occurs through mediated transport processes (Chirigos et al., 1960; Lajtha, 1964; Blasberg and Lajtha, 1966). The existence of a blood–brain barrier for amino acids is indicated by competition among amino acids for entry into the brain, various degrees of restriction for entry into the brain for different amino acids, and stereospecificity of uptake (Oldendorf, 1973; Richter and Wainer, 1971; McKean et al., 1968; Roberts and Morelos, 1965).

Competition among groups of amino acids led to the postulate that several systems exist, each specific for a certain group of amino acids. One or more of these systems may be associated with γ-glutamyl transpeptidase, and it is tempting to speculate that the enzyme functions in the transfer of amino acids at the barrier between blood and brain and at the barrier between blood and cerebrospinal fluid. Supporting this idea is the observation that methionine, a good substrate for the transpeptidase, is rapidly taken up by the brain (Battistin et al., 1971), while glycine, aspartate, and glutamate, which are poor substrates, are hardly taken up at all. Studies cited previously indicate that the γ-glutamyl cycle functions in the brain. Both the enzymes and intermediates of the γ-glutamyl cycle have been found in the brain. Glutathione is present at a concentration of about 2 mM. L-Pyrrolidone carboxylate is normally present in human cerebrospinal fluid and in the brain of several laboratory animals at concentrations similar to those in other tissues (Wilk and Orlowski, 1973; Orlowski and Wilk, 1975b). Small amounts of γ-glutamyl derivatives of several amino acids have been found in the brain.

Operation of the γ-glutamyl cycle would predict that the administration of amino acids will cause increased transpeptidation reactions with glutathione, formation of γ-glutamyl amino acids, and possibly also an increase in the concentration of pyrrolidone carboxylate. Experiments (Orlowski and Wilk, 1975b) have shown that, after administration of methionine, glycine, or phenylalanine, small amounts of the corresponding γ-glutamyl derivatives can be detected in the kidney.

None of these derivatives could be detected in the brain; this is, however, not surprising in view of the limited distribution of γ-glutamyl transpeptidase in the CNS. Administration of single amino acids did not cause an increase in the concentration of pyrrolidone carboxylate in mouse tissues, however, a significant increase was observed in the brain, liver, and kidney after administration of a mixture containing all protein amino acids (Orlowski and Wilk, 1975b). Administration of L-2-imidazolidone-4-carboxylic acid (an inhibitor of L-pyrrolidone carboxylate hydrolase), together with several amino acids, provoked a much higher increase in the level of pyrrolidone carboxylate in mouse tissues than administration of the inhibitor alone (Van der Werf *et al.*, 1974). These findings suggest that administration of amino acids leads to increased transpeptidations with glutathione. However, in view of the low activity of pyrrolidone carboxylate hydrolase in mouse tissues, and the rather small increase in pyrrolidone carboxylate after amino acid loading, it is unlikely that the transport of each amino acid results in the formation of one molecule of pyrrolidone carboxylate, as has been suggested (Meister, 1973). It seems more likely that the γ-glutamyl amino acids formed are generally not released as free intermediates into the cytoplasm.

Several studies seem to support the idea that the γ-glutamyl cycle may be involved in the transport of amino acids. Although these studies relate to tissues other than the CNS, they are worth mentioning here because their validity can probably be extended to the CNS. It is reasonable to predict that transport activity of tissues will be reflected in the turnover of glutathione. Since transport activity is one of the main functions of the kidney, a high turnover of glutathione is expected in this organ. It is of interest in this respect that Lajtha *et al.* (1959) found that, 2 minutes after administration of [14C]glutamate to mice, the specific activity of kidney glutathione exceeded many times the specific activity of the peptide in other tissues. Sekura and Meister (1974) reported recently that the turnover of glutathione in the kidney is five times more rapid than in the liver. Although further studies are needed on the quantitative aspects of this relationship between amino acid transport and glutathione turnover, the high turnover in the kidney is consistent with the existence of such a relationship.

Recent studies have shown that maleate modifies the activity of γ-glutamyl transpeptidase, in that it stimulates the hydrolytic function of the enzyme and inhibits the transpeptidase activity (Curthoys and Kuhlenschmidt, 1975; Tate and Meister, 1975). As a result, amino acids cannot be used as acceptors in the transpeptidation reaction. It has long been known that maleate produces amino aciduria after administration to rats (Harrison and Harrison, 1954; Angielski et al., 1958). Rosenberg and Segal (1964) showed that maleate inhibits uptake of amino acids by kidney cortex slices. The inhibition is reversible and apparently does not involve the formation of a covalent bond between thiol groups and maleate. This action of maleate is consistent with the function of γ-glutamyl transpeptidase in amino acid transport (Tate and Meister, 1974b). It should, however, be noted that maleate may react with sulfhydryl groups of glutathione and proteins and inhibit other enzymes. Furthermore, the action of maleate in vivo is not limited to producing amino aciduria, since glycosuria and phosphaturia are also observed.

A unique system for the transport of phenylalanine via the γ-glutamyl cycle was described by Bodnaryk (1974) and Bodnaryk et al. (1974) in larvae of the housefly.

The possibility must also be considered that γ-glutamyl transpeptidase functions in the uptake and transport of γ-glutamyl amino acids and γ-glutamyl peptides. This function would be analogous to the postulated function of dipeptidases in the transport of dipeptides in the intestine and kidney (Smyth, 1972; Matthews, 1972; Ugolev, 1972).

Recent studies in our laboratory (M. Orlowski and S. Wilk, unpublished data) have shown that the kidney has a very high capacity for uptake of γ-glutamyl peptides. When L-γ-glutamyl-L-α-aminobutyrate, an analog of γ-glutamylcysteine, is administered to mice, there is a rapid accumulation of the peptide in the kidney, along with a high accumulation of metabolites derived from it. Thus 30 minutes after administration of the peptide there is a great increase in the concentration of glutamate, aspartate, glutamine, and ophthalmic acid in the kidney. The accumulation of these metabolites is very rapid and can be demonstrated as early as 3 minutes after administration of the peptide. It is of interest that a similar accumulation of metabolites is seen in the kidney after administration of other γ-glutamyl compounds, e.g., γ-glutamylphenylalanine and γ-glutamylglycylglycine. When methionine is administered together with L-γ-glutamyl-L-α-aminobutyrate, there is a strong inhibition of accumulation of the metabolites derived from the dipeptide (Table VI). It seems reasonable to assume that methionine competes with γ-glutamyl-L-α-aminobutyrate for uptake into the kidney. That this competition occurs at the level of γ-glutamyl transpeptidase is made likely by the observation that no such competition or accumulation of metabolites is seen in the liver, where the activity of γ-glutamyl transpeptidase is very low.

The need for a system for uptake of γ-glutamyl compounds seems justified by the presence of a definite, although low, level of free glutathione in

TABLE VI

EFFECT OF METHIONINE ON THE ACCUMULATION OF METABOLITES IN THE KIDNEY
AFTER ADMINISTRATION OF γ-L-GLUTAMYL-L-α-AMINOBUTYRATE[a]

Treatment	Dose (μmoles/ gm)	Time after adminis- tration (min- utes)	γ-L-Glut- amyl-L- α-amino- butyrate (μmoles/ gm)	Ophthal- mic acid (μmoles/ gm)	Gluta- mate (μmoles/ gm)	Gluta- mine (μmoles/ gm)	Aspar- tate (μmoles/ gm)
L-γ-Glutamyl- L-α-amino- butyrate (A)	2.5	30	0.35	2.60	3.15	1.01	2.25
A + L-meth- ionine	2.5 + 2.5	30	0.34	1.19	1.86	0.08	2.20

[a] The values given in the table are in excess of those found in normal controls.

plasma (about 1.5μg/ml) (Tietze, 1969). This concentration of glutathione, if filtered in the glomeruli, would present more than 0.5 μmoles of glutathione per minute to the proximal tubules of the kidney for reabsorption. The origin of free extracellular glutathione is not known, however, the finding that red blood cells actively eliminate oxidized glutathione (Srivastava and Beutler, 1969) and that a similar system operates in porcine liver (Sies, 1973) may provide an adequate answer to this question.

Evidence was presented that reduced glutathione disappears from plasma, probably by forming mixed disulfides with protein sulfhydryl groups (Lieben-son and Jena, 1967; Tietze, 1969). The metabolic fate of such bound gluta-thione is not known; it can, however, be assumed that at some stage the action of γ-glutamyl transpeptidase has to be involved in its degradation. Kidney γ-glutamyl transpeptidase may also be involved in the handling of γ-glutamyl amino acids formed by transpeptidation in other tissues and then transported to the kidney in the plasma. Such a possibility deserves explor-ation. Among the natural amino acids, glutamine, which constitutes approxi-mately 25% of all the plasma amino acids and is a very good substrate for γ-glutamyl transpeptidase is the most likely substrate for this enzyme *in vivo*.

VI. Inherited Disorders of Glutathione Metabolism

A. "PYROGLUTAMIC ACIDURIA" AND GLUTATHIONE SYNTHETASE DEFICIENCY

In 1970 Jellum *et al.*, in Norway, described a new inborn error of metab-olism in a 19-year-old mentally retarded patient and called it pyroglutamic aciduria. The patient excreted about 30 gm daily of pyroglutamic acid (pyrrolidone carboxylate) in the urine and suffered from metabolic acidosis. Neurological examination revealed the presence of spastic tetraparesis and signs of cerebellar damage with ataxic gait and intentional tremor. The level of pyrrolidone carboxylate in the plasma was approximately 50–60 mg/100 ml (normally less than 0.1 mg/100 ml). Somewhat lower levels (30 mg/100 ml) were found in the cerebrospinal fluid. The patient had an elevated level of proline in the plasma (5 mg/100 ml). The levels of other amino acids in the plasma and urine were generally normal, except for slightly elevated levels of aspartate, serine, glutamate, citrulline, glycine, and leucine. The excretion of urea in the urine was diminished. It was first thought that the patient had a deficiency of ATP-dependent pyrrolidone carboxylate hydrolase (5-oxo-L-prolinase) limited to the kidney and was therefore unable to convert pyrrolidone carboxylate into glutamate in the kidney (Eldjarn et al., 1972). Fibroblasts cultured from skin biopsies of the patient and normal controls, however, metabolized pyrrolidone carboxylate at about the same rate (Stromme and Eldjarn, 1972). It is of interest that, when the patient was given an infusion of a mixture of amino acids, massive amino aciduria developed and an approximately twofold increase in urinary excretion of pyrrolidone carboxylate occurred simultaneously. These results were interpreted as evidence that infusion of amino acids caused increased transpeptidation with glutathione, and formation of γ-glutamyl amino acids, followed by their conversion to pyrrolidone carboxylate.

Two sisters, one a newborn, the other 3 years old, with chronic metabolic acidosis and pyroglutamic aciduria were soon thereafter found in Sweden (Hagenfeldt et al., 1974; Larsson et al., 1974). The patients leukocytes converted [^{14}C]pyrrolidone carboxylate to $^{14}CO_2$ at a normal rate. No neurological damage was observed.

Subsequent studies on the Norwegian patient have shown that the excessive excretion of pyrrolidone carboxylate is not due to a block in its metabolism. Instead, the defect appeared to be due to its increased formation (Eldjarn et al., 1973). Similar conclusions were derived from studies of the Swedish patients (Larsson et al., 1974). Both patients showed, in addition, signs of increased hemolysis and had a markedly reduced level of glutathione in their erythrocytes. Enzyme studies on erythrocytes, placenta, and a culture of skin fibroblasts showed a markedly reduced activity of glutathione synthetase. The activities of γ-glutamylcysteine synthetase, γ-glutamyl cyclotransferase, and pyrrolidone carboxylate hydrolase were all normal (Wellner et al., 1974). The activity of glutathione synthetase in erythrocytes of the patients' parents was higher than in the erythrocytes of the two patients, but lower than in normal controls. These results indicated that it may be possible to detect heterozygotes for glutathione synthetase deficiency. The discovery of glutathione synthetase deficiency in the two Swedish patients with pyrogluta-mic aciduria seemed to provide an adequate explanation for the metabolic dis-order. Thus, in the absence of glutathione synthetase, γ-glutamylcysteine is apparently continuously converted into pyrrolidone carboxylate and free cys-teine by the action of γ-glutamyl cyclotransferase. The amount of pyrroli-done carboxylate formed exceeds the capacity of pyrrolidone carboxylate hydrolase to convert it into glutamate. The result is an accumulation of pyrrolidone carboxylate and its excretion in the urine. It is also likely that more γ-glutamylcysteine is synthesized than normally, because of the low concentration of glutathione in tissues, which probably exerts feedback inhibi-tion on the activity of γ-glutamylcysteine synthetase (Jackson, 1969; Rich-man and Meister, 1975). The absence of amino aciduria in the patients was explained by the ability of γ-glutamylcysteine to substitute for glutathione in the transpeptidation reactions with amino acids (Wellner et al., 1974).

It is not known whether the Norwegian patient has a glutathione syn-thetase deficiency also, although such a defect is likely. Further studies are needed to account for the increased excretion of pyrrolidone carboxylate in this patient after an amino acid infusion. Is the "extra" pyrrolidone carboxy-late derived from excessive synthesis of γ-glutamylcysteine or is it derived from γ-glutamyl amino acids formed in a transpeptidation reaction between γ-glutamylcysteine and the infused amino acids? The answers to these ques-tions will be of importance to our understanding of the function of the γ-glutamyl cycle and its significance in the renal handling of amino acids.

It is notable that several other cases of erythrocyte glutathione synthetase deficiency have been described, however, no metabolic acidosis or pyroglu-tamic aciduria has been observed in these patients (Prins et al., 1966; Mohler et al., 1970). They suffer from mild, compensated nonspherocytic hemolytic anemia. Heterozygotes have glutathione synthetase activity levels half those in erythrocytes of normal controls. It is not known whether these patients also have increased excretion of pyrrolidone carboxylate and metabolic aci-dosis which have escaped detection. The possibility must, however, be con-sidered that the glutathione synthetase deficiency in these patients is limited only to erythrocytes. Such a possibility, if confirmed, would indicate that a deficiency of glutathione synthetase is not a uniform disorder and that it may have various metabolic and clinical manifestations. Further metabolic and biochemical studies in these patients are indicated.

B. γ-GLUTAMYLCYSTEINE SYNTHETASE DEFICIENCY

Two patients, a sister (35 years old) and a brother (37 years old) were described who have nonspherocytic hemolytic anemia and less than 5% of the normal level of glutathione in their erythrocytes. Biochemical studies have shown a deficiency of γ-glutamylcysteine synthetase in erythrocytes (Konrad et al., 1972). The patients showed signs of spinocerebellar degeneration, absent reflexes in the lower extremities, and ataxia. The older patient developed an irregular staccato speech, dysdiadochokinesis, and decreased vibratory and position sensation in both the upper and lower extremities. A reduction in glutathione, although of a lower degree, was also observed in their leukocytes and skeletal muscles. Studies of the amino acids in the urine showed the presence of amino aciduria. The excretion of both neutral amino acids (alanine, valine, asparagine, glutamine, cystine, and threonine) and basic amino acids (arginine and lysine) was increased. It was concluded that "patients with autosomal recessive forms of spinocerebellar degeneration should be examined for disorders of glutathione metabolism" (Richards et al., 1974). The finding of amino aciduria in the two patients is consistent with the function of glutathione in amino acid transport, probably through the γ-glutamyl cycle as shown in Fig. 1. It also supports the idea that the nonoccurrence of amino aciduria in patients with low glutathione levels and glutathione synthetase deficiency is probably due to the presence of γ-glutamylcysteine which can substitute for glutathione in transpeptidation reactions and in reactions in which the sulfhydryl group of the tripeptide takes part.

C. SERUM γ-GLUTAMYL TRANSPEPTIDASE DEFICIENCY

In a letter to *The Lancet*, Goodman et al. (1971) described a 33-year-old, moderately retarded, white male who excreted in the urine an abnormal ninhydrin-positive compound. Acid hydrolysis of the isolated material yielded equimolar amounts of glutamate, glycine, and cysteine, consistent with its identification as glutathione. The patient had lower-than-normal serum γ-glutamyl transpeptidase activity. The concentration of glutathione in the plasma was 2.43 μg/ml, and in the urine, 125.4 μg/ml. Normal urine contains little if any glutathione. These investigators assume the existence of a generalized γ-glutamyl transpeptidase deficiency. No other data were presented to support this generalization. The activity of γ-glutamyl transpeptidase in the urine, which is several times higher than in the serum and is derived from the kidney, was not determined. Nor were any enzyme determinations made for cells or tissues. The concentration of glutathione in red blood cells, leukocytes, or muscle biopsies also was not determined, and the results of amino acid analysis in the blood and urine were not reported. In the absence of these data the existence of a generalized γ-glutamyl transpeptidase deficiency remains in doubt. The discovery of such a defect would be expected to provide important information related to the function of glutathione and to the significance of the γ-glutamyl transpeptidase-catalyzed reaction in its metabolism.

D. GLUTATHIONE REDUCTASE DEFICIENCY

Many cases of glutathione reductase deficiency with a variety of clinical syndromes have been reported. These disorders do not represent a uniform clinical entity, and it is rather unlikely that they all can be attributed to a deficiency of the enzyme. Among the reported clinical findings were drug-induced anemias (Carson et al., 1961), congenital hemolytic anemia, pancy-topenia, and thrombomytopenia with a positive Heinz-body test (Lohr and Waller, 1962; Waller et al., 1965). The cause-and-effect relationship in these disorders has not been adequately established. A significant finding in the explanation of these disorders was that glutathione reductase, which is a flavoprotein, is only partially saturated in red blood cells with FAD. Addi-tion of FAD to hemolysates increases the activity of the enzyme. Similar in-creases are obtained by feeding riboflavin, since red blood cells have the capability to synthesize FAD (Beutler, 1973). Thus many of the cases of glutathione reductase deficiency can be attributed to a nutritional ribo-flavin deficiency. The activity of the enzyme in red blood cells is not rate limiting, and a decrease of more than 50% is needed before impairment of glutathione reduction can be demonstrated (Beutler, 1975). It therefore seems that the significance of glutathione reductase deficiency as a cause of hemolytic anemia needs reevaluation.

E. GLUTATHIONE PEROXIDASE DEFICIENCY

A 50% decrease in glutathione peroxidase activity was described in the red blood cells of newborns (Necheles et al., 1968) with hemolysis following exposure to sulfonamides or nitrofurantoin. A presumably homozygous pa-tient having 30% of normal activity was also described. The patient de-veloped an acute hemolytic episode after the infusion of autologous red cells. Numerous cells with Heinz bodies were detected (Necheles et al., 1969). Hemolytic states have been attributed to a deficiency of this enzyme (Necheles et al., 1970), however, a cause-and-effect relationship has not been estab-lished. The clinical importance of common mild deficiencies of this enzyme is not known. Selenium deficiency causes severe induced deficiency of the enzyme (Smith et al., 1974).

In three patients with Glanzmann's thrombastenia markedly reduced activity of glutathione peroxidase was reported in the platelets (Karpatkin and Weiss, 1972). In two of these patients a twofold increase in glutathione was found. The relationship of these abnormalities to the defect in the function of the platelets of the patients remains to be determined.

VII. Conclusions

A considerable body of new information has been accumulated concerning the metabolism of glutathione in the nervous system. The enzymes of the γ-glutamyl cycle, which control the synthesis and degradation of glutathione, have all been found in the CNS. The presence of intermediates of the cycle (e.g., glutathione, γ-glutamyl amino acids, and pyrrolidone carboxylate) indicate that the cycle functions in the brain. Similarly, the brain contains the enzymes that catalyze reactions in which the sulfhydryl group of glutathione is involved. The significance of glutathione in brain function is suggested by the finding of mental retardation in a patient with pyroglutamic aciduria and in another patient believed to have a deficiency of γ-glutamyl transpeptidase. Evidence of central nervous disease, including signs of spinocerebellar degeneration, has also been found in two patients with a γ-glutamylcysteine synthetase deficiency.

There is good evidence that glutathione is needed for maintaining both the integrity of cell membranes and the thiol-disulfide status of cells. A reduction in glutathione concentration in red blood cells renders these cells vulnerable to hemolysis, especially when subjected to oxidation stress. Other cells are probably also affected under such conditions.

There are indications that glutathione also functions in transport processes, through involvement of the γ-glutamyl group or the sulfhydryl group or both. Amino aciduria was described in patients with a γ-glutamylcysteine synthetase deficiency and in experiments with rats after administration of maleic acid. Reagents that block sulfhydryl groups of membranes, including heavy metals, generally inhibit transport of amino acids in tissue slices and also across the blood-brain barrier (Steinwall, 1968). The *in vivo* administration of sulfhydryl-blocking agents causes amino aciduria. Diamide, which oxidizes intracellular glutathione, inhibits the uptake of amino acids by kidney cortex slices (Hewitt *et al.*, 1974).

The mechanisms by which glutathione affects transport are not yet sufficiently understood. Part of this glutathione function may be mediated through the γ-glutamyl transpeptidase reaction. The role of this enzyme in transport processes needs further exploration. The topography of the enzyme in the cell membrane and the directionality of its function should be investigated. It is conceivable that the enzyme performs a secretory function for amino acids. Such a function would be consistent with the localization of the enzyme in glandular epithelia, where secretion occurs. The specificity of the γ-glutamyl transpeptidase reaction under conditions similar to those that exist *in vivo* also requires exploration. The concentration of this enzyme in the choroid plexus and in brain capillaries suggests that its function in the nervous system is limited to these sites. The finding, however, of the enzyme in some groups of neurons in the brainstem suggests that the enzyme has significance in some neuronal functions.

REFERENCES

Adamson, E. D., Szewczuk, A., and Connell, G. E. (1971). *Can. J. Biochem.* **49**, 218.
Agrawal, H. C., Davis, J. M., and Himwich, W. A. (1966). *J. Neurochem.* **13**, 607.
Albert, Z., Orlowski, M., and Szewczuk, A. (1961). *Nature (London)* **191**, 767.
Albert, Z., Orlowska, J., Orlowski, M., and Szewczuk, A. (1964). *Acta Histochem.* **18**, 78.
Albert, Z., Orlowski, M., Rzucidlo, Z., and Orlowska, J. (1966). *Acta Histochem.* **25**, 312.
Alevizos, B., Vassilopoulos, D., Spengos, M., and Stefanis, C. (1975). *Br. Med. J.* **2**, 443.
Al-Kassab, S., Boyland, E., and Williams, K. (1963). *Biochem. J.* **87**, 4.
Angielski, S., Niemiro, R., Makarewicz, W., and Rogulski, J. (1958). *Acta Biochim. Pol.* **5**, 396.
Ansorage, S., Bohley, P., Kirschke, H., Langner, J., Marquardt, I., Wiederanders, B., and Hanson, H. (1973). *FEBS Lett.* **37**, 238.
Askelof, P., Axelsson, K., Eriksson, S., and Mannervik, B. (1974). *FEBS Lett.* **38**, 263.
Ball, E. G., Cooper, O., and Clarke, E. C. (1953). *Biol. Bull.* **105**, 369.
Battistin, L., Grynbaum, A., and Lajtha, A. (1971). *Brain Res.* **29**, 85.
Beck, W. S. (1958). *J. Biol. Chem.* **232**, 271.
Bentley, E., McDermott, E. E., Moran, T., Pace, J., and Whitehead, J. K. (1950). *Proc. R. Soc. London, Ser. B* **137**, 402.
Berl, S., and Purpura, D. P. (1963). *J. Neurochem.* **10**, 237.
Berl, S., and Purpura, D. P. (1966). *J. Neurochem.* **13**, 293.
Berl, S., Lajtha, A., and Waelsch, H. (1961). *J. Neurochem.* **7**, 186.
Berl, S., Purpura, D. P., Girado, M., and Waelsch, H. (1959). *J. Neurochem.* **4**, 311.
Beutler, E. (1973). *Hoppe-Seyler's Z. Physiol. Chem.* **354**, 830.
Beutler, E. (1975). *Life Sci.* **16**, 1499.
Beutler, E., and Yeh, M. K. Y. (1963). *Blood* **21**, 573.
Binkley, F. (1951). *Nature (London)* **167**, 888.
Binkley, F. (1961). *J. Biol. Chem.* **236**, 1075.
Binkley, F., and Nakamura, K. (1948). *J. Biol. Chem.* **173**, 411.
Black, S. (1963). *Annu. Rev. Biochem.* **32**, 399.
Blasberg, R., and Lajtha, A. (1966). *Brain Res.* **1**, 86.
Bloch, K. (1949). *J. Biol. Chem.* **179**, 1245.
Bodnaryk, R. P. (1974). *Insect Biochem.* **4**, 439.
Bodnaryk, R. P., Bronskill, J. F., and Fetterly, J. R. (1974). *J. Insect. Physiol.* **20**, 167.
Booth, J., Boyland, E., and Sims, P. (1960). *Biochem. J.* **74**, 117.
Booth, J., Boyland, E., and Sims, P. (1961). *Biochem. J.* **79**, 516.
Boyland, E. (1971). *Handb. Exp. Pharmakol.* **28**, 585.
Boyland, E., and Chasseaud, L. F. (1967). *Biochem. J.* **104**, 95.
Boyland, E., and Chasseaud, L. F. (1968). *Biochem. J.* **109**, 651.

114   MARIAN ORLOWSKI, AND ABRAHAM KARKOWSKY

Boyland, E., and Chasseaud, L. F. (1969). *Adv. Enzymol.* 32, 173.
Boyland, E., and Williams, K. (1965). *Biochem. J.* 94, 190.
Boyne, A. F., and Ellman, G. L. (1972). *Anal. Biochem.* 46, 639.
Braunstein, A. E., Shamshikova, G. A., and Ioffe, A. L. (1948). *Biokhimiya* 13, 95.
Buchanan, D. L., Haley, E. E., and Markiw, R. T. (1962). *Biochemistry* 1, 612.
Carson, P. E., Brewer, G. J., and Ickes, C. E. (1961). *J. Lab. Clin. Med.* 58, 804.
Chandler, M. L., and Varandani, P. T. (1972). *Biochim. Biophys. Acta* 286, 136.
Chandler, M. L., and Varandani, P. T. (1973). *Biochim. Biophys. Acta* 320, 258.
Chang, S. H., and Wilken, D. R. (1966). *J. Biol. Chem.* 241, 4251.
Chasseaud, L. F. (1973). *Drug Metab. Rev.* 2, 185.
Chirigos, M. A., Greengard, P., and Udenfriend, S. (1960). *J. Biol. Chem.* 235, 2075.
Christensen, H. N., Aspen, A. J., and Rice, E. G. (1956). *J. Biol. Chem.* 220, 287.
Christophersen, B. O. (1966). *Biochem. J.* 100, 95.
Cliffe, E. E., and Waley, S. G. (1958). *Biochem. J.* 69, 649.
Cliffe, E. E., and Waley, S. G. (1961). *Biochem. J.* 79, 118.
Cohen, G., and Hochstein, P. (1963). *Biochemistry* 2, 1420.
Colowick, S., Lazarow, A., Racker, E., Schwarz, D. R., Stadtman, E., and Waelsch, H., eds., (1954). "Glutathione." Academic Press, New York.
Combes, B., and Stakelum, G. S. (1961). *J. Clin. Invest.* 40, 981.
Connell, G. E., and Hanes, C. S. (1956). *Nature (London)* 177, 377.
Crook, E. M., ed. (1959). "Glutathione." Cambridge Univ. Press, London and New York.
Crook, E. M., and Law, K. (1950). *Biochem. J.* 46, XXXVII.
Csaky, T. Z., and Rigor, B. M. (1968). *Prog. Brain Res.* 29, 147.
Curthoys, N. P., and Kuhlenschmidt, T. (1975). *J. Biol. Chem.* 250, 2099.
Curtis, D. R., and Watkins, J. C. (1965). *Pharmacol. Rev.* 17, 343.
Dakin, H. D., and Dudley, H. W. (1913a). *J. Biol. Chem.* 14, 155.
Dakin, H. D., and Dudley, H. W. (1913b). *J. Biol. Chem.* 15, 463.
Davidson, B. E., and Hird, F. J. R. (1964). *Biochem. J.* 93, 232.
De Lorenzo, F., and Molea, G. (1967). *Biochim. Biophys. Acta* 146, 593.
De Lorenzo, F., Goldberger, R. F., Steers, E., Givol, D., and Anfinsen, C. B. (1966). *J. Biol. Chem.* 241, 1562.
De Marchena, O., Guarnieri, M., and McKhann, G. (1974). *J. Neurochem.* 22, 773.
de Rey-Pailhade, J. (1888a). *C. R. Hebd. Seances Acad. Sci.* 106, 1683.
de Rey-Pailhade, J. (1888b). *C. R. Hebd. Seances Acad. Sci.* 107, 43.
De Robertis, E., Sellinger, O. Z., De Lores Arnaiz, G. R., Alberici, M., and Zieher, L. M. (1967). *J. Neurochem.* 14, 81.
De Ropp, R. S., and Snedeker, E. H. (1961). *J. Neurochem.* 7, 128.
Dimant, E., Landsberg, E., and London, I. M. (1955). *J. Biol. Chem.* 213, 769.
DiNamarca, M. L., Saavedra, I., and Valdés, E. (1969). *Comp. Biochem. Physiol.* 31, 269.
DiNamarca, M. L., Levenbook, L., and Valdés, E. (1971). *Arch. Biochem. Biophys.* 147, 374.
Douglas, G. W., and Mortensen, R. A. (1956). *J. Biol. Chem.* 222, 581.
Edwards, S. W., and Knox, W. E. (1956). *J. Biol. Chem.* 220, 79.
Eldjarn, L., Jellum, E., and Stokke, O. (1972). *Clin. Chim. Acta* 40, 461.
Eldjarn, L., Jellum, E., and Stokke, O. (1973). *Clin. Chim. Acta* 49, 311.
Eriksson, S., Guthenberg, C., and Mannervik, B. (1974). *FEBS Lett.* 39, 296.
Ewen, L. M., and Griffiths, J. (1971). *Clin. Chem.* 17, 642.
Ewen, L. M., and Griffiths, J. (1973). *Am. J. Clin. Pathol.* 59, 2.

Fjellstedt, T. A., Allen, R. H., Duncan, B. K., and Jakoby, W. B. (1973). *J. Biol. Chem.* **248**, 3702.

Flohe, L., Eisele, B., and Wendel, A. (1971a). *Hoppe-Seyler's Z. Physiol. Chem.* **352**, 151.

Flohe, L., Gunzler, W., Jung, G., Schaich, E., and Schneider, F. (1971b). *Hoppe-Seyler's Z. Physiol. Chem.* **352**, 159.

Flohe, L., Schaich, E., Voelter, W., and Wendel, A. (1971c). *Hoppe-Seyler's Z. Physiol. Chem.* **352**, 170.

Flohe, L., Gunzler, W. A., and Schock, H. H. (1973). *FEBS Lett.* **32**, 132.

Flohe, L., Benohr, H. C., Sies, H., Waller, H. D., and Wendel, A., eds. (1974). "Glutathione." Thieme, Stuttgart.

Fodor, J. P., Miller, A., and Waelsch, H. (1953). *J. Biol. Chem.* **202**, 551.

Folbergova, J. (1963). *J. Neurochem.* **10**, 775.

Fuchs, S., De Lorenzo, F., and Anfinsen, C. B. (1967). *J. Biol. Chem.* **242**, 398.

Garfinkel, D. (1962). *J. Theor. Biol.* **3**, 412.

Garfinkel, D. (1966). *J. Biol. Chem.* **241**, 3918.

Geiger, A. (1935). *Biochem. J.* **29**, 811.

Gibinski, K., Nowak, A., and Kochanska, D. (1967). *Gastroenterologia* **108**, 219.

Glenner, G. G., and Folk, J. E. (1961). *Nature (London)* **192**, 338.

Glenner, G. G., Folk, J. E., and McMillan, P. J. (1962). *J. Histochem. Cytochem.* **10**, 481.

Goldbarg, J. A., Friedman, D. M., Pineda, E. P., Smith, E. E., Chatterji, R., Stein, E. H., and Rutenburg, A. M. (1960). *Arch. Biochem. Biophys.* **91**, 61.

Goodman, J. I., and Tephly, T. R. (1971). *Biochim. Biophys. Acta* **252**, 489.

Goodman, S. I., Mace, J. W., and Pollak, S. (1971). *Lancet* **1**, 234.

Green, M. L., and Elliott, W. H. (1964). *Biochem. J.* **92**, 537.

Greenberg, E., Wollaeger, E. E., Fleisher, G. A., and Engstrom, G. V. (1967). *Clin. Chim. Acta* **16**, 79.

Habig, W. H., Pabst, M. J., and Jakoby, W. B. (1974a). *J. Biol. Chem.* **249**, 7130.

Habig, W. H., Pabst, M. J., Fleischner, G., Gatmaitan, Z., Arias, I. M., and Jakoby, W. B. (1974b). *Proc. Natl. Acad. Sci. U.S.A.* **71**, 3879.

Hagenfeldt, L., Larsson, A., and Zetterström, R. (1974). *Acta Paediatr. Scand.* **63**, 1.

Hais, I. M., Chmelar, V., Stransky, Z., and Tomana, M. (1965). *Bull. Inst. Int. Froid, Annexe* **4**, 627.

Hanes, C. S., Hird, F. J. R., and Isherwood, F. A. (1950). *Nature (London)* **166**, 288.

Hanes, C. S., Hird, F. J. R., and Isherwood, F. A. (1952). *Biochem. J.* **51**, 25.

Harrison, H., and Harrison, H. (1954). *Science* **120**, 606.

Haugaard, N. (1968). *Physiol. Rev.* **48**, 311.

Hayakawa, T., LeMahieu, R. A., and Udenfriend, S. (1974). *Arch. Biochem. Biophys.* **162**, 223.

Henriques, O. B., Henriques, S. B., and Neuberger, A. (1955). *Biochem. J.* **60**, 409.

Heppel, L. A., and Hilmoe, R. J. (1950). *J. Biol. Chem.* **183**, 129.

Hewitt, J., Pillion, D., and Leibach, F. H. (1974). *Biochim. Acta* **363**, 267.

Hird, F. J. R. (1950). Doctoral Dissertation, Cambridge University, England.

Holmberg, N. J. (1968). *Exp. Eye Res.* **7**, 570.

Hopkins, F. G. (1921). *Biochem. J.* **15**, 286.

Hosoda, S., and Nakamura, W. (1970). *Biochim. Biophys. Acta* **222**, 53.

Hotta, S. S. (1962). *J. Neurochem.* **9**, 43.

Hotta, S. S. (1966). *Arch. Biochem. Biophys.* **113**, 395.

Hotta, S. S. (1967). *Arch. Biochem. Biophys.* **122**, 524.
Hotta, S. S. (1970). *Arch. Biochem. Biophys.* **139**, 200.
Hotta, S. S., and Seventko, J. M. (1968). *Arch. Biochem. Biophys.* **123**, 104.
Icen, A. (1967). *Scand. J. Clin. Lab. Invest., Suppl.* **96**, 1.
Ichio, I. I., and Sakai, H. (1974). *Biochim. Biophys. Acta* **350**, 141.
Jackson, R. C. (1969). *Biochem. J.* **111**, 309.
Jacob, H. S., and Jandl, J. H. (1966). *J. Biol. Chem.* **241**, 4243.
Jellinck, P. H., Lewis, J., and Boston, F. (1967). *Steroids* **10**, 329.
Jellum, E., Kluge, T., Borrensen, H. C., Stokke, O., and Eldjarn, L. (1970). *Scand. J. Clin. Lab. Invest.* **26**, 327.
Jerzykowski, T., Winter, R., and Matuszewski, W. (1973). *Biochem. J.* **135**, 713.
Jocelyn, P. C., ed. (1972). "Biochemistry of the SH Group." Academic Press, New York.
Johnson, M. K. (1966a). *Biochem. J.* **98**, 38.
Johnson, M. K. (1966b). *Biochem. J.* **98**, 44.
Jowett, M., and Quastel, J. H. (1934). *Biochem. J.* **28**, 162.
Kakimoto, Y., Nakajima, T., Kanazawa, A., Takesada, M., and Sano, I. (1964). *Biochim. Biophys. Acta* **93**, 333.
Kakimoto, Y., Kanazawa, A., Nakajima, T., and Sano, I. (1965). *Biochim. Biophys. Acta* **100**, 426.
Kanazawa, A., and Sano, I. (1967). *J. Neurochem.* **14**, 596.
Kanazawa, A., Kakimoto, Y., Nakajima, T., Shimizu, H., Takesada, M., and Sano, I. (1965a). *Biochim. Biophys. Acta* **97**, 460.
Kanazawa, A., Kakimoto, Y., Nakajima, T., and Sano, I. (1965b). *Biochim. Biophys. Acta* **111**, 90.
Kaplan, J. C. (1968). *Nature (London)* **217**, 256.
Kaplowitz, N., Percy-Robb, I. W., and Javitt, N. B. (1973). *J. Exp. Med.* **138**, 483.
Karpatkin, S., and Weiss, H. J. (1972). *N. Engl. J. Med.* **287**, 1062.
Katzen, H. M., and Stetten, D. (1962). *Diabetes* **11**, 271.
Katzen, H. M., and Tietze, F. (1966). *J. Biol. Chem.* **241**, 3561.
Kern, H. L., and Ho, C. K. (1973). *Exp. Eye Res.* **17**, 455.
Kester, M. V., and Norton, S. J. (1975). *Biochim. Biophys. Acta* **391**, 212.
Knox, E. (1960). *In* "The Enzymes" (P. D. Boyer, H. A. Lardy, and K. Myrbäck, eds.), Vol. 2, p. 253. Academic Press, New York.
Kohno, K., Noda, K., Mizobe, M., and Utsumi, I. (1969). *Biochem. Pharmacol.* **18**, 1685.
Kokot, F., and Sledzinski, Z. (1974). *Z. Klin. Chem. Klin. Biochem.* **12**, 374.
Kokot, F., Kuska, J., and Grzybek, H. (1965). *Arch. Immunol. Ther. Exp.* **13**, 549.
Kolousek, J., Horak, F., and Miracek, V. (1959). *J. Neurochem.* **4**, 175.
Konrad, P. N., Richards, F., Valentine, W. N., and Paglia, D. E. (1972). *N. Engl. J. Med.* **286**, 557.
Kosower, E. M., and Kosower, N. S. (1969). *Nature (London)* **224**, 117.
Kosower, E. M., Correa, W., Kinon, B. J., and Kosower, N. S. (1972). *Biochim. Biophys. Acta* **264**, 39.
Kuss, E. (1967). *Hoppe-Seyler's Z. Physiol. Chem.* **348**, 1707.
Lack, L. (1961). *J. Biol. Chem.* **236**, 2835.
Lajtha, A. (1956). *J. Neurochem.* **3**, 358.
Lajtha, A. (1964). *Int. Rev. Neurobiol.* **6**, 1.
Lajtha, A. (1968). *Prog. Brain Res.* **29**, 20.
Lajtha, A., Berl, S., and Waelsch, H. (1959). *J. Neurochem.* **3**, 322.

Lamar, C., and Sellinger, O. (1965). *Biochem. Pharmacol.* **14**, 489.

Larsson, A., Zetterström, R., Hagenfeldt, L., Andersson, R., Dreborg, S., and Hörnell, H. (1974). *Pediat. Res.* **8**, 852.

Lawinski, M., Szacki, J., Grzebieluch, M., and Rzucidlo, Z. (1969). *Arch. Immunol. Ther. Exp.* **17**, 649.

Lawrence, R. A., Sunde, R. A., Schwartz, G. L., and Hoekstra, W. G. (1974). *Exp. Eye Res.* **18**, 563.

Leibach, F. H., and Binkley, F. (1968). *Arch. Biochem. Biophys.* **127**, 292.

Levi, A. J., Gatmaitan, Z., and Arias, I. M. (1969). *J. Clin. Invest.* **48**, 2156.

Libenson, L., and Jena, M. (1967). *Cancer Res.* **27**, 1196.

Lipke, H., and Kearns, C. W. (1959a). *J. Biol. Chem.* **234**, 2123.

Lipke, H., and Kearns, C. W. (1959b). *J. Biol. Chem.* **234**, 2129.

Little, C., and O'Brien, P. J. (1968). *Biochem. Biophys. Res. Commun.* **31**, 145.

Litwack, G., Ketterer, B., and Arias, I. M. (1971). *Nature (London)* **234**, 466.

Lohr, G. W., and Waller, H. D. (1962). *Med. Klin.* **57**, 1521.

Lorenzo, A. V., and Cutler, R. W. P. (1969). *J. Neurochem.* **16**, 577.

McIlwain, H., and Tresize, M. A. (1957). *Biochem. J.* **65**, 288.

McKean, C. M., Boggs, D. E., and Peterson, N. A. (1968). *J. Neurochem.* **15**, 235.

Majerus, P. W., Branner, M. J., Smith, M. B., and Minnich, V. (1971). *J. Clin. Invest.* **50**, 1637.

Mandeles, S., and Bloch, K. (1955). *J. Biol. Chem.* **214**, 639.

Mannervik, B., Lindström, L., and Bártfai, T. (1972). *Eur. J. Biochem.* **29**, 276.

Mannervik, B., Persson, G., and Eriksson, S. (1974). *Arch. Biochem. Biophys.* **163**, 283.

Marks, N. (1970). *Handb. Neurochem.* **3**, 133–171.

Martin, H., and McIlwain, H. (1959). *Biochem. J.* **71**, 275.

Matthews, D. M. (1972). *Pept. Transp. Bact. Mamm. Gut, Ciba Found. Symp., 1971* pp. 71–92.

Meister, A. (1973). *Science* **180**, 33.

Meister, A. (1974a). *In* "The Enzymes" (P. D. Boyer, ed.), 3rd ed., Vol. 10, pp. 671–698. Academic Press, New York.

Meister, A. (1974b). *Ann. Intern. Med.* **81**, 247.

Meister, A. (1974c). *Life Sci.* **15**, 177.

Mellanby, E. (1946). *Br. Med. J.* **2**, 885.

Metz, E. N., Balcerzak, S. P., and Sagone, A. L. (1974). *Blood* **44**, 691.

Mills, G. C. (1957). *J. Biol. Chem.* **229**, 189.

Mills, G. C. (1959). *J. Biol. Chem.* **234**, 502.

Mills, G. C. (1960). *Arch. Biochem. Biophys.* **86**, 1.

Minard, F. N., and Mushahwar, I. K. (1966). *J. Neurochem.* **13**, 1.

Minnich, V., Smith, M. B., Brauner, M. J., and Majerus, P. W. (1971). *J. Clin. Invest.* **50**, 507.

Mize, C. E., and Langdon, R. G. (1962). *J. Biol. Chem.* **237**, 1589.

Mohler, D. N., Majerus, P. W., Minnich, V., Hess, C. E., and Garrick, M. D. (1970). *N. Engl. J. Med.* **283**, 1253.

Mooz, E. D., and Meister, A. (1967). *Biochemistry* **6**, 1722.

Mooz, E. D., and Meister, A. (1971). *In* "Methods in Enzymology" (H. Tabor and C. W. Tabor, eds.), Vol. 17B, p. 483. Academic Press, New York.

Moran, T. (1947). *Lancet* **2**, 289.

Nakamura, W., Hosoda, S., and Hayashi, K. (1974). *Biochem. Biophys. Acta* **358**, 251.

118   MARIAN ORLOWSKI AND ABRAHAM KARKOWSKY

Necheles, T. F., Boles, T. A., and Allen, D. M. (1968). *J. Pediatr.* **72**, 319.
Necheles, T. F., Maldonado, N., Barquet-Chediak, A., and Allen, D. M. (1969). *Blood* **33**, 164.
Necheles, T. F., Steinberg, M. H., and Cameron, D. (1970). *Br. J. Haematol.* **19**, 605.
Neuberg, C. (1913). *Biochem. Z.* **49**, 502.
Neubert, D., Wojtczak, A. B., and Lehninger, A. L. (1962). *Proc. Natl. Acad. Sci. U.S.A.* **48**, 1651.
Oh, S. H., Ganther, H. E., and Hoekstra, W. G. (1974). *Biochemistry* **13**, 1825.
Ohkawa, H., and Casida, J. E., (1971). *Biochem. Pharmacol.* **20**, 1708.
Okonkwo, P. O., Orlowski, M., and Green, J. P. (1974). *J. Neurochem.* **22**, 1053.
Oldendorf, W. H. (1973). *Am. J. Physiol.* **224**, 967.
Ondarza, R. N., and Martinez, J. (1966). *Biochim. Biophys. Acta* **113**, 409.
Ondarza, R. N., Escamilla, E., Guttiérrez, J., and De la Chica, G. (1974). *Biochim. Biophys. Acta* **341**, 162.
O'Neal, R. M., and Koeppe, R. E. (1966). *J. Neurochem.* **13**, 835.
Orlowski, M. (1963). *Arch. Immunol. Ther. Exp.* **11**, 1.
Orlowski, M., and Meister, A. (1963). *Biochim. Biophys. Acta* **73**, 679.
Orlowski, M., and Meister, A. (1965). *J. Biol. Chem.* **240**, 338.
Orlowski, M., and Meister, A. (1970a). *Proc. Natl. Acad. Sci. U.S.A.* **67**, 1248.
Orlowski, M., and Meister, A. (1970b). In "Methods in Enzymology" (H. Tabor and C. W. Tabor, eds.), Vol. 17A, p. 863. Academic Press, New York.
Orlowski, M., Meister, A. (1971a). *Biochemistry* **10**, 372.
Orlowski, M., and Meister, A. (1971b). In "Methods in Enzymology" (H. Tabor and C. W. Tabor, eds.), Vol. 17B, p. 495. Academic Press, New York.
Orlowski, M., and Meister, A. (1971c). *J. Biol. Chem.* **246**, 7095.
Orlowski, M., and Meister, A. (1971d). In "The Enzymes" (P. D. Boyer, ed.), 3rd ed., Vol. 4, p. 123. Academic Press, New York.
Orlowski, M., and Meister, A. (1973). *J. Biol. Chem.* **248**, 2836.
Orlowski, M., and Szewczuk, A. (1961). *Acta Biochim. Pol.* **8**, 189.
Orlowski, M., and Szewczuk, A. (1962). *Clin. Chim. Acta* **7**, 755.
Orlowski, M., and Wilk, S. (1975a). *J. Neurochem.* **25**, 601.
Orlowski, M., and Wilk, S. (1975b). *Eur. J. Biochem.* **53**, 581.
Orlowski, M., Richman, P. G., and Meister, A. (1969). *Biochemistry* **8**, 1048.
Orlowski, M., Okonkwo, P. D., and Green, J. P. (1973). *FEBS Lett.* **31**, 237.
Orlowski, M., Sessa, G., and Green, J. P. (1974). *Science* **184**, 66.
Pabst, M. J., Habig, W. H., and Jakoby, W. B. (1974). *J. Biol. Chem.* **249**, 7140.
Pace, J., and McDermott, E. E. (1952). *Nature (London)* **169**, 415.
Peters, E., and Tower, D. B. (1959). *J. Neurochem.* **5**, 80.
Pisano, J. L. (1969). *Handb. Neurochem.* **1**, 53.
Prins, H. K., Oort, M., Loos, J. A., Zurcher, C., and Beckers, T. (1966). *Blood* **27**, 145.
Purpura, D. P., Berl, S., Gonzales-Monteagudo, O., and Wyatt, A. (1960). In "Inhibition in the Nervous System and Gamma-Aminobutyric Acid" (E. Roberts, ed.), p. 331. Macmillan, New York.
Racker, E. (1951). *J. Biol. Chem.* **190**, 685.
Racker, E. (1953). *Fed. Proc., Fed. Am. Soc. Exp. Biol.* **12**, 711.
Racker, E. (1955). *J. Biol. Chem.* **217**, 867.
Rall, T. W., and Lehninger, A. L. (1952). *J. Biol. Chem.* **194**, 119.

Ramakrishna, M., Krishnaswamy, P. R., and Rao, R. D. (1970). *Biochem. J.* **118**, 895.

Rathbun, W. (1967). *Arch. Biochem. Biophys.* **122**, 62.

Ray, L. E., and Prescott, J. M. (1975). *Proc. Soc. Exp. Biol. Med.* **148**, 402.

Reddy, V. N., and Unakar, N. J. (1973). *Exp. Eye Res.* **17**, 405.

Reed, P. W. (1969). *J. Biol. Chem.* **244**, 2459.

Reichelt, K. L. (1970). *J. Neurochem.* **17**, 19.

Reichelt, K. L., and Fonnum, F. (1969). *J. Neurochem.* **16**, 1409.

Revel, J. P., and Ball, E. G. (1959). *J. Biol. Chem.* **234**, 577.

Richards, F., Cooper, M. R., Pearce, L. A., Cowan, R. J., and Spurr, C. L. (1974). *Arch. Intern. Med.* **134**, 534.

Richman, P. G. (1975). Ph.D. Dissertation, Cornell University, Ithaca, New York.

Richman, P. G., and Meister, A. (1975). *J. Biol. Chem.* **250**, 1422.

Richman, P. G., Orlowski, M., and Meister, A. (1973). *J. Biol. Chem.* **248**, 6684.

Richter, J. J., and Wainer, A. (1971). *J. Neurochem.* **18**, 613.

Richter, R. (1969). *Arch. Immunol. Ther. Exp.* **17**, 476.

Roberts, E., ed. (1960). "Inhibition in the Nervous System and Gamma-Aminobutyric Acid." Pergamon, Oxford.

Roberts, S., and Morelos, B. S. (1965). *J. Neurochem.* **12**, 373.

Romano, A. H., and Nickerson, W. J. (1954). *J. Biol. Chem.* **208**, 409.

Ronzio, R. A., and Meister, A. (1968). *Proc. Natl. Acad. Sci. U.S.A.* **59**, 164.

Ronzio, R. A., Rowe, B. W., and Meister, A. (1969). *Biochemistry* **8**, 1066.

Rosalki, S. B. (1975). *Adv. Clin. Chem.* **17**, 53–107.

Rosalki, S. B., Tarlow, D., and Rau, D. (1971). *Lancet* **2**, 376.

Rosenberg, L. E., and Segal, S. (1964). *Biochem. J.* **92**, 345.

Ross, L. L., Barber, L., Tate, S. S., and Meister, A. (1973). *Proc. Natl. Acad. Sci. U.S.A.* **70**, 2211.

Rush, E. A., and Starr, J. L. (1970). *Biochim. Biophys. Acta* **199**, 41.

Rutenburg, A. M., Kim, H., Fischbein, J. W., Hanker, J. S., Wasserkrug, H. L., and Seligman, A. M. (1969). *J. Histochem. Cytochem.* **17**, 517.

Sanders, A. P., Currie, W. D., and Woodhall, B. (1969). *Proc. Soc. Exp. Biol. Med.* **130**, 1021.

Sano, I. (1970). *Int. Rev. Neurobiol.* **12**, 235.

Sano, I., Kakimoto, Y., Kanazawa, A., Nakajima, T., and Shimizu, H. (1966). *J. Neurochem.* **13**, 711.

Sass, M. D. (1968). *Clin. Chim. Acta* **22**, 207.

Schroeder, E. F., Munro, M. P., and Weil, L. (1935). *J. Biol. Chem.* **110**, 181.

Scott, E. M., Duncan, I. W., and Ekstrand, V. (1963). *J. Biol. Chem.* **238**, 3928.

Sekura, R., and Meister, A. (1974). *Proc. Natl. Acad. Sci. U.S.A.* **71**, 2969.

Seltzer, S. (1972). *In* "The Enzymes" (P. D. Boyer, ed.), 3rd ed., Vol. 6, p. 381. Academic Press, New York.

Semenza, G. (1957). *Biochim. Biophys. Acta* **24**, 401.

Sies, H. (1973). *Hoppe-Seyler's Z. Physiol. Chem.* **354**, 837.

Small, C. W., and Watkins, W. B. (1974). *Nature (London)* **251**, 237.

Smith, J. E. (1971). *Biochim. Biophys. Acta* **242**, 36.

Smith, P. J., Tappel, A. L., and Chow, C. K. (1974). *Nature (London)* **247**, 392.

Smyth, D. H. (1972). *Pept. Transp. Bact. Mamm. Gut, Ciba Found. Symp., 1971* pp. 59–70.

Snoke, J. E. (1955). *J. Biol. Chem.* **213**, 813.

Snoke, J. E., and Bloch, K. (1952). *J. Biol. Chem.* **199**, 407.

120   MARIAN ORLOWSKI AND ABRAHAM KARKOWSKY

Snoke, J. E., and Bloch, K. (1955). *J. Biol. Chem.* **213**, 825.
Srivastava, S. K. (1971). *Exp. Eye Res.* **11**, 294.
Srivastava, S. K., and Beutler, E. (1969). *J. Biol. Chem.* **244**, 9.
Srivastava, S. K., and Beutler, E. (1970). *Biochem. J.* **119**, 353.
Staal, G. E. J., Visser, J., and Veeger, C. (1969). *Biochim. Biophys. Acta* **185**, 39.
Stark, M. J., Thompson, B., and Frenkel, R. (1975). *Arch. Biochem. Biophys.* **166**, 174.
States, B., and Segal, S. (1969). *Biochem. J.* **113**, 443.
Steinwall, O. (1968). *Prog. Brain Res.* **29**, 357.
Sternburg, J. G., Vinson, E., and Kearns, C. W. (1954). *J. Econ. Entomol.* **46**, 513.
Strittmatter, P., and Ball, E. G. (1955). *J. Biol. Chem.* **213**, 445.
Stromme, J. H., and Eldjarn, L. (1972). *Scand. J. Clin. Lab. Invest.* **29**, 335.
Strumeyer, D. H. (1959). Ph.D. Dissertation, Harvard University, Cambridge, Massachusetts.
Suga, T., Ohata, I., Kumaoka, H., and Akagi, M. (1967). *Chem. Pharm. Bull.* **15**, 1059.
Swinnen, J. (1967). *Clin. Chim. Acta* **17**, 255.
Szent-Györgyi, A., Egyud, L. G., and McLaughlin, J. A. (1967). *Science* **155**, 539.
Szewczuk, A., and Baranowski, T. (1963). *Biochem. Z.* **338**, 317.
Szewczuk, A., and Connell, G. E. (1965). *Biochim. Biophys. Acta* **105**, 352.
Szewczuk, A., and Orlowski, M. (1960). *Clin. Chim. Acta* **5**, 680.
Takahashi, Y., and Akabane, Y. (1961). *J. Neurochem.* **7**, 89.
Taniguchi, N. (1974). *J. Biochem. (Tokyo)* **75**, 473.
Tappel, A. L. (1974). *Am. J. Clin. Nutr.* **27**, 960.
Tarantino, L. M., and Hotta, S. S. (1974). *Proc. Soc. Exp. Biol. Med.* **147**, 887.
Tate, S. S., and Meister, A. (1974a). *J. Biol. Chem.* **249**, 7593.
Tate, S. S., and Meister, A. (1974b). *Proc. Natl. Acad. Sci. U.S.A.* **71**, 3329.
Tate, S. S., and Meister, A. (1975). *J. Biol. Chem.* **250**, 4619.
Tate, S. S., Ross, L. L., and Meister, A. (1973). *Proc. Natl. Acad. Sci. U.S.A.* **70**, 1447.
Tews, J. K., Carter, S. H., Roa, P. D., and Stone, W. E. (1963). *J. Neurochem.* **10**, 641.
Tietze, F. (1969). *Anal. Biochem.* **27**, 502.
Tietze, F., (1970a). *Arch. Biochem. Biophys.* **138**, 177.
Tietze, F. (1970b). *Biochim. Biophys. Acta* **220**, 449.
Tietze, F., Bradley, K. H., and Schulman, J. D. (1972). *Pediatr. Res.* **6**, 649.
Tomizawa, H. H. (1962). *J. Biol. Chem.* **237**, 428.
Ugolev, A. M. (1972). *Pept. Transp. Bact. Mamm. Gut Ciba Found. Symp., 1971* pp. 123–143.
Uotila, L. (1975). *Biochemistry* **12**, 3944.
Uotila, L., and Koivusalo, M. (1974a). *J. Biol. Chem.* **249**, 7653.
Uotila, L., and Koivusalo, M. (1974b). *J. Biol. Chem.* **249**, 7664.
Uotila, L., and Koivusalo, M. (1975). *Eur. J. Biochem.* **52**, 493.
Vander Jagt, D. L., and Han, L. P. B. (1973). *Biochemistry* **12**, 5161.
Vander Jagt, D. L., Han, L. P. B., and Lehman, C. H. (1972). *Biochemistry* **11**, 3735.
Van Der Werf, P., Orlowski, M., and Meister, A. (1971). *Proc. Natl. Acad. Sci. U.S.A.* **68**, 2982.
Van Der Werf, P., Stephani, R. A., Orlowski, M., and Meister, A. (1973). *Proc. Natl. Acad. Sci. U.S.A.* **70**, 759.

Van Der Werf, P., Stephani, R. A., and Meister, A. (1974). *Proc. Natl. Acad. Sci. U.S.A.* **71,** 1026.

Varandani, P. T. (1973). *Biochim. Biophys. Acta* **304,** 642.

Varandani, P. T., and Nafz, M. A. (1974). *Biochim. Biophys. Acta* **371,** 577.

Varma, R. R., Khuteta, K. P., and Dandiya, P. C. (1968). *Psychopharmacologia* **12,** 170.

Waelsch, H., and Rittenberg, D. (1942). *J. Biol. Chem.* **144,** 53.

Waley, S. G. (1956). *Biochem. J.* **64,** 715.

Waley, S. G. (1957). *Biochem. J.* **67,** 172.

Waley, S. G. (1958). *Biochem J.* **68,** 189.

Waley, S. G. (1966). *Adv. Protein Chem.* **21,** 2.

Waller, H. D., Lohr, G. W., Zysno, E., Gerok, W., Voss, D., and Strauss, G. (1965). *Klin. Wochenschr.* **43,** 413.

Wellner, V. P., Sekura, R., Meister, A., and Larsson, A. (1974). *Proc. Natl. Acad. Sci. U.S.A.* **71,** 2505.

Wendel, A., Schaich, E., Weber, U., Flohe, L. (1972). *Hoppe-Seyler's Z. Physiol. Chem.* **353,** 514.

Wendel, A., Heinle, A., and Wiest, E. (1975a). *Hoppe-Seyler's Z. Physiol. Chem.* **356,** 867.

Wendel, A., Flugge, U. I., and Jenke, H. S. (1975b). *Hoppe-Seyler's Z. Physiol. Chem.* **356,** 881.

Wendel, A., Pilz, W., Ladenstein, R., Sawatzki, G., and Weser, U. (1975c). *Biochim. Biophys. Acta* **377,** 211.

Wendell, P. L. (1968). *Biochim. Biophys. Acta* **159,** 179.

Werman, R., Carlen, P. L., Kushnir, M., and Kosower, E. M. (1971). *Nature (London) New Biol.* **233,** 120.

Wilk, S., and Orlowski, M. (1973). *FEBS Lett.* **33,** 157.

Williams, C. D., and Haugaard, N. (1970). *J. Neurochem.* **17,** 709.

Wood, J. L. (1970). *Metab. Conjugation Metab. Hydrolysis* **2,** 261.

Woodward, G. E., and Reinhart, F. E. (1942). *J. Biol. Chem.* **145,** 471.

Woodward, G. E., Munro, M. P., and Schroeder, E. F. (1935). *J. Biol. Chem.* **109,** 11.

Worthington, D. J., and Rosemeyer, M. A. (1974). *Eur. J. Biochem.* **48,** 167.

Zelazo, P., and Orlowski, M. (1975). *Eur. J. Biochem.* **53,** 581.

NEUROCHEMICAL CONSEQUENCES OF ETHANOL ON THE NERVOUS SYSTEM

By Arun K. Rawat

Departments of Psychiatry and Biochemistry
Medical College of Ohio, Toledo, Ohio

123

124 ARUN K. RAWAT

I. Introduction

The central nervous system (CNS) is highly sensitive to the pharmacological effects of a wide variety of drugs including ethanol and its metabolic product acetaldehyde. Ethanol is a primary and continuous depressant of the CNS and reversibly inhibits a variety of cellular functions. In general, the effects of ethanol are proportional to its concentration in the blood and are very marked and dramatic on the CNS in spite of the fact that the liver is the principal organ of ethanol metabolism in the body.

A significant increase in the number of persons abusing ethanol has faced basic and clinical scientists with the problem of understanding the fundamental action of ethanol on biochemical processes. Although considerable effort was devoted in the past to understanding the metabolic consequences of ethanol in the liver, as reviewed elsewhere (Rawat, 1969a, 1973), relatively few attempts were made to demonstrate the mechanism of ethanol action on the CNS. However, from investigations made so far on the CNS a picture is emerging which indicates that the familiar changes in behavior observed during ethanol intoxication and during ethanol withdrawal periods are reflections of biochemical and biophysical changes in the CNS (Rawat, 1975a).

This article deals with the biochemical and biophysical effects of ethanol on the CNS.

II. Possible Metabolism of Ethanol in the Brain

An indication of the ability of brain tissue to oxidize ethanol was given in some early *in vivo* studies made by Himwich *et al.* (1933), which showed that the respiratory quotient of the cerebral cortex fell after ethanol administration. In subsequent studies, Dewan (1943) observed that brain slices from several species including ox, dog, cat, cow, and pig formed acetaldehyde and acetate from added ethanol. It was further shown that the oxidation of ethanol required nicotinamide-adenine dinucleotide (NAD). Furthermore, studies with [¹⁴C]ethanol showed the production of $^{14}CO_2$ on incubation with brain slices (Sutherland *et al.*, 1958). However, most efforts to demonstrate ethanol utilization by cerebral tissue or the existence of alcohol dehydrogenase (ADH: alcohol NAD oxidoreductase; EC 1.1.1.1) in the brain were unsuccessful (Beer and Quastel, 1958; Towne, 1964) and, until recently, it was believed that brain tissue is incapable of oxidizing ethanol (Wallgren, 1966). Since the most dramatic pharmacological actions of ethanol are observed on the CNS, there have been several investigations of the activity of alcohol-oxidizing systems in the brain.

A. ALCOHOL DEHYDROGENASE

Since much of the information regarding the mechanism of action and kinetics of a alcohol oxidation has come from studies on liver ADH (Sund and Theorell, 1963), this kinetic information has been put to use recently to ascertain whether or not small amounts of ADH are present in the brain. For the studies on liver, NADH formation was used as a parameter for ethanol oxidation. However, the measurement of NADH formation in the brain to determine ethanol oxidation by ADH, especially by unpurified preparations of brain tissue, is inherently difficult, if not impossible. One specific problem is the high rate of production and utilization of endogenous NADH by other dehydrogenases in the brain. Employing a more sensitive assay system, Raskin and Sokoloff (1968, 1970) demonstrated the capacity of brain tissue to oxidize ethanol and showed that the reaction is catalyzed by ADH. The activity of ADH in the brain can be assayed on the basis of ADH-catalyzed, coupled oxidation of ethanol to acetaldehyde and propanediol (Gupta and Robinson, 1960).

$$\text{Ethanol} + \text{L-lactaldehyde} \xrightleftharpoons{\text{ADH}+\text{NAD}} \text{2-propanediol} + \text{acetaldehyde}$$

ADH from the brain has been isolated, and its kinetics studied. Several kinetic properties, pH optimum, and the response to pyrazole of this enzyme are similar to those of liver ADH. However, it cannot be overemphasized that the activity of ADH in the brain is very low as compared to that in the liver. In fact the rate of ethanol metabolism by the brain is only 1/4000 of that observed for the liver (Raskin and Sokoloff, 1970). In view of this, the contribution of the brain in the disposal of an ethanol load would be insignificant. As in the case of the liver, the presence of ADH in the brain for the local oxidation of ethanol would, however, have important consequences for local biochemical pathways in the brain (Rawat and Kuriyama, 1972a; Rawat et al., 1973). This has, in fact, been observed, as discussed in Section III, D. Chronic administration of ethanol for a prolonged period does not have a significant effect on the rate of ethanol utilization by the brain or on the activity of ADH in the brain. The rate of ethanol metabolism and the activity of ADH in the brain of normal mice, and the effect of chronic and prolonged ethanol administration on these parameters are given in Table I.

Although brain tissue can be demonstrated to metabolize ethanol, using a technique involving coupled oxidation with L-lactaldehyde, as shown by

TABLE I

RATES OF ETHANOL UTILIZATION AND ADH ACTIVITY IN BRAINS FROM
CONTROL MICE AND MICE CHRONICALLY FED ETHANOL[a]

Treatment	Metabolism of ethanol (μmoles per gm wet weight of brain per hour)	ADH (μmoles per gm wet weight of brain per hour)
Control	26.0 ± 2.5 (12)	1.87 ± 0.02 (10)
Chronic ethanol	27.2 ± 3.0 (12)	1.90 ± 0.03 (10)

[a] Brains from mice fed on an ethanol or sucrose diet for 4 weeks were homogenized in phosphate buffer (pH 7.6). Samples of brain homogenates were incubated at 37°C for varying intervals of time to determine the rate of ethanol metabolism; the complete reaction mixture contained 250 mM ethanol, 0.7 NAD$^+$, 13 mM L-lactaldehyde, and 90 mM potassium phosphate (pH 7.60) brought to a final volume of 1.0 ml with glass-distilled water. For the assay of ADH samples of the 105,000 g supernatant fraction were prepared. The propanediol formed was measured enzymically. The ethanol-dependent activity has been corrected for ethanol-free blank activity. Results are expressed as means ± S.E.M. for the number of animals given in parentheses. From Rawat et al. (1973).

Raskin and Sokoloff (1972) and later confirmed by Rawat et al. (1973), one problem remains with such a technique. Namely, this system can only be used to study oxidation in vitro, and the extrapolation of in vitro studies to the in vivo metabolism of ethanol is rather difficult. Such a system also does not permit the study of any possible rate-limiting step in the brain in vivo. Although the brain enzyme has been observed to be inhibited by pyrazole, several characteristics of the enzyme obtained under the coupled assay conditions need further exploration.

B. CATALASE

Catalase preparations from the liver and kidney have long been known to convert ethanol to acetaldehyde through peroxidation (Keilin and Hartree, 1936, 1945). Catalase activity has also been demonstrated in the brain (Feinstein et al., 1967). Since the availability of hydrogen peroxide determines whether or not catalase-mediated ethanol metabolism occurs in the brain, the presence of catalase alone does not provide evidence for ethanol metabolism by this pathway. Based on studies using high concentrations of externally added glucose in the incubation medium, Burbridge et al. (1959) suggested that catalase activity may account for as much as 70 μg/minute per gram of brain of ethanol metabolism. However, there was no evidence of direct catalase involvement in ethanol metabolism in this study.

Recently, a preliminary report by Hoffman and Schulman (1973) has proposed the involvement of catalase in the observed disappearance of alcohol. In this study also, glucose was found necessary for the maintenance of ethanol metabolism. Although catalase-mediated metabolism of ethanol in the brain has not been established, it remains an intriguing possibility. Monoamine oxidase (MAO) (Aebi et al., 1963) present in the brain may provide peroxide-generating systems. Anderson and Schulman (1974) in a preliminary report recently suggested such MAO-dependent ethanol metabolism in the brain.

However, the contribution of such a mechanism in catalase-mediated ethanol metabolism would be exceedingly small in view of the other endogenous substrates that would compete with ethanol.

C. Oxidation of Acetaldehyde

Although the metabolism of acetaldehyde in the brain has not been studied extensively, there is evidence to show that a NAD-dependent dehydrogenase system exists which converts acetaldehyde to acetate in vivo (Ridge, 1963). Acetaldehyde can be produced by the direct oxidation of ethanol in the brain, or it can be derived from ethanol oxidation in liver. The acetaldehyde molecule is small, readily soluble in body fluids and lipids, and can easily pass through the blood-brain barrier (Ridge, 1963). Besides acetaldehyde arising from ethanol, several aldehydes occur in brain tissue (Blaschko, 1952). It has been suggested that these aldehydes arise in brain tissue through oxidation deamination of monoamines (Quastel, 1965). It has also been suggested that the brain contain the small amounts of enzymes necessary to oxidize these aldehydes to their corresponding acids.

1. Aldehyde Dehydrogenase (Aldehyde NAD Oxidoreductase EC 1.2.1.3)

This enzyme has been studied in the brain (Deitrich, 1966; Raskin and Sokoloff, 1972). It has broad substrate specificity and several aliphatic aldehydes ranging from formaldehyde to palmitic aldehyde and aldehydes derived from serotonin, epinephrine, and dopamine (3,5-dihydroxyphenylethylamine) are substrates for the enzyme (Erwin and Deitrich, 1966). This enzyme is specific for NAD and NAD analogs. These observations suggest the possible heterogeneity of aldehyde dehydrogenase in the brain. A palmitic aldehyde dehydrogenase requiring $NADP^+$ as a cofactor has also been reported in the brain (Brady et al., 1958). Although a major portion of the aldehyde-oxidizing activity is found in the mitochondrial fraction, the cytoplasmic fraction also contains a substantial amount of activity. In contrast to the broad specificity of aldehyde dehydrogenase, brain also contains a specific NAD-dependent succinic semialdehyde dehydrogenase (Albers and Salvador, 1958; Albers and Koval, 1961). Succinic semialdehyde is a product of γ-aminobutyric acid (GABA) metabolism in the brain.

2. *Aldehyde Reductase* (*Alcohol NADP Oxidoreductase, EC 1.1.1.2*)

Oxidation of aldehyde intermediates to their corresponding acid metabolites has long been considered the primary route of degradation. However, now it is known that in some mammals the major pathway in brain tissue for the disposition of naturally occurring aldehydes is through reduction to their respective alcohol derivatives (Glowinski *et al.*, 1965). Recently, the enzyme systems responsible for the conversion of aldehydes to alcohols in the brain have been studied in detail. Reductases capable of reducing hydroxypyruvate (Kohn and Jakoby, 1968) and lactaldehyde have been described (Gupta and Robinson, 1966). The presence of nonspecific NADPH-linked aldehyde reductases has also been reported (Tabaloff and Erwin, 1970; Bronough and Erwin, 1973). The enzyme catalyzes the following reversible reaction.

$$RCHO + NADH \text{ or } NADPH + H^+ \rightleftharpoons RCHOH + NAD \text{ or } NADP$$

This enzyme is localized in the cytoplasmic fraction of the brain and differs from ADH. It is not active on short-chain aliphatic aldehydes like acetaldehyde. In contrast to ADH from the brain (Raskin and Sokoloff, 1970), aldehyde reductase is not inhibited by pyrazole.

D. LIVER AS THE MAJOR SITE OF ALCOHOL METABOLISM

Since no organ in the body functions as an independent entity, the effects of ethanol on one organ may influence its action throughout the body. Therefore, to be able to outline the metabolic consequences of ethanol and its metabolites, it is important to discuss the major site of alcohol metabolism in the body.

As discussed at the beginning of this section, although the brain may be capable of metabolizing small amounts of alcohol, it is widely realized that the liver is the principal organ involved in the initial oxidation of ethanol. As early as 1938, the classical studies of Leloir and Munoz (1938) and of Lundsgaard (1938) showed that the liver of the rat, pigeon, and cat was mainly involved in the metabolism of ethanol. It is generally agreed that 90–95% ethanol is metabolized in the liver.

1. *Liver ADH*

The enzyme ADH is the principal enzyme of alcohol metabolism and catalyzes the transfer of hydrogen from alcohol to NAD, thus generating acetaldehyde. The enzyme was purified by Lutwak-Mann (1938), and has been studied in detail by Bonnichsen an Wassén (1948), Dalziel (1958), Åkeson (1964), and Theorell (1967), among others. For a detailed discussion the reader is referred to a review by Rawat (1969a).

2. Action of Catalase

Keilin and Hartree (1945) suggested the possibility of oxidation of alcohol to acetaldehyde through catalase in the liver. This involves peroxidation by means of hydrogen peroxide formed from autoxidizable flavoproteins. The addition of alcohol and catalase results in the formation of hydrogen peroxide and its reduction to water. Chance (1947) studied the kinetics of this reaction in detail.

$$E + H_2O_2 \rightleftharpoons E(H_2O_2) \tag{1}$$

$$E(H_2O_2) + C_2H_5OH \rightleftharpoons E(H_2O_2)(C_2H_5OH) \tag{2}$$

$$E(H_2O_2)(C_2H_5OH) \rightleftharpoons E + CH_3CHO + 2H_2O \tag{3}$$

Here E represents the enzyme catalase, reactions (1) and (2) are rapid processes, and the $E(H_2O_2)(C_2H_5OH)$ complex is rapidly dissociable. Chance and Oshino (1971) utilized measurements of catalase intermediates for further documentation of hepatic alcohol oxidation. For detailed studies on this topic the reader is referred to Chance and Oshino 1971 and Oshino et al. (1973).

Besides the oxidation of alcohol by ADH and catalase, the possibility of ethanol oxidation by hepatic microsomes has also been suggested by the original findings of Orme-Johnson and Ziegler (1965). It was shown that ethanol oxidation by hepatic microsomes is NADPH-dependent and requires oxygen. It was subsequently hypothesized (Lieber and DeCarli, 1968) that ethanol in the microsomes is metabolized by the so-called microsomal ethanol-oxidizing system. However, this hypothesis has been found to be controversial. By using selective enzyme inhibitors in carefully controlled studies, it has been shown (Isselbacher and Carter, 1970; Thurman et al., 1972) that the liver microsomal fraction is contaminated with other enzymes, e.g., catalase, NADPH oxidase, and ADH. Involvement of the hepatic microsomal ethanol-oxidizing system as a single enzyme system responsible for alcohol metabolism in the microsomes has also been ruled out by the studies of Rawat and Kuriyama (1972b). In this study and others a lack of correlation between the blood alcohol clearance and the microsomal ethanol-oxidizing system was observed (Mezey and Tobon, 1971). For a review on this subject, the reader is referred to the "Alcohol and Aldehyde Metabolizing Systems" (Thurman et al., 1974).

E. Fate of Acetaldehyde Arising from Hepatic Metabolism

Acetaldehyde produced by the oxidation of ethanol has several possibilities for subsequent metabolism, among which oxidation to acetate is perhaps the most obvious (Lundquist, 1960). Although the liver is the main site of acetaldehyde oxidation (Lubin and Westerfeld, 1945), certain amounts of acetaldehyde also reach the brain through the circulation. Acetaldehyde, whether produced in the liver and then transported to the brain, or produced directly in the brain, must undergo very rapid metabolism in the brain. Although a definite increase in acetaldehyde concentration after alcohol ingestion have been observed (Freund and O'Hollaren, 1965), demonstrable quantities of acetaldehyde have not been found in the brain. This again suggests that the metabolism of acetaldehyde in the brain is very high. Other details of acetaldehyde metabolism in the brain were discussed earlier in this section.

III. Effects of Ethanol on Cerebral Metabolism

With the availability of new knowledge regarding the presence of ADH in the brain and the capability of this tissue to metabolize ethanol, the task of offering explanations for at least some of the metabolic effects of ethanol in the brain has become somewhat easier. Although knowledge of such alterations could facilitate our understanding of the mode of action of alcohol in the brain, it by no means offers a complete explanation of the multiple actions of alcohol on the brain. It is, however, important to remember that, in view of the low level of ethanol metabolism in the brain, the magnitude of changes in the steady-state concentration of several metabolites in the brain is not as great as that observed in the liver. It is not surprising therefore that several investigators have overlooked these changes. Furthermore, in view of the special susceptibility of brain tissue to anoxia, hypoxia, and hyperthermia, many precautions are required to prevent such conditions while determining the changes produced by ethanol.

A. Oxidative Metabolism in the Brain

During the metabolism of ethanol it has been observed in the liver that the oxidation of other substrates such as lipids and carbohydrates decreases. Oxidation of ethanol in the liver monopolizes 75% of the oxidative capacity of this tissue. As early as 1938 Lundsgaard, in liver perfusion experiments, observed that the total carbon dioxide production decreased during ethanol metabolism. The ethanol administered was oxidized only to acetate, and the respiratory quotient (RQ) decreased. Before the addition of ethanol, the RQ was 0.69, and after ethanol addition it fell to 0.37. The earlier studies of Leloir and Munoz (1938) with rat liver slices showed that the oxygen consumption of the tissue decreased. The calculation from the liver slice studies showed that the oxidation of alcohol to acetate accounted for three-fourths of normal oxygen consumption. These studies lend support to the idea that ethanol interferes with oxidative metabolism in the liver. For a detailed review on the effects of ethanol on oxidative metabolism in the liver, the reader is referred to Rawat (1969a). To a certain extent, similar effects of ethanol are observed on oxidative metabolism in the brain. In this section only the effects of ethanol on oxidative metabolism in the brain are discussed.

Effects on Oxygen Metabolism

In the past, several *in vitro* studies were carried out with brain cortex slices to observe the effect of ethanol on oxidative metabolism. These studies were conducted both in the presence and absence of potassium in the incubation medium. It has long been known that changes in the concentration of cations affect the consumption of oxygen by mammalian brain-cortex slices (Ashford and Dixon, 1935). An increase in potassium ion concentration in the incubation medium results in stimulation of oxygen consumption by rat brain-cortex slices (Buchel, 1953). This phenomenon is termed potassium-stimulated respiration. Similar stimulation of oxygen consumption can be obtained by electrical impulses. This stimulated respiration roughly equals the *in vivo* respiration in the brain. It seems rather clear that ethanol has little effect on unstimulated respiration in brain-cortex slices (Beer and Quastel, 1958; Wallgren and Kulonen, 1960) and brain mitochondria. A low ethanol concentration (0.5–1%) produces a small, transient stimulation of respiration in unstimulated tissue. This action of ethanol is compatible with the reversible action *in vivo*. Such observations have also been made with human brain tissue (Wallgren and Kulonen, 1960). However, with high concentrations of ethanol (0.05 M) in the incubation medium, respiration in potassium-stimulated brain-cortex slices is depressed. (Majchrowicz, 1965). Furthermore, the inhibitory effect of alcohols on these potassium-stimulated brain cortex slices increases markedly as the carbon-chain length of the alcohol increases. Thus pentanol has a greater inhibitory effect as compared to ethanol, propanol, or butanol. It has also been observed in these studies that aldehydes at concentrations several times lower than those of the corresponding alcohols severely inhibit oxygen consumption.

Electrically stimulated cerebral cortex tissue is more sensitive to ethanol than potassium-stimulated preparations. In cell-free brain preparations, only lethal concentrations of ethanol, about 0.11 M in humans and 0.2 M in rats, affect oxygen consumption. However, in brain homogenates low concentrations of ethanol (0.1 M) have been found to cause only an insignificant decrease in oxygen consumption (Grenell, 1957).

Since most alcohols do not interfere with the oxidative phosphorylation of brain mitochondria (Beer and Quastel, 1958; Truitt *et al.*, 1956) but suppress oxygen consumption in brain-cortex slices, it has been suggested that the site of alcohol inhibition is probably associated with part of the oxidative system that is dependent on the normal functioning of the cell membrane (Beer and Quastel, 1958; Wallgren, 1966). The interference of alcohols with nerve cell function appears to result from the inhibition of active transport of sodium across the cell membrane, which in turn causes suppression of the sodium-dependent ATPase of brain microsomes (Jarnefelt, 1961; Skou, 1957). The diminished rate of sodium concentration gradient across the membrane would consequently lead to a lowering of the membrane resting potential (Jarnefelt, 1961). Studies on the effect of alcohol on membrane potential (Armstrong and Binstock, 1964) are in agreement with observed changes in membrane excitability and in metabolism in the brain *in vivo* (Battey *et al.*, 1953).

B. EFFECTS ON CARBON DIOXIDE METABOLISM

The effects of ethanol, other aliphatic alcohols, and aldehydes on the formation of respiratory carbon dioxide and the production of $^{14}CO_2$ from [U-^{14}C]glucose have been studied in potassium-stimulated brain-cortex slices (Majchrowicz, 1965). Ethanol produces only a slight suppression of respiratory carbon dioxide. The inhibitory effect increases with increasing carbon-chain length of the alcohol. Aldehydes produce a much more pronounced inhibitory effect on both respiratory carbon dioxide and $^{14}CO_2$ formation. The effects of alcohols and aldehydes on the formation of total respiratory carbon dioxide are parallel to those observed for $^{14}CO_2$ production. An inhibitory effect of ethanol on the production of $^{14}CO_2$ has also been observed with other substrates such as [1-^{14}C]palmitate and [3-^{14}C]pyruvate in brain slice preparations (Rawat *et al.*, 1973). However, this effect can be abolished if the slices are incubated with pyrazole, an inhibitor of ADH.

A slight isotopic dilution occurs in determinations of the effect of ethanol on $^{14}CO_2$ production from labeled substrates; however, the fact that the effect of ethanol is not a mere isotopic dilution is further supported by the inhibition of respiratory carbon dioxide. The more pronounced inhibitory effect of aldehydes on the production of carbon dioxide compared to their corresponding alcohols is due to the aldehydes per se (Majchrowicz, 1965). The inhibitory effect of acetaldehyde on respiration in brain mitochondria (Beer and Quastel, 1958) is greatest in the presence of pyruvate and malate, suggesting that aldehydes interfere in energy metabolism via the citric acid cycle. Previously, it was considered that acetaldehyde in the brain arises from metabolism of ethanol in the liver, however, with the demonstration of the ability of the brain to metabolize ethanol, it is now apparent that acetaldehyde can also be produced locally in the brain. The ability of pyrazole to abolish the effects of ethanol in brain slices further supports the concepts of acetaldehyde production in the brain through the metabolism of ethanol (Rawat et al., 1973). The effect of ethanol on the rate of $^{14}CO_2$ production from various substrates is given in Table II.

C. Functioning of the Tricarboxylic Acid (TCA) Cycle

Decreased production of carbon dioxide also indicates decreased activity of the TCA cycle which is the major pathway for the production of carbon dioxide in the brain (Fig. 1). Inhibition of the TCA cycle in the liver during ethanol metabolism has been attributed to an increased NADH/NAD ratio (Forsander, 1966; Rawat, 1968, 1972). At present it is not clear, however, whether the increases in the NADH/NAD ratio in the brain alone is able to inhibit the activity of the TCA cycle or whether additional mechanisms are involved. Veloso et al. (1972) have suggested that some of the

TABLE II

RATE OF SUBSTRATE OXIDATION BY SLICES OF BRAIN FROM CONTROL
MICE AND MICE CHRONICALLY FED ETHANOL[a]

		(Micromoles of substrate converted to $^{14}CO_2$ per gm per hour)		
Substrate	Dietary treat- ment	No pyrazole		With 2 mM pyrazole
10 mM [U-^{14}C]glucose	Sucrose	2.0 ± 0.05 (10)	$P < .001$	2.1 ± 0.05 (10)
	Alcohol	1.3 ± 0.02 (10)		2.0 ± 0.06 (10)
10 mM [1-^{14}C]palmitate	Sucrose	0.76 ± 0.02 (12)	$P < .001$	0.80 ± 0.03 (12)
	Alcohol	0.51 ± 0.01 (12)		0.78 ± 0.03 (12)
10 mM [3-^{14}C]pyruvate	Sucrose	3.0 ± 0.06 (10)	$P < .001$	3.1 ± 0.08 (10)
	Alcohol	2.1 ± 0.08 (10)		3.1 ± 0.08 (10)

[a] Slices of brain from control sucrose-fed mice or mice chronically fed ethanol were incubated without or with 2 mM pyrazole in 5 ml of Krebs–Henseleit bicarbonate-buffered (pH 7.6) medium. Radioactive substrates were added at concentrations of 10 mM (0.5 μCi/flask). After incubation for 60 minutes, 0.3 ml of hyamine (10×) was injected into the hanging cups, followed by 0.5 ml of 1 N H_2SO_4 into the medium to stop the reaction and release CO_2. After 40 minutes further incubation, the contents of cups were transferred to vials containing scintillation fluid and counted in a liquid scintillation counter. Values are means ± S.E.M. for the number of animals given in parentheses. From Rawat et al. (1973).

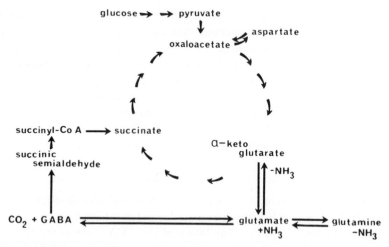

Fɪɢ. 1. Metabolic relationship of the TCA cycle to glutamate and its precursors. (Rawat, 1975a).

changes in the steady-state concentration of the metabolites of the TCA cycle may be caused by an elevation in pCO_2 during ethanol intoxication. Another possibility of TCA cycle inhibition is increased ammonia concentration in the brain (Recknagel and Potter, 1951; Katunuma *et al.*, 1966). However, in liquid nitrogen–frozen mouse brain preparations neither acute nor chronic administration of ethanol results in altered ammonia concentrations (Rawat *et al.*, 1973). Besides changes in the steady-state concentration of components of malate dehydrogenase and glutamate dehydrogenase, a sharp decrease in brain acetyl-CoA concentration is also observed during ethanol metabolism (Rawat *et al.*, 1973). A decrease in the acetyl-CoA content of the brain caused by ethanol is further suggestive of interference in the functioning of the TCA cycle. Acetaldehyde, produced by ethanol metabolism, has been suggested to be involved in the inhibitory effect of ethanol on acetyl-CoA in the brain. At high concentrations acetaldehyde can bind with the sulfhydryl groups of Coenzyme A sulfhydryl (CoASH), converting it into inactive thiohemiacetal which is unable to participate in transacetylation reactions (Ammon *et al.*, 1969). Although the hypothesis advanced by Ammon *et al.* (1965) is a logical one, we do not have experimental evidence to support it. In livers from normal-fed animals ethanol decreases the steady-state concentration of acetyl-CoA (Rawat, 1968). The concentration of acetaldehyde is about 0.2 μmole/gm in the presence of 10 mM ethanol in the liver; however, the concentration of acetaldehyde in the brain was not measured in experiments in which acetaldehyde was injected (Rawat *et al.*, 1973). The concentration of glutathione in the tissue is about 0.8 mM, which makes it somewhat difficult to visualize that acetaldehyde selectively attacks the sulfhydryl groups of CoA and not other sulfhydryl groups. However, further investigation is needed to clarify this point. The effects of ethanol on the steady-state concentration of certain metabolites of the TCA cycle are shown in Table III.

D. REDOX CHANGES IN THE BRAIN

As in the liver, if either ethanol or acetaldehyde is metabolized by ADH or acetaldehyde dehydrogenase in the brain, changes in the redox potentials will become evident. Since cytoplasmic NADH/NAD ratios are linked to other metabolites near equilibrium (Rawat, 1968, 1969a, 1970a), other redox couples in the brain should also be observed. Earlier attempts to measure the steady-state levels of NAD and NADH in the brain after ethanol administration suffered severe technical setbacks. In one such study, Cherrick and Leevy (1965) reported that they could not find any changes in the NAD/NADH ratios in the brain after ethanol administration. However, no attempts to expedite the measurement of nucleotides were made in this study, and consequently the effects of hyperthermia, anoxia, and other postmortem changes were included. In another study, Veloso et al. (1972), using a freeze-blown technique in which two holes were drilled in the skull of a living rat, did not find any significant changes due to ethanol in the NADH/NAD ratio in the brain. Using a less drastic technique of total immersion in liquid nitrogen, Rawat et al. (1973) observed very small but statistically

TABLE III

EFFECT OF CHRONIC ADMINISTRATION OF ETHANOL ON VARIOUS
METABOLITES IN MOUSE BRAIN[a]

| Metabolite | Metabolite level (μmoles per gm wet weight of brain) | | |
	Control	Chronically ethanol-fed	
Malate	0.298 ± 0.03	0.310 ± 0.03	$P < .02$
Oxaloacetate	0.006 ± 0.001	0.005 ± 0.001	$P < .02$
Glutamate	8.60 ± 0.98	9.0 ± 1.0	$P < .02$
α-Ketoglutarate	0.440 ± 0.06	0.400 ± 0.07	$P < .02$
Ammonia	0.330 ± 0.04	0.330 ± 0.04	N.S.
Aspartate	2.81 ± 0.23	2.88 ± 0.24	N.S.

[a] The levels of the various metabolites were determined enzymically in brains from control mice and mice fed ethanol for 4 weeks. The animals were dropped in liquid nitrogen, and their brains were powdered in a mortar with the addition of liquid nitrogen. The powdered tissue was treated with $HClO_4$, and the metabolites in the neutralized supernatant fluid were determined. Results are expressed as averages $\pm$ S.E.M. for 12 animals in each case. From Rawat et al. (1973).

significant changes in NADH/NAD ratios in mouse brain after ethanol administration. These changes were partially prevented by pretreatment of the animals with pyrazole, an inhibitor of ADH (Rawat, 1973). However, in contrast to the observations of Raskin and Sokoloff (1970), Mushahwar and Koeppe (1972), and Rawat et al. (1973), Veloso et al. (1972) were unable to observe the oxidation of ethanol by cerebral tissue. ADH in the brain, like that in the liver, is a cytoplasmic enzyme, and "H shuttles" have not been found to operate in brain tissue to any significant extent (Rawat et al., 1973). A valid question arises then: How does ethanol metabolism in the brain increase the NADH/NAD ratio in the mitochondrial compartment? This problem, however, can be solved by the presence of ADH both in the cytoplasm and in the mitochondria. Since in these two studies different species of animals, different routes of administration, and different techniques of tissue preparation were used, a direct comparison may be difficult. Since the inhibition of ethanol metabolism by pyrazole only partially prevented the changes in the redox state, it is quite possible that some of the observed changes were caused by the metabolism of acetaldehyde in the brain. Acetaldehyde metabolism has been shown to change the redox state of the liver at a higher (6.4 mM) acetaldehyde concentration (Lindros et al., 1972).

IV. Effects of Ethanol on Energy Metabolism in the Brain

It has been well established by now that during the metabolism of ethanol in liver there is a significant decrease in the production of carbon dioxide. Since carbon dioxide is mainly produced in the citric acid cycle, blockage during ethanol metabolism has been suggested (Rawat, 1969a, 1972). In spite of the fact that large quantities of ethanol are not metabolized by the brain, significant inhibition of the citric acid cycle in the brain has been shown (Rawat et al., 1973). Since the citric acid cycle is also the producer of high-energy compounds such as ATP, it would be of interest to examine the effect of ethanol on the levels of high-energy compounds in the brain.

A. ENERGY-RICH PHOSPHATES

In contrast to the great number of investigations conducted with hypnotics, tranquilizers, and anesthetics, only a few in vivo studies have dealt with the effects of ethanol on brain adenine nucleotides (Ammon et al., 1965; Redetzki, 1967; Rawat and Kuriyama, 1972a; Veloso et al., 1972; Rawat et al., 1973).

In vivo studies by Ammon et al. (1965) showed that ethanol (4.1 gm/kg) increased cerebral concentrations of creatine phosphate (CP) and AMP and decreased the concentration of ADP. A decline in cerebral ADP content resulting in an increased ATP/ADP ratio has also been found in the rat (Redetzki, 1967). These findings have been interpreted as suggestive of decreased utilization of ATP and CP in brain secondary to the depressant effect of ethanol. Support of this possibility is also provided by the *in vitro* studies of Wallgren (1963). In electrically stimulated brain slices, ethanol (0.4%) strongly retarded the breakdown of CP and ATP, which normally occurs on application of electrical impulses.

While considering the effect of ethanol on energy metabolism in the brain, it is rather important that its dose and the duration of its action also be taken into consideration. With the use of small doses of ethanol it has been observed that, in *in vivo* studies with liquid nitrogen–frozen brain preparations (Rawat and Kuriyama, 1972a; Veloso *et al.*, 1972; Rawat *et al.*, 1973), acute ethanol intoxication does not produce significant changes in the cerebral concentration of CP, ATP, ADP, or AMP. Observations made both *in vivo* and *in vitro* suggest that ethanol has no apparent effect on the synthesis of energy-rich phosphates, at least in acute ethanol-treated animals. The situation in long-term alcohol-fed animals may be different. Chronic and continuous feeding of ethanol has been observed to increase mitochondrial ATPase activity in the brain (Israel and Kuriyama, 1971), which would result in an increased breakdown of ATP, in turn resulting in a decrease in ATP and a subsequent increase in ADP and AMP. This has been in fact observed using liquid nitrogen–frozen brain preparations (Rawat *et al.*, 1973). Brains from chronic ethanol-fed mice showed a significant decrease in cerebral ATP and CP concentrations. The effect of ethanol administration on cerebral CP and adenine nucleotides in mouse brain is given in Table IV. While ethanol intoxication is associated with alterations in the activity of ATPase both in the microsomal and mitochondrial fractions of the brain, interference with enzymes specifically associated with neural and synaptic transmission is also involved. Israel *et al.* (1965) observed that ethanol inhibits Na^+-K^+-ATPase. It is reasonable to assume that this inhibition of ATPase may result in alterations in the membranes of nerve cells. Alterations in brain cell membranes could also lead to a decrease in oxygen consumption by the brain after ethanol intoxication. It has been also commonly observed that general depressants such as halothane, cyclopropane, and diethyl ether also inhibit brain Na^+-K^+-ATPase.

B. Effects of Ethanol on cAMP

The relatively high concentration of cAMP in the CNS, and higher activity in neural tissue than in somatic tissue (Robinson *et al.*, 1971), sug-

ARUN K. RAWAT

TABLE IV

Effect of Acute or Chronic Administration of Ethanol on Levels of
Creatine Phosphate and Adenine Nucleotides in Mouse Brain

| | Micromoles per gram wet weight of brain | | | | |
| | Acutely treated mice | | Chronically treated mice | | |
	Control	Alcohol	Control	Alcohol	
CP	3.35 ± 0.20	3.32 ± 0.23	3.40 ± 3.0	2.90 ± 0.20	$P < .01$
ATP	2.2 ± 0.08	2.1 ± 0.07	2.3 ± 0.09	1.85 ± 0.05	$P < .01$
ADP	0.40 ± 0.02	0.43 ± 0.02	0.40 ± 0.02	0.78 ± 0.03	$P < .001$
AMP	0.27 ± 0.03	0.28 ± 0.02	0.27 ± 0.02	0.42 ± 0.02	$P < .001$

[a] Brain levels of creatine phosphate (CP) and adenine nucleotides from acutely and chronically treated mice and controls were determined fluorimetrically. The animals were dropped into liquid nitrogen, and their brains powdered in a mortar with the addition of liquid nitrogen. The powdered tissue was treated with $HClO_4$, and the metabolites in the neutralized supernatant fluid were determined enzymically. The values were means ± S.E.M. for 6 animals in each case. From Rawat *et al.* (1973).

gest that cAMP may have an important function in the CNS. Although the definite role of cAMP in the CNS is not completely understood, an increasing amount of evidence indicates that it may be involved in metabolic regulation in the brain. There is evidence to suggest that cAMP is involved in synaptic transmission (Greengard *et al.*, 1972). Increased cAMP levels have been observed in cat superior cervical ganglia after orthodromic but not after antidromic stimulation. Since adenylate cyclase in the ganglia is dopamine-sensitive, it was suggested that dopamine is released by inhibitory interneurons in the ganglia. Neurophysiological evidence indicates that increased levels of cAMP mediate slow inhibitory postsynaptic potentials (McAfee and Greengard, 1972). A role of cAMP in the basal ganglia has also been suggested, since dopamine-sensitive adenylate cyclase has been found in the basal ganglia. Some indirect evidence is available, which indicates that cAMP may be involved in at least some of the actions of ethanol on the brain. The respiratory depression and anesthestic effect of ethanol was observed to be inhibited by α-methyl-*p*-tyrosine (Blum, 1972) and propranolol (Smith *et al.*, 1970) in mice, although in humans it was found to show no effect of even to potentiate the behavioral effects of ethanol (Noble *et al.*, 1973). Ethanol-induced depression of behavioral performance in rats is inhibited by several antihistamines. All these drugs prevent a rise in cAMP levels.

Recently, two opposing observations have been made regarding the effect of ethanol on the level of cAMP in the brain. In a recent study with the rat, Volicer and Gold (1973) showed that ethanol administration resulted in a decrease in the level of cAMP in the brain. This effect of ethanol was found to be dose-dependent. In contrast to this, studies on mice (Kuriyama and Israel, 1973) showed that acute administration of ethanol was without significant effect on the steady-state concentration of cAMP in brain. It was further observed in this study that chronic ethanol consumption for up to 3 weeks resulted in an increase in cAMP levels. Besides the contradictory observations regarding the effect of ethanol on cAMP levels in the brain, the mechanism by which ethanol affects the cAMP system also has not been explained. It seems from these observations that further investigation is required to resolve the existing contradictory observations in the literature regarding cAMP levels in the brain.

1. Effects of Ethanol on Adenylate Cyclase

It is possible that a compound like ethanol affects both the formation and degradation of cAMP in the brain. These two opposing effects can be obtained by the action of alcohol on adenylate cyclase and phosphodiesterase. This is observed in gastric mucosa where administration of 20% ethanol inhibits both enzymes, leaving the levels of cAMP unchanged (Tague and Shanbour, 1974). In studies on mouse brain (Kuriyama and Israel, 1973) it was observed that acute ethanol administration did not affect the activity of adenylate cyclase either in the absence or presence of sodium fluoride. However, chronic ethanol administration resulted in a significant increase in the activity of adenylate cyclase in the absence of sodium fluoride. Unfortunately, there is not enough experimental evidence conclusively to show the effects of acute and chronic ethanol administration on the activity of adenylate cyclase in the brain.

2. Effects of Ethanol on Phosphodiesterase

Phoshodiesterase is an enzyme responsible for the catabolism of cAMP. The enzyme hydrolyzes cAMP at the 3-position to yield 5′-monophosphate. There have been few reports indicating an effect of ethanol on the activity of phosphodiesterase. In vitro addition of ethanol to phosphodiesterase from rat gastric mucosa was observed to inhibit this enzyme (Tague and Shanbour, 1974). However, acute or chronic administration of ethanol was found to be without an effect on phosphodiesterase activity in the brain (Kuriyama and Israel, 1973). In vitro addition of ethanol was found not to affect the activity of this enzyme in the brain. One weakness of this experimental design was that the activity of phosphodiesterase was tested at only one substrate concentration. This makes it difficult to detect the activity of other phosphodiesterases which may have different substrate affinities. The observations of Volicer and Gold (1975) indicated that, in the pons, phosphodiesterase activity was inhibited in the rat by ethanol pretreatment. The effects of ethanol on the activity of brain phosphodiesterase are, however, contradictory, and there is a need for further investigation in this area.

V. Active in Transport as Affected by Ethanol in the Brain

Interference by alcohol with nerve cell function appears to result from the inhibition of Na^+-K^+-ATPase (Skou, 1957; Armstrong and Binstock, 1964), thus blocking the active transport of sodium across the cell membrane. The diminished rate of sodium transport is followed by a lowering of the sodium concentration gradient across the membrane, which leads to a lowering of the membrane resting potential (Skou, 1957). Studies on the effects of alcohol on membrane potential (Armstrong and Binstock, 1964) are in agreement with the above changes in the metabolism of the brain *in vivo* (Battey *et al.*, 1953).

The action potential in the neuron is generated by maintaining a constant low intracellular concentration of sodium and high intracellular potassium. This is believed to be accomplished (Hokin, 1969) by an active transport system involving magnesium-dependent Na^+-K^+-ATPase and low sodium permeability in all excitable membranes.

A. TRANSPORT OF SODIUM AND POTASSIUM

Several studies have been conducted to investigate the *in vitro* effects of alcohol on the transport of sodium and potassium. Aerobic incubation of rat brain slices promoted potassium uptake from the medium, however, in the presence of 0.11 M ethanol this uptake of potassium was inhibited by about 70% within 10 minutes of incubation (Israel *et al.*, 1966). There was a progressive decrease in the degree of inhibition with an increase in incubation time. Alcohols with longer chain lengths produced the same effects, but at lower concentrations. A retarded uptake of potassium by ethanol (0.11 M) was also observed in brain slices recovering from electrical stimulation (Wallgren *et al.*, 1974). However, the efflux of sodium during this time was unaffected.

In rat and guinea pig cortex, ethanol has been observed to inhibit microsomal and synaptosomal Na^+-K^+-ATPase at a 0.05–0.22 M ethanol concentration; this inhibition is competitive with respect to potassium and can be enhanced by an increase in the concentration of sodium (Sun and Somorajski, 1970). A serious problem with studies involving Na^+-K^+-ATPase and the transport of ions is that they can be performed only in an *in vitro* system. Therefore the extrapolation of such results to the *in vivo* system is always questionable. If the inhibition of Na^+-K^+-ATPase were to be considered an important mechanism by which alcohols produce depression of the CNS, it would be of value to examine the effects of different experimental conditions resulting in inhibition of Na^+-K^+-ATPase *in vivo*. At the moment it is not clear what potential alterations in the excitability of nerve tissue occur as a consequence of inhibition of the sodium pump. Although in some species the sodium pump appears to regulate the resting potential directly (Carpenter, 1970), in others it seems to have no effect (Hodgkin and Keynes, 1955). The effect of the sodium pump in regulating the resting potential in humans is relatively unclear at the moment.

Several drugs are capable of inhibiting ion transport, and consequently Na^+–K^+-ATPase activity. A well-known depolarizing agent is ouabain (Swanson and McIlwain, 1965). Increased leakage of potassium into the cerebral spinal fluid was observed along with the occurrence of convulsions after direct administration of ouabain into the brain (Bignami and Palladini, 1966). An accumulation of extracellular potassium further stimulates neurons by reducing their resting membrane potential, thus producing a hyperexcitable condition (Gross and Woodbury, 1972). Thus present evidence indicates that inhibition of Na^+–K^+-ATPase activity generally leads to hyperexcitability. This suggests at least that the mechanism of action of acute doses of alcohol is not mediated through these systems and that these may be secondary in nature.

B. Effect on Calcium and Magnesium Transport

The mechanism of the involvement of calcium and magnesium in membrane function is not clearly understood. However, two fairly well-known functions of calcium in the nervous system are its involvement in the release of transmitters (Rubin, 1970) and in maintaining a permeability barrier to sodium influx (Rothstein, 1968). Calcium is mostly an extracellular ion, as a result of its ionic and electrical properties. In order to maintain a low intracellular concentration of calcium, there appears to be a large number of ATP-dependent mechanisms, including active extraction of calcium by exchange with sodium. Although the role of magnesium as a cofactor for several enzymes and its involvement in potassium permeability are known, its role in membrane function is not fully understood (Hoffman, 1962).

Relatively few investigations have been made of the interaction of alcohol and calcium metabolism. Ethanol in concentrations of 0.11–0.87 M is capable of blocking inward currents in the neurons of *Aplysia* (Bergman *et al.*, 1974), although the mechanism by which this blockage occurs is not clear. Studies with erythrocyte ghost cell membranes indicate that ethanol in a concentration range above 0.02 M increases calcium binding in the membranes (Seeman *et al.*, 1971). However, studies by Ross *et al.* (1974) demonstrated that nonintoxicating doses of ethanol significantly decreased calcium levels in several areas of the brain. Interestingly, a similar effect of morphine on the levels of calcium in the brain may lead one to assume that the mechanism of action of alcohol and morphine on the brain are similar. However, the great variation in the other metabolic effects of ethanol and morphine on the brain exclude such a possibility.

Both in the rat and dog, ethanol was observed to produce hypocalcemia in an oral dose of 2–8 gm/kg body weight, which lasted for at least 5 hours (Peng et al., 1972). This peripheral effect of ethanol does not seem to be mediated through either the thyroid or parathyroid gland. Although hypocalcemia and hypomagnesimia have been observed after alcohol withdrawal in humans (Victor and Adams, 1953), sometimes resulting in seizures (Simpson, 1968), it is not clear how hypocalcemia and hypomagnesimia affect the action of alcohol.

C. Effect on Membranes and Membrane Lipids

It has long been considered that one of the mechanisms of the intoxication effect of ethanol may involve interference with membrane structure and function in the brain. Alcohols are analogous to anesthetics in several ways. Anesthetics generally follow the Meyer–Overton hypothesis which states that the narcosis is directly related to the concentration of the anesthetic in the cell membrane and to its lipid solubility (Meyer, 1937). It has been observed that alcohols as well as anesthetics block the generation of action potentials at concentrations that have little effect on resting membrane potentials (Seeman, 1972). This suggests that, like anesthetics, alcohols exert their effect on membranes. In an attempt to understand the effect of prolonged ethanol consumption on brain structure and function, a large number of specific neurolipids was studied (Rawat, 1974a), e.g., cerebrosides, gangliosides, sulfatides, and phospholipids which contribute to the structure of some brain cell membranes. It was observed in this study that chronic ethanol feeding in mice resulted in a significant increase in gangliosides and sulfatides. The observed changes in the cerebral ganglioside content in chronic ethanol-fed animals may be of importance in explaining some of the actions of ethanol on the CNS (Table V). It was particularly of interest in view of the fact that a direct relationship between the excitability of nervous tissue and the extractable ganglioside content (measured by their N-acetylneuraminic acid moiety) has been observed (McIlwain, 1961). Furthermore, the decreased metabolic response of brain-cortex slices to electrical stimulation during ethanol intoxication has been explained (Wallgren and Kulonen, 1960) on the basis of a decrease in N-acetylneuraminic acid groups. N-Acetylneuraminic acid has been suggested to form a hydrophilic path for cations through the lipid membrane (McIlwain, 1961). An increase in the extractability of gangliosides in rat brain during

TABLE V

EFFECTS OF CHRONIC ETHANOL ADMINISTRATION ON GANGLIOSIDE, SULFATIDE,
AND CEREBROSIDE/SULFATIDE CONCENTRATION IN BRAIN[a]

Treatment	Cerebral lipids (mg/gm fresh brain)		
	Gangliosides	Sulfatides	Cerebrosides/ Sulfatides
Sucrose-fed, chronic	0.92 ± 0.2 (6)	0.84 ± 0.16 (6)	9.7 ± 1.1 (6)
Ethanol-fed	1.23 ± 0.3 (6)	1.16 ± 0.20 (6)	10.3 ± 1.0 (6)

[a] Results are expressed as means ± S.E.M. for the number of animals given in parentheses. From Rawat (1974a).

acute alcohol intoxication was also observed previously (Hakkinen and Kulonen, 1963).

In addition to such biochemical explanations of the interference of alcohols with membrane structure and function, certain biophysical aspects of membrane structure also are involved. Several studies have shown that alcohols are capable of causing membrane expansion. They have been observed to expand monolayers of stearic acid, phospholipids, and cholesterol, and nerve lipid films (Gatenbeck and Ehrenberg, 1953; Skou, 1958).

Generally, studies involving the biophysical interactions of membranes and alcohols have been inconclusive so far. In most cases the concentrations of alcohol required to produce a significant change would be lethal in most species, and therefore the physiological relevance of such studies is questionable.

VI. Effects of Ethanol on Neurotransmitters

Presumptive neurotransmitters such as acetylcholine, GABA, and biogenic amines [e.g., norepinephrine, dopamine, and serotonin (5-hydroxytryptamine)] play an important role in the CNS by acting as transmitters of neuronal functions. In view of the importance of neurotransmitter substances a large number of studies has been conducted to investigate the effects of ethanol or acetaldehyde on their metabolism, uptake, turnover, and storage. In this section the relationship between ethanol and neurotransmitters is discussed.

A. Steady-State Levels of Neurotransmitters

The effects of ethanol and its metabolite acetaldehyde have been studied in the past in several species. However, the results obtained by various investigators are quite often not directly comparable. However, it is clear from these studies that the observed variation in the effects of ethanol can be largely attributed to differences in dosage, route of administration, duration of the study, and areas of the brain studied.

1. Effect on Norepinephrine and Serotonin

Intravenous administration of 2 gm/kg of ethanol to rabbits was reported (Gursey and Olson, 1960) to cause a significant decrease in norepinephrine and serotonin content in the brainstem up to 8 hours later. In rat whole brain, however, an increase in serotonin content was observed 1 hour after ethanol administration (Bonnycastle et al., 1962). Studies by Duritz and Truitt (1966) attempted to resolve this controversy by conducting experiments with rats and rabbits. This study showed that intraperitoneal administration of ethanol (2–4 gm/kg body weight) had no effect on norepinephrine and serotonin levels in either rat or rabbit brain 90 minutes later. It was also observed in this study that, when aldehyde dehydrogenase was inhibited by pretreatment with disulfiram before ethanol administration, a significant decrease was observed in the norepinephrine content in both rats and rabbits. This however, had no effect on the serotonin content. These results suggest that, while acetaldehyde is capable of causing partial depletion of norepinephrine in the brain, ethanol alone has no significant effect.

Since the steady-state concentration of neurotransmitters in the brain is very susceptible to postmortem changes such as hyperthemia and anoxia, a study was designed to rule out such possibilities (Rawat, 1974b). The effects of intraperitoneally administered ethanol (3 gm/kg) on whole-brain norepinephrine and serotonin levels were studied (Table VI). Control animals were given saline solution, and after 15 minutes of ethanol administration the animals were sacrificed by total immersion in liquid nitrogen. Studies on such frozen brain preparations showed that ethanol did not result in a significant change in the steady-state concentration of serotonin and norepinephrine. It appears from these studies that intraperitoneally or orally administered ethanol has little effect on steady-state concentrations of serotonin and norepinephrine.

In a study by Jofre de Breyer et al. (1972), in which ethanol was given for over a period of 2 months as a 10% solution ad libitun, it was observed that serotonin increased significantly in the cerebellum, mesencephalon, and rhombencephalon. It was also observed in this study that, whereas dopamine levels did not change significantly in any of the above-mentioned areas of the

TABLE VI

EFFECT OF ACUTE AND CHRONIC ADMINISTRATION OF ETHANOL ON THE CONCENTRATION OF NOREPINEPHRINE, SEROTONIN, AND γ-AMINOBUTYRATE IN MOUSE BRAIN[a]

Metabolite	Acute treatment			Chronic treatment		
	Control	Ethanol		Sucrose	Ethanol	
Norepinephrine (μg/gm)[b] (8)	1.23 ± 0.10	1.20 ± 0.10	N.S.	1.35 ± 0.12	1.10 ± 0.12	$P < .02$
Serotonin (μg/gm) (8)	0.97 ± 0.08	1.0 ± 0.08	N.S.	0.98 ± 0.09	1.00 ± 0.09	N.S.
GABA (μmole/gm) (8)	3.00 ± 0.30	3.80 ± 0.30	$P < .02$	3.00 ± 0.30	3.95 ± 0.30	$P < .02$

[a] Brain preparations frozen in liquid nitrogen were used for these estimations. Serotonin and norepinephrine were determined fluorimetrically. GABA was determined either enzymically or chromatographically. The values are means ± S.E.M. for the number of animals given in parentheses. From Rawat (1974b).
[b] Per gram fresh weight of brain.

brain, the norepinephrine content decreased. In another study on mice (Rawat, 1974b) the effect of chronic ethanol administration on the steady-state concentrations of norepinephrine and serotonin was investigated. It was found that, whereas chronic ethanol administration did not significantly alter the concentration of serotonin in the brain, the norepinephrine content showed a significant decrease. The levels of norepinephrine returned to control values after 4 days of ethanol withdrawal. A consistent observation in the above-mentioned studies was a decrease in the content of norepinephrine in the brain as a result of chronic ethanol administration.

2. Effect on GABA

Both acute (3 gm/kg) and chronic prolonged (4 weeks, 6% w/v) administration of ethanol resulted in a significant increase in the concentration of GABA in the adult mouse (Rawat, 1974b). The observed increase in the content of GABA in the brain has been suggested to be due to an increase in the content of glutamate, since these two amino acids are metabolically interrelated. However, in some studies a decrease in rat brain GABA content was observed (Gordon, 1967). However, the results of this study cannot be attributed to the action of ethanol, since the GABA content was determined in the brains of rats decapitated at room temperature. As mentioned earlier, the steady-state concentration of neurotransmitters is very susceptible to postmortem hypoxia and hyperthermia, and therefore in determining *in vivo* levels of GABA the use of rapid freezing of the tissue is essential.

3. Effect on Dopamine

The role of dopamine as a neurotransmitter in the CNS has been discussed in detail by Hornykiewicz (1966). Although inhibition of MAO by alcohol has been studied (Heim, 1950), not much work has been done in this regard on the metabolism of dopamine as a substrate for MAO. Homovanillic acid (HVA) is the major metabolic product of dopamine. Ethanol administration has been observed to decrease the excretion of HVA without causing a significant effect on excretion of the alcohol derivative of this metabolite, namely, 3-methoxy-4-hydroxyphenyl ethanol (MOPET). However, there is not much information on the effects of ethanol on the levels of dopamine *in vivo* in the brain.

Unfortunately, the work done regarding the effect of ethanol on dopamine turnover in the brain is not quite consistent. Chronic administration of ethanol for 5 days has been observed to cause a decrease in dopamine turnover in the brain. No significant effect of ethanol on dopamine turnover was reported by Corrodi et al. (1966). It seems that contrasting observations have been made in this regard as a result of the use of different doses of ethanol and differences in the duration of the experiment. Carlson and

Lindquist (1973) observed a dose-dependent effect of ethanol on brain levels of dopa. Since no effect of ethanol was observed on the levels of serotonin in this study, it is suggested that ethanol may have a specific action on the catecholamine-metabolizing systems.

4. Effect on Acetylcholine

The role of acetylcholine in central synaptic transmission has been well documented, and most studies are highly suggestive of a role as a central neurohumoral transmitter. It is also well known that the levels of acetylcholine in the brain vary with the functional activity of the organ (Richter and Crossland, 1949) and are affected by a variety of drugs.

Our studies on mouse brain showed that acute administration of either ethanol (3 gm/kg, intraperitoneally) or acetaldehyde (40 mg/kg, intravenously) resulted in a decrease in the cerebral concentration of acetylcholine 15 minutes after administration. Chronic (4 weeks, 6% v/v administration of alcohol also resulted in a decrease in whole-brain acetylcholine content in the mouse (Rawat, 1974b). The effects of ethanol or acetaldehyde on cerebral acetylcholine content are consistent with the effect of these substances on cerebral acetyl-CoA and CoA content. The levels of both these compounds are decreased (Table VII) in the brain by ethanol or acetaldehyde. Acetylcholine content in the brain was also observed to decrease after ethanol administration (Moss et al., 1967). However, it is difficult, to ascertain whether the observed changes seen in this study can be attributed to ethanol or to the ether anesthesia and the technique of sacrificing the animals at room temperature by cervical dislocation. In contrast to the in vivo effects of ethanol, incubation of brain cell preparations or potassium-stimulated brain slices does not affect acetylcholine concentration or its release (Kalant et al., 1967).

Ethanol intoxication also interferes with the incorporation of choline into acetylcholine. Although the steady-state concentration of cerebral choline is not affected by acute or chronic administration of ethanol, a decreased incorporation of [^{3}H]choline into cerebral acetylcholine from acute ethanol-treated (3 gm/kg) mice was observed as shown in Fig. 2. Although acute ethanol administration did not affect the activity of the enzymes involved in acetylcholine synthesis and degradation, chronic (4 weeks, 6% v/v) ethanol feeding of mice resulted in a decrease in cerebral acetyl choline transferase activity (Rawat, 1974b).

B. EFFECTS ON RATE OF TURNOVER OF NEUROTRANSMITTERS

Studies on the rate of turnover of serotonin have produced conflicting results regarding the effects of ethanol on this presumptive neurotransmitter.

TABLE VII

EFFECTS OF ACUTE ADMINISTRATION OF ETHANOL OR ACETALDEHYDE, OR CHRONIC ADMINISTRATION OF ETHANOL, ON ACETYLCHOLINE, CHOLINE, CoA, ACETYL CoA, AND ATP IN MOUSE BRAIN[a]

Metabolite	Acute treatment					Chronic treatment		
	Control	Ethanol		Acetaldehyde		Sucrose	Ethanol	
Acetylcholine (8)	0.013 ± 0.002	0.008 ± 0.001	$P < .001$	0.006 ± 0.001	$P < .001$	0.014 ± 0.001	0.009 ± 0.001	$P < .001$
Acetyl CoA (6)	0.040 ± 0.005	0.027 ± 0.003	$P < .001$	0.020 ± 0.003	$P < .001$	0.044 ± 0.004	0.025 ± 0.002	$P < .001$
Choline (8)	0.115 ± 0.020	0.109 ± 0.040	N.S.	0.115 ± 0.020	N.S.	0.125 ± 0.03	0.121 ± 0.03	N.S.
CoA (6)	0.412 ± 0.04	0.310 ± 0.04	$P < .02$	0.268 ± 0.03	$P < .02$	0.420 ± 0.05	0.300 ± 0.05	$P < .02$
ATP (6)	2.2 ± 0.08	2.1 ± 0.07	N.S.			2.3 ± 0.09	1.85 ± 0.05	$P < .02$

[a] Brain levels of metabolites were determined in preparations frozen in liquid nitrogen. Acetylcholine was determined either by gas chromatography or enzymically. Acetyl CoA, CoA, choline, and ATP were determined spectrophotometrically. The values are means ± S.E.M. for the number of animals given in parentheses. From Rawat (1974b).

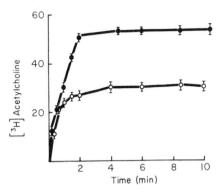

FIG. 2. Effect of ethanol on acetylcholine turnover. *In vivo* turnover rates in mouse brain were studied after [³H]choline administration in control (solid circles) and ethanol-treated (open circles) animals (Rawat, 1974b).

It was observed in the studies of Tyce *et al.* (1970) that ethanol administration (3.3 gm/kg, intraperitoneally) resulted in a small decrease in serotonin turnover. Using mice as experimental animals, Kuriyama *et al.* (1971) found that acute ethanol administration (4 gm/kg, intraperitoneally) did not result in a significant change in serotonin turnover. However, chronic administration of ethanol in a liquid diet (2 gm/kg per day) in mice was found to result in a significant increase in serotonin turnover at 8 and 14 days. An increase in the activity of tryptophan hydroxylase activity was also observed in this study. However, a decrease was observed in serotonin turnover after acute and chronic ethanol administration in intoxicated rat brains by Hunt and Majchrowicz (1974). From the observations cited above it seems that the effects of ethanol on serotonin turnover are totally inconclusive, and no sound conclusions can be drawn from the existing data.

The effects of ethanol on the turnover of norepinephrine are less controversial and there is greater agreement that acute or chronic ethanol administration results in an increased turnover of norepinephrine. However, it is not clear whether this effect is a direct or an indirect one.

1. Uptake of Neurotransmitters

A large number of studies has been conducted to investigate the effects of ethanol or acetaldehyde on the uptake of various neurotransmitters by brain tissue *in vitro*. When a very high ethanol concentration (0.22 M) was used, it was observed that norepinephrine uptake by brain slices decreased (Israel *et al.*, 1973). The uptake of several presumptive neurotransmitters by synapsis was studied by Roach *et al.* (1973). It was found that only the uptake of glutamate was affected and that the uptake of norepinephrine, serotonin, and GABA was unaffected. However, it is difficult to offer an explanation regarding the mechanism of the action of ethanol.

2. Effect on Neurotransmitter Enzymes

In an attempt to understand the effects of ethanol on the steady-state levels of neurotransmitters in the brain activities of enzymes involved in the synthesis and degradation of the neurotransmitters have been investigated. The effect of chronic ethanol administration on L-glutamic 1-carboxylyase (EC 4.1.1.15) and 4-aminobutyrate 2-oxoglutarate aminotransferase (EC 2.6.1.19) was studied by Rawat (1974b). Only the activity of L-glutamic decarboxylase was observed to show any measurable decrease after chronic ethanol administration. The activity of GABA transaminase did not show any significant change after ethanol administration (Figs. 3 and 4); it was also observed to remain unaffected after chronic ethanol administration, according to a recent report by Sytinsky et al. (1975).

From the experimental evidence presented it is apparent that ethanol, or its metabolite acetaldehyde, exerts a profound effect on the normal metabolism of biogenic amines in the peripheral nervous system. This effect is achieved by a shift from oxidative pathways to reductive pathways. The mechanism by which this effect is exerted appears to be through competition for aldehyde dehydrogenase between acetaldehyde and the aldehydes derived from biogenic amines. This is achieved through an increase in the NADH/NAD ratios which shifts the metabolism from an oxidative to a reductive

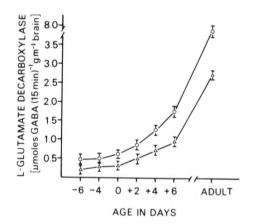

FIG. 3. Developmental changes in L-glutamate decarboxylase activity in the brain. The effect of ethanol feeding on the developmental pattern of this enzyme in pregnant or lactating rats was studied in the fetal, neonatal, and adult brain. The activity of this enzyme was significantly inhibited in alcoholic brains (triangles) as compared to the controls (circles) throughout the developmental stage.

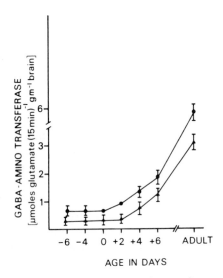

Fig. 4. Developmental changes in GABA aminotransferase activity in the brain. Effect of ethanol feeding on the developmental pattern of this enzyme in pregnant or lactating rats was studied in the fetal, neonatal, and adult brain. The activity of this enzyme was significantly inhibited in alcoholic brains (triangles) as compared to the controls (circles) throughout the developmental stage.

pathway. In spite of these investigations on biogenic amine catabolism, the mechanism of ethanol action leading to intoxication or ethanol dependence remains unclear.

The effects of ethanol or acetaldehyde on MAO, on catechol-O-methyltransferase (COMT), and on the uptake of various presumptive neurotransmitters by brain tissue have been proven to be very weak or nonexistent and provide no positive insight into the mechanism(s) of ethanol action.

C. Urinary Excretion of Biogenic Amines

Several studies have demonstrated that the ingestion of ethanol by humans results in alterations in the urinary excretion of certain biogenic amines and their metabolites, although in such studies the concentrations of biogenic amines were determined in the urine, representing an overall picture of biogenic amine metabolism in the brain. It was observed that ingestion of 0.71 gm/kg of ethanol resulted in a significant increase in the urinary excretion of norepinephrine, metanephrine, and dopamine (Anton, 1965). A significant decrease in the excretion of 5-hydroxyproline acetic acid was observed. Other studies have shown that ethanol produces an increase in the urinary excretion of catecholamines and their metabolites in animals (von Wartburg et al., 1961).

It seems safe to assume that there is increased excretion of certain bio-genic amines (Davis *et al.*, 1967). This increased excretion may result from adrenal activation. The question that remains to be answered is: What is the relation of this increased excretion of biogenic amines to intoxication, alcohol addiction, and alcohol withdrawal?

VII. Ethanol Tolerance and Physical Dependence

Recently it has been stated that alcoholism is a disease. Alcoholism is generally defined as a condition in which alcohol is consumed to such an extent that it interferes with a person's physical health, mental health, and adequate functioning in society. Voluntary consumption of alcohol, or any other drug for that matter, appears to be a psychological disorder which may result in a variety of diseases ranging from liver dysfunction to physical dependence. Many different physiological, sociological, and psychological factors appear to play a role in the initial excessive consumption of alcohol. Although the human physiological and sociological factors involved cannot be understood through animal experimentation, animal research may, how-ever, be of interest in understanding the neurochemical and pharmacological sequence of events that lead to symptoms of physical dependence and of withdrawal (Table VIII).

In patients with a history of prolonged ethanol consumption a wide variety of subjective symptoms and objective signs of ethanol withdrawal appears (Mendelson, 1964). Some of these symptoms include nervousness, hallucinatory psychosis, convulsive seizures, and delirium tremens. These conditions may be accompanied by agitation, gross tremor, perceptual dis-orders, and increased psychomotor and autonomic nervous system activity. The underlying biochemical mechanisms of such conditions are not fully known. Just as in the case of the withdrawal syndrome, the biological basis of physical dependence is also unclear. However, it is generally assumed that the presence of alcohol in nerve tissue results in a gradual development of adaptive changes in the functional state of the CNS. Withdrawal of ethanol results in a functional imbalance, thus producing what is called the withdrawal reaction.

A. POSSIBLE ROLE OF RNA AND PROTEIN IN TOLERANCE

Although a precise neurochemical mechanism for either physical depen-dence or the withdrawal reaction cannot be offered at the present time, learned behavior has been found to be correlated at physiological and chemi-cal levels. In the case of morphine tolerance, Ungar and his associates

TABLE VIII

EFFECT OF ETHANOL WITHDRAWAL ON PRESUMPTIVE NEUROTRANSMITTERS IN MOUSE BRAIN[a]

Neurotransmitter	Days after withdrawal from ethanol							
	0	1		2		4	
Norepinephrine (μg/gm)[b] (6)	1.10 ± 0.12	1.30 ± 0.10	$P < .02$	1.34 ± 0.10	$P < .02$	1.35 ± 0.10	$P < .02$
Acetylcholine (μmole/gm) (6)	0.009 ± 0.001	0.009 ± 0.001	N.S.	0.01 ± 0.001	N.S.	0.013 ± 0.002	$P < .02$
GABA (μmole/gm) (6)	3.95 ± 0.30	3.85 ± 0.30	N.S.	3.20 ± 0.32	$P < .02$	3.20 ± 0.32	$P < .02$

[a] Brain preparations frozen in liquid nitrogen were used for determination of the levels of neurotransmitters. The values are means ± S.E.M. for the number of animals given in parentheses. From Rawat (1974b).
[b] Per gram fresh weight of brain.

demonstrated that morphine tolerance, which they call "an elementary form of memory" could be transferred from one animal to another. This hypothesis could be valid if the information pertaining to tolerance is recorded in a chemical code as suggested by Ungar (1966). Support of this kind of hypothesis also comes from the work of Cox and Osman (1970), in which they suggest that the synthesis of new RNA and protein in the brain is essential to the development of tolerance of morphine in rats.

In a recent study we observed that the brains of some alcohol-dependent mice showed an additional band of protein when subjected to polyacrylamide gel electrophoresis either in the presence or absence of sodium dodecyl sulfate (Fig. 5). This band of protein was not observed in the brains of control pair-fed animals, and was not found in the brain of all ethanol-dependent animals. The comparative electrophoretic migration of standard bovine serum albumin (BAS) suggests that this protein has a molecular weight of 80,000.

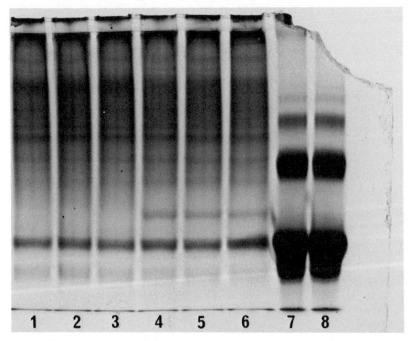

Fig. 5. Electrophoretic pattern of brain proteins from control and alcohol-fed mice. The brains from chronic ethanol-fed (4 weeks) and corresponding controls were homogenized, and after sedimentation of nuclei and mitochondria the supernatant fraction was subjected to polyacrylamide gel electrophoresis. Bands 4–6 represent alcohol brains, and bands 1–3, control brains. The three alcohol strips showed an additional band which was not seen in the three control strips. Bands 7 and 8 represent BSA standards.

At the moment, however, we have no evidence indicating that it is involved in the development of alcohol dependence. It is interesting in this connection that several agents that interfere with RNA or protein synthesis, such as actinomycin cyclohexamide, puromycin, and 5-flurouracil, have been found to abolish or reduce the development of tolerance to morphine (Cox and Osman, 1970).

B. Possible Role of Neurotransmitters in Addiction

A hypothesis has recently been put forth by Alivisatos and Arora (1975), according to which alkaloid formation occurs *in vivo* at the membrane level *in situ* through interaction of indolamines and/or catecholamines with the products of polypeptide chains, and thereby modifies the properties of plasmalemmal membranes. This hypothesis has been advanced in view of the presence of an enzyme in beef and mouse brain. This enzyme is capable of oxidizing lysyl residues of the polypeptide chain, at receptor sites, to corresponding aldehydes or semialdehydes. Serotonin binding involves the formation of a Schiff's base at the binding site. The formation of an aldehyde or semialdehyde by lysyl oxidase at the receptor protein interferes with the tertiary configuration of the protein, thereby modifying the properties of the membrane. It has been suggested that this kind of molecular mechanism plays some part in the development of tolerance. One must remember that this is only a working hypothesis and, before any conclusions can be drawn regarding its validity, such a mechanism will have to be demonstrated to occur *in vivo*.

C. Possible Role of False Neurotransmitters

The concept of false adrenergic transmitters can be most clearly expressed in terms of nonspecific amine substitution at nerve endings. Kopin (1971) explored this concept in detail. The major criteria for the indentification of false transmitters are similar to those for transmitters per se. False transmitters, although not normally present in significant quantities in nerve endings, can be made to accumulate at the same site in nerve endings as physiological transmitters. Muscholl and Maitre (1963) demonstrated that γ-methylnorepinephrine is released by sympathetic nerve stimulation from isolated rabbit hearts pretreated with γ-methyldopa. Studies by Murphy (1972) showed the possibility of a "physiological" exchange of transmitter in platelets obtained from mentally depressed and normal humans.

Some evidence has started to accumulate relating to the possible role of false neurotransmitters in physical dependence on alcohol (Robbins, 1968; Davis and Walsh, 1970). As mentioned earlier, ethanol is primarily con-

verted to acetaldehyde which is further metabolized through aldehyde dehydrogenase. Saturation of this system leads to an excessive accumulation
of aromatic aldehydes (biogenic aldehydes), which are normally produced
from endogenous catecholamines or indolamines such as dopamine and
serotonin. Condensation of either biogenic aldehydes or acteladehyde with
catecholamines and/or indolamines leads to the production of a variety of
substituted alkaloids, mostly tetrahydropapaveroline, tetrahydrocarboline, or
tetrahydroisoquinoline. Biosynthesis of such alkaloids in humans during alcohol intake, and the functioning of these substances as false transmitters, may
be possible but have never been documented. By interfering with adrenergic
mechanisms in the brain and in the periphery, the biosynthesis of alkaloids
could then be capable of altering mood and behavior, thus suggesting a possible role in alcohol intoxication and alcohol dependence. Although suggestions of a cause-effect relationship between the possible metabolic products
of biogenic amine and addiction have been put forth, the current evidence is
somewhat preliminary. An alternative hypothesis has been proposed by
Alivisatos and Arora (1975), according to which alkaloid formation occurs
in vivo at sites at the membrane level through interaction of indolamines
and/or catecholamines with the products of polypeptide chains, thereby
modifying the properties of plasmalemmal membranes.

VIII. Neurochemical Aspects of the Fetal Alcohol Syndrome

Greek and Roman mythology recorded the association between heavy
drinking by pregnant mothers and developmental defects in their offspring.
In the early nineteenth century increased rates of abortions and stillbirths were
reported (cf. Jones and Smith, 1973) among mothers who chronically abused
alcohol. It was also observed in these studies that the frequency of epilepsy
in the surviving offspring also increased. Since then more clinical reports have
appeared, which suggest an association between chronic alcohol consumption
by mothers and serious physical abnormalities in their children.

Recently there has been a new surge of interest in the effects of chronic
ethanol consumption by pregnant mothers and its effects on their offspring
both in animals (Sandor and Amels, 1971) and in humans (Jones and
Smith, 1973; Jones *et al.*, 1973, 1974). Human studies have shown that
children born in chronic alcoholic mothers show developmental delay and
a prenatal-onset growth deficiency. Cardiovascular defects along with mental deficiency have also been observed in these offspring.

Although morphological and behavioral abnormalities have been observed
in the offspring of alcoholic mothers, the precise biochemical and neurochemical mechanisms of the so-called fetal alcohol syndrome are not known.

In an attempt to elucidate the neurochemical mechanisms responsible for the mental deficiency observed in the offspring of chronic alcoholic mothers, the animal model has been employed in our laboratory.

A. Effect of Maternal Ethanol Intake on Fetal Protein Metabolism

Studies with ethanol showed that its acute or chronic administration causes alterations in cerebral intermediary metabolism (Rawat and Kuriyama, 1972a; Veloso et al., 1972; Rawat et al., 1973) and neurotransmitter metabolism (Rawat, 1974b). Recently it was noted that acute or chronic ethanol administration resulted in an alteration in the rate of protein synthesis in adult mouse and rat brain (Kuriyama et al., 1971; Noble and Tewari, 1973). Prolonged ethanol consumption by pregnant women has led to several abnormalities in childbirth, in neurological signs in the fetus, and even in the morphology of the newborn baby (Jones et al., 1973, 1974). These symptoms have been collectively described as the fetal alcohol syndrome. A precise biochemical mechanism which might lead to such alterations is not known at present. Recently, it (Rawat, 1975a) was shown that chronic ethanol consumption by pregnant rats resulted in a decrease in the rate of cerebral protein synthesis in the fetus. In this study, two groups of pregnant albino rats were fed a liquid Metrecal diet consisting of 61% (v/v) commercial Metrecal and 6% (v/v) ethanol or isocaloric sucrose. The animals were pair-fed. Chronic ethanol feeding resulted in about 30% decrease in the rate of [14C]leucine incorporation by fetal cerebral ribosomes. The inhibitory effect of ethanol on protein synthesis was found to be concentration-dependent. It was further observed that the capacity of both ribosomes and pH-5 enzymes to synthesize proteins was decreased in fetal brains from alcohol-fed mothers as compared to those from corresponding sucrose-fed mothers (Table IX).

Effect on Neonatal Protein Synthesis

The effect of chronic ethanol consumption (for 2 weeks) by lactating mothers on the rate of [14C]leucine incorporation into the brains of suckling neonates has been investigated. These rates were compared with protein synthesis from control neonatal brains. The experimental results showed (Rawat, 1975b) that the rates of [14C]leucine incorporation into neonatal brains in alcoholic groups were about 60% lower than in the corresponding controls. The defect was found in both ribosomal and pH-5 enzyme fractions. In order to ensure that under these conditions actual rates of [14C]leucine incorporation were being studied, several omission experiments were performed. Pretreatment of the neonates with cycloheximide, an inhibitor of

TABLE IX

EFFECT OF MATERNAL ETHANOL CONSUMPTION ON [14C]LEUCINE
INCORPORATION IN FETAL AND NEONATAL RIBOSOMES
AND pH-5 ENZYME FRACTIONS[a]

	[14C]Leucine incorporation	
	Picomoles per minute per milligram of pH-5 enzyme and ribosomal protein	Picomoles per minute per milligram of pH-5 enzyme protein
Control, fetus	5.76 ± 0.8 (8)	9.8 ± 1.0 (8)
Alcohol, fetus	3.90 ± 0.7 (8)	4.8 ± 0.5 (8)
Control, neonate	8.07 ± 1.0 (8)	15.9 ± 1.0 (8)
Alcohol, neonate	3.40 ± 0.9 (8)	6.2 ± 0.5 (8)

[a] Incorporation of [14C]leucine into cerebral ribosomes in the presence of its corresponding pH-5 enzyme is shown in the second column; incorporation without ribosomes, only in the presence of pH-5 enzyme is shown in the third column. The results are expressed as means ± S.E.M. for the number of observations in parentheses. From Rawat (1975c).

protein synthesis, resulted in inhibition of the rate of cerebral protein synthesis. The inhibitory effect of ethanol on the rate of protein synthesis in the neonatal brain is shown in Table X.

B. EFFECT OF MATERNAL ETHANOL INTAKE ON NEONATAL BRAIN RNA AND DNA

The effect of chronic ethanol consumption (for 2 weeks) by lactating mothers on steady-state concentrations of RNA and DNA was investigated

TABLE X

EFFECT OF MIXING VARIOUS BRAIN FRACTIONS FROM FETUSES
FROM ETHANOL-FED AND CONTROL RATS

	Picomoles of [14C]leucine incorporated per milligram of protein per 30 minutes	
Source of cerebral pH-5 enzyme	Control	Ethanol
Control	173.6 ± 15 (12)	123 ± 11 (12)
Ethanol	110.0 ± 10 (12)	92 ± 8 (12)

[a] Cerebral pH enzyme fractions and ribosomes were prepared from control and ethanol fetuses. The rates of [14C]leucine incorporation by ribosomes from both control and ethanol-fed groups were studied in the presence of pH-5 enzyme fractions from control fetuses and ethanol fetuses. The results are expressed as means ± S.E.M. for the number of observations in parentheses. From Rawat (1975c).

in the brains of suckling neonates. Ethanol consumption by lactating mothers resulted in a decrease in both RNA and DNA content in the brains of newborns when compared with the corresponding controls. The mean content of total DNA phosphate (DNA-P) in the brains of newborn rats suckling on sucrose-fed mothers was 96 μg/gm of brain, and in the ethanol-fed group it was 55 μg/gm of brain. The mean content of ribonucleic acid phosphate (RNA-P) in the sucrose-fed group was 100 μg/gm of brain and decreased to 78 μg/gm of brain in the alcoholic group. The already observed inhibition of tRNA formation in the ethanol-fed group is in accord with the decreased in total RNA content in the brain.

C. Effect of Maternal Ethanol Consumption on Fetal and Neonatal Neurotransmitters

One of the frequently observed occurrences in alcoholic women is breech birth. It seems that, because of alterations in brain inhibitory and excitatory neurotransmitters, the neurological signs in the baby become abnormal. This leads to a breech birth, in which the baby is born feet first instead of head first. In an attempt to understand the mechanism at the molecular level that might result in such abnormal neurological signs, a study was undertaken in our laboratory (Rawat, 1976a). It was observed that chronic ethanol feeding of pregnant rats resulted in alterations in the steady-state concentration of several neurotransmitters in the fetal brain. Chronic ethanol consumption by pregnant animals on a Metrecal diet resulted in a significant increase in the cerebral content of GABA in the fetal brain at various ages of gestation. The cerebral glutamate content was also found to be increased in this study. Although the cerebral serotonin content was not significantly altered, the norepinephrine concentration showed a significant increase in the ethanol-fed group.

Ethanol consumption by lactating mothers also resulted in significant changes in the steady-state concentration of several presumptive neurotransmitters in the neonatal brain. Neonates suckling on alcohol-fed mothers were examined from 0 to 12 days after birth. As in the case of fetuses, in neonates also, ethanol led to an increase in the cerebral content of GABA, glutamic acid, and norepinephrine. However, in contrast to the results obtained with fetal brains, in neonatal brains the steady-state concentration of serotonin was increased until 10 days after birth, after which time it started to return to normal (Table XI). Chronic ethanol consumption by pregnant or lactating animals resulted in a significant decrease in the steady-state concentration of acetylcholine in the brains of both fetuses and neonates. In addition to measurements of the steady-state concentration of neurotransmitters in fetal and neonatal brains, the effects of ethanol on some of the enzymes involved in the synthesis and breakdown of neurotransmitters were

TABLE XI

EFFECTS OF MATERNAL ETHANOL CONSUMPTION ON THE CONCENTRATION OF SEROTONIN, NOREPINEPHRINE, AND ACETYLCHOLINE IN FETAL AND NEONATAL BRAINS[a]

	Fetal, 3 days		Neonatal, 6 days	
Metabolite	Control	Ethanol	Control	Ethanol
Serotonin (μg/gm brain)	0.21 ± 0.03	0.20 ± 0.03 (6)	0.71 ± 0.07	0.90 ± 0.08 (8)
Norepinephrine (μg/gm brain)	0.09 ± 0.008	0.13 ± 0.009 (6)	0.68 ± 0.05	0.79 ± 0.05 (8)
Acetylcholine (μmole/gm brain)	4.0 ± 0.008	3.0 ± 0.007 (6)	8.0 ± 0.01	6.0 ± 0.01 (8)

[a] Brain levels of serotonin, norepinephrine, and acetylcholine were determined in preparations frozen in liquid nitrogen. Acetylcholine was determined enzymically. Serotonin and norepinephrine were determined fluorimetrically. The values are means ± S.E.M. for the number of experiments given in parentheses. From Rawat (1976a).

also examined. The activity of glutamate decarboxylase and GABA transferase in fetal as well as neonatal brains was significantly decreased in the alcohol-fed group as compared to the sucrose-fed group.

The decrease in the activity of these enzyme is in accordance with a decrease in the rate of protein synthesis. In the brains of neonates suckling on alcohol-fed mothers, it was previously observed that numerous drugs including minor tranquilizers, alcohol, and nicotine, are excreted in the maternal milk (Vorherr, 1974). The development changes in ADH activity are shown in Fig. 6.

In addition to changes in brain metabolism, other changes in hepatic intermediary metabolism were also observed in fetuses and neonates of chronically ethanol-fed rats (Rawat, 1976b). The details of such changes in the liver are beyond the scope of this article but may have severe consequences for the total picture of the fetal alcohol syndrome.

In the new and developing field of fetal alcohol syndrome there is urgent need for further biochemical studies to understand the neurological defects in the offspring of alcoholic mothers. The observed prenatal growth deficiency in these babies shows that factors other than simple nutritional deprivation are involved in "fetal alcohol syndrome." It is suggested that alcohol exerts a direct effect on the fetus.

IX. Factors That Affect the Metabolism of Alcohol

Since alcohol intoxication and alcohol withdrawal symptoms are closely related to the presence or absence of alcohol, it will be important to under-

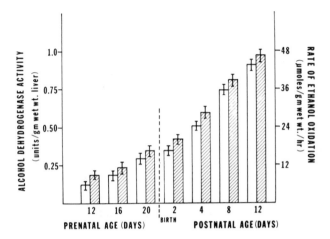

Fig. 6. Developmental changes in hepatic ADH activity. The developmental changes in the activity of ADH and the capacity of the liver to oxidize ethanol were studied in rats. Rat fetuses were removed from pregnant animals by an abdominal operation at different times of gestation. ADH activity was assayed on liver homogenates, and the rate of ethanol oxidation was determined by incubating rat liver slices. The open bars represent ADH activity, and the shaded bars represent the rate of ethanol oxidation (Rawat, 1976b).

stand the factors that influence the metabolism of ethanol. Furthermore, the symptoms of alcohol withdrawal also seem to be closely related to the intoxicant effect, because the more profound the intoxication the more severe the withdrawal symptoms.

For more than half a century, clinicians and basic scientists have been interested in testing and evaluating a large number of chemical compounds, hormones, and physical measures to accelerate the rate at which ethanol is metabolized in the body. For a detailed discussion the reader is referred to an earlier review by Rawat (1969a). It is generally the clinician who quite frequently comes across cases in which rapid removal of ethanol from the systems of patients is imperative for their physical well-being. However, before listing the compounds that have been tested for this purpose, it would be helpful to understand the factors that act as rate-limiting steps in the metabolism of ethanol.

A. Rate-Limiting Steps in Alcohol Metabolism

In spite of extensive investigation of the problem of alcohol metabolism, there does not seem to exist general agreement regarding rate-limiting steps in the intact organism. Since three separate entities, namely, ethanol, NAD, and ADH, participate in the oxidation of ethanol to acetaldehyde, it would be expected that the availability of any one of the reaction components, or the removal of the reaction product would limit the reaction.

Several investigations have pointed to the possibility that, under *in vivo* conditions, the activity of ADH is not the sole factor that determines the rate of alcohol oxidation (Smith *et al.*, 1957), nor does the removal of acetaldehyde limit the reaction (Rawat, 1973).

At the present time it seems probable that the enzyme systems responsible for the transport of hydrogen equivalents from NADH (generated during ethanol metabolism in the cytoplasmic compartment) to the mitochondria may be rate-limiting (Rawat and Kuriyama, 1972b). A more likely possibility is the oxidation capacity of the mitochondrial chain, perhaps because of the limited availability of ADP. Further exploration of the latter probability is needed to understand the rate-limiting step in alcohol metabolism.

B. EFFECT OF HORMONES ON ALCOHOL METABOLISM

The substances that have been employed over the last several years to accelerate the rate of ethanol metabolism in the body can be broadly classified either as hormones or chemical substances. Several of the hormones, including insulin, thyroxine, glucagon, and epinephrine, have been used with different degrees of success.

1. *Effect of Insulin*

Reports that insulin accelerates alcohol metabolism have attracted considerable attention, especially with respect to a possible relationship between alcohol and carbohydrate metabolism. However, the literature on the influence of insulin on alcohol oxidation is controversial. Insulin has been reported to no effect on the disappearance of alcohol in dogs, normal human subjects, rabbits, and diabetic patients. However, some data have indicated that insulin increases alcohol metabolism in rabbits, dogs, and humans (cf. Rawat, 1969a). In our laboratory, administration of insulin was observed to increase significantly the metabolism of ethanol in slices of rat liver. It was also observed in this study that a deficiency of insulin results in an increase in free fatty acids (FFA) which inhibit ADH activity (Rawat, 1969a). A decrease in the level of circulating FFA after insulin administration would relieve the inhibition of ADH, and this would consequently increase the metabolism of alcohol.

2. *Effect of Thyroxine*

Claims have been made repeatedly that administration of thyroid hormone accelerates the metabolism of ethanol. Recent studies on the effect of thyroid hormones at the level of enzymes in the liver made reinvestigation of this problem desirable (Rawat and Lundquist, 1968). The observation that the activity of mitochondrial α-glycerophosphate dehydrogenase (Lee and Lardy, 1965) increases markedly after thyroid hormone administration was of special interest. This change is assumed to facilitate the oxidation of extra-mitochondrial hydrogen in the mitochondrial respiratory chain, through the proposed α-glycerophosphate cycle. However, it was observed that neither the administration of thyroxine nor its deficiency resulted in a change in the rate of alcohol oxidation. This suggests that either the rate of hydrogen transport into the mitochondria, or the α-glycerophosphate cycle, is of little importance in the oxidation of ethanol. On the basis of these observations the use of thyroid hormone for the treatment of alcohol intoxication or to accelerate alcohol metabolism does not seem to be very effective (Table XII).

3. Effect of Glucagon

Glucagon is another hormone capable of making gross alterations in carbohydrate metabolism. Although glucagon was found to increase the rate of alcohol oxidation in rat liver slices, the increase was not very significant (Rawat, 1970b). In view of this, the use of glucagon as a therapeutic agent for intoxicated persons and to accelerate alcohol metabolism is not very promising. Two other hormones, epinephrine and glucocorticoids, have been tested, but without much success (Rawat, 1969a).

TABLE XII

EFFECTS OF HORMONE ADMINISTRATION AND THEIR DEFICIENCIES ON THE RATE OF HEPATIC ALCOHOL OXIDATION IN LIVER SLICES[a]

Treatment	Addition	Rate of ethanol oxidation (μmoles per gm per hour)
Control		43.5 ± 1.8 (15)
Thyroxine		38.8 ± 4.4 (15)
Thiouracil-treated		42.1 ± 3.0 (6)
Glucagon, 35 mg		65.0 ± 6.5 (4)
Control (saline-injected)		43.8 ± 1.3 (6)
	Glucose (11 mM)	44.9 ± 1.8 (6)
	Fructose (11 mM)	51.0 ± 2.5 (6)
Insulin, 5U		59.6 ± 2.8 (6)
Alloxan diabetic, 60 mg/kg		35.4 ± 1.7 (6)
AIS		35.1 ± 1.5 (6)

[a] Livers were taken from animals with either the hyper- or the hypo-condition of the hormone. In the hyper-condition one of the hormones is injected, and in the hypo-condition compounds are given that decrease the level of the hormone in the body. Incubation medium consisted of Krebs/Henseliet bicarbonate buffer, ethanol (4 mM), and glucose or fructose. Samples of incubation medium were analyzed for alcohol at 15-minute intervals. From Rawat (1969a).

C. Effect of Chemical Substances on Alcohol Metabolism

Much indirect evidence has been presented over the past several years to suggest a possible relationship between alcohol and carbohydrate metabolism. Animals kept on a high-carbohydrate diet and consequently having a higher carbohydrate metabolism generally have a higher metabolic rate as compared to animals kept on a low-carbohydrate diet. It has also been suggested that blood sugar levels have an effect on the rate of blood alcohol disappearance. However, a direct relationship has not been established.

1. *Effect of Glucose*

As early as 1958 Lundquist and Wolthers observed that administration of glucose had a very slight effect on the rate of alcohol metabolism. It was observed that glucose administration led to a small increase in the rate of blood alcohol elimination. In an attempt to test the effectiveness and possible mechanism of action of glucose on the rate of alcohol metabolism, studies were performed with slices of liver (Rawat, 1969b). In these studies liver preparations from animals with a different hormonal status were incubated with glucose (11 mM). The rate of alcohol disappearance in liver slices from normal, insulin-treated, alloxan-diabetic, and antiinsulin serum-treated rats was studied at 15 minute intervals for 1 hour. Observations showed that the addition of glucose did not have a significant effect on the rate of ethanol oxidation in the liver slices.

We recently investigated the effect of glucose on alcoholic patients. In this study the effect of oral glucose administration on the rate of blood alcohol disappearance was investigated in both normal and alcoholic subjects. It was observed that glucose (0.5–1.0 gm/kg body weight) had no significant accelerating effect on the rate of blood alcohol disappearance after the blood alcohol level reached a peak. The ineffectiveness of glucose in increasing the rate of alcohol disappearance was observed in undernourished patients as well as in well-nourished patients.

2. *Effect of Fructose*

Of the substances investigated to obtain an accelerating effect on the rate of alcohol oxidation, fructose was found to be most effective. It was observed that the addition of fructose to normal rat liver slices resulted in a significant increase in the rate of alcohol metabolism (Thieden and Lundquist, 1967; Rawat, 1969b). Some studies have been reported in which this effect was not observed, perhaps as a result of insufficient quantities of fructose being employed. In most studies, including that of Lundquist and Walthers (1958), oral administration of fructose was observed to increase the rate of blood alcohol disappearance. In our alcohol ward, in a recent study on the effect of fructose on the rate of blood alcohol disappearance, we observed that fructose was very effective in bringing intoxicated persons to sobriety. The effect of oral fructose administration (0.5–1.0 gm/kg body weight) was studied in about 100 patients, some of whom had been admitted in an intoxicated state. Oral administration of fructose resulted in an increase of about 40–50% in the rate of alcohol disappearance from the blood in 96% of the patients. Orally administered fructose showed a lag period of 30 minutes in its accelerating effect. Presumably, this time was required for its absorption from the intestine. In all our studies, the effect of fructose was studied after blood alcohol levels reached a peak. The effect of fructose is exerted largely on the oxidation–reduction state of the liver (Rawat and Menahan, 1975). In accordance with the observed effect of fructose on the liver, in patients with alcoholic fatty liver or liver cirrhosis, fructose was found either to be ineffective or to have a minimum effect on the rate of alcohol disappearance. The effect of fructose on the rate of blood alcohol disappearance is shown in Fig. 7.

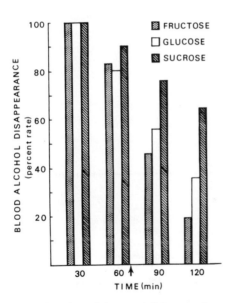

Fig. 7. Effect of orally administered fructose, glucose, and sucrose on blood alcohol disappearance. The effect of the above-mentioned compounds on the rate of blood alcohol clearance was studied in humans. Blood alcohol disappearance was measured with and without the administration of any of the above-mentioned compounds. After the blood alcohol levels reached a peak, fructose, glucose, or sucrose, was given orally. Blood samples were taken at 30-minute intervals, and the rate of blood alcohol disappearance was compared in the same individual with or without administration of the chemical compound.

Mechanism of the Fructose Effect. Various suggestions have been put forward to explain in biochemical terms the effect of fructose in accelerating alcohol metabolism. Fructose may exert a direct effect by acting as an hydrogen acceptor through the reaction of sorbitol dehydrogenase. Fructose would be reduced to sorbitol, leading to oxidation of NADH and thus generating NAD for alcohol oxidation.

However, the effect of fructose in accelerating alcohol metabolism can not be fully explained on the basis of sorbitol formation. Holzer and Schneider (1955) reported that the formation of glycerol from glyceraldehyde may be mediated by an ADH–NADH complex formed during the oxidation of ethanol. As mentioned before, it was shown that the dissociation of this complex may be the rate-limiting step in the oxidation of ethanol. This step would be circumvented by the reduction of glyceraldehyde to glylcerol by the ADH-NADH complex. The effectiveness of fructose is partially due to the formation of free glyceraldehyde (Fig. 8.).

3. Effect of Pyruvate and Amino Acids

The possibility of a coupled oxidation-reduction of alcohol and pyruvate in a coenzyme-linked reaction has been suggested. In such a mechanism the oxidation of alcohol and the reduction of pyruvate would take place through

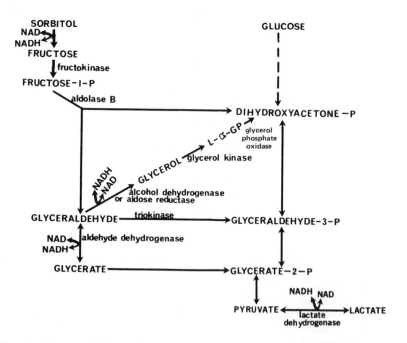

Fig. 8. The metabolic pathway of fructose in the liver (Rawat and Menahan, 1975).

NAD. In the presence of both these substrates, their respective enzymes, and NAD, hydrogen would transfer from alcohol to pyruvate via enzymes until an equilibrium is reached. The net result of such a reaction would be the oxidation of alcohol to acetaldehyde and the reduction to lactate. In our laboratory, pyruvate in moderate amounts increases the metabolism of alcohol (Rawat, 1972). However, the suitability of this compound for increasing alcohol metabolism in human subjects still remains to be tested.

The production of pyruvate through transamination of alanine in the liver is the main reason for employing alanine for rapid alcohol detoxification. Although in our animal studies we found both pyruvate and alanine to be quite effective in accelerating the rate of alcohol metabolism, in human studies oral alanine administration was found to be without any significant effect.

D. Effect of Various Substances on Withdrawal

Several of the chemical compounds that have been tested to accelerate alcohol metabolism have also been recently employed in our laboratory to study their effects on the alcohol withdrawal as measured by several target symptoms, e.g., agitation, confusion, convulsive episodes, sweating, hallucinations, and delirium. Withdrawal symptoms were found to be pronounced in withdrawal patients who were malnourished. In well-nourished patients, the severity of withdrawal symptoms was not so great. It was found in this study that, both in undernourished and well-nourished patients, oral administration of glucose, sucrose, or alanine did not have a significant effect on any of the above-mentioned symptoms.

Effect of Fructose in the Management of Delirium Tremens

In a recent study on about 50 male patients we observed that alcohol withdrawal symptoms were much more severe in patients who were chronic alcoholics and were undernourished. This observation led us to test the effect of oral fructose administration on alcohol withdrawal symptoms and delirium tremens. Our studies indicated that the administration of fructose (1 gm/kg body weight, orally) resulted in a significantly faster recovery of the patient from withdrawal. Overall symptoms, such as shakes, time taken for full orientation, fits, and delirium tremens, showed much less severity, and faster recovery of the patient was observed, as compared either to no treatment or to glucose treatment. This apparent contradiction that fructose, on the one hand, accelerates the rate of removal of alcohol in an intoxicated patient and, on the other hand, prevents the severity of alcohol withdrawal symptoms led us to investigate the nature of the fructose effect on delirium tremens. It was observed that fructose accelerated the rate of acetaldehyde removal from the blood. It seems to us that the ability of fructose to prevent severe alcohol withdrawal symptoms may be related to the possibility that it accelerates the removal of residual acetaldehyde from the system of patients in withdrawal. Fructose in combination with oral thiamine hydrochloride administration was found to be more effective in the management of delirium tremens than fructose alone. A therapeutic effect of fructose on delirium tremens has also been observed by Dalton and Duncan (1970).

X. Summary

From the detailed evidence presented in this article on various aspects of the effects of alcohol on the CNS, it is evident that the most profound effects are on the nerve cell membrane. Although there is no generally agreed neurochemical mechanism which directly explains the intoxication effect of alcohol on the brain, it seems probable that the interference of alcohol in the normal functioning of the sodium-potassium pump leads to changes in the transmembrane potential.

However, the other major possibility is that alcohol impairs the normal functioning of the brain by interfering with metabolic processes in the neurons. This could be caused either by disturbing the homeostasis of the metabolic pathways or by impairing the transmission of nerve impulses by interference in the release, storage, and metabolism of neurotransmitters.

Before definite answers can be provided regarding the mechanism of alcohol addiction and withdrawal and the treatment of alcoholism, it is important that fundamental knowledge regarding the mechanism of intoxication be obtained. Although the existing methodology is limiting, further organized efforts will have to be made to resolve this basic problem.

ACKNOWLEDGMENTS

The original studies reported in this paper from the author's laboratory were supported by grants from the Ohio State Department of Health and the National Institute of Mental Health. The author wishes to express his sincere thanks to the postdoctoral fellows, students, and research assistants who have collaborated on different aspects of this study. The secretarial assistance of Barbara A. Cheney and Joan Andrews is gratefully acknowledged.

REFERENCES

Aebi, H., Stocker, F., and Eberhardt, M. (1963). *Biochem. Z.* **336,** 526–544.
Åkeson, Å. (1964). *Biochem. Biophys. Res. Commun.* **17,** 211–214.
Albers, R. W., and Koval, G. J. (1961). *Biochim. Biophys. Acta* **52,** 29–35.
Albers, R. W., and Salvador, R. A. (1958). *Science* **128,** 359–360.
Alivisatos, S. G. A., and Arora, R. C. (1975). *Adv. Exp. Med. Biol.* **56,** 255–261.
Ammon, H. P. T., and Estler, C. (1968). *J. Pharm. Pharmacol.* **20,** 164–165.

Ammon, H. P. T., Estler, C., and Heim, F. (1965). *Arch. Int. Pharmacodyn. Ther.* **154**, 108–121.

Ammon, H. P. T., Estler, C., and Heim, F. (1969). *Biochem. Pharmacol.* **18**, 29–33.

Anderson, R. A., and Schulman, M. P. (1974). *Trans. Am. Soc. Neurochem.* **5**, 91 (abstr).

Anton, A. H. (1965). *Clin. Pharmacol. Ther.* **6**, 462–469.

Armstrong, C. M., and Binstock, L. (1964). *J. Gen. Physiol.* **48**, 265–277.

Ashford, C. P., and Dixon, K. C. (1935). *Biochem. J.* **29**, 157–168.

Battey, L. L., Heyman, A., and Patterson, J. L., Jr. (1953). *J. Am. Med. Assoc.* **152**, 6–10.

Beer, C. T., and Quastel, J. H. (1958). *Can. J. Biochem. Physiol.* **36**, 548–556.

Bergman, M. C., Klee, M. W., and Faber, D. S. (1974). *Pfluegers Arch.* **348**, 139–153.

Bignami, A., and Palladini, G. (1966). *Nature (London)* **209**, 413–414.

Blaschko, H. (1952). *Pharmacol. Rev.* **4**, 415–458.

Blum, K. (1972). *Curr. Ther. Res.* **14**, 415–458.

Bonnichsen, R. K., and Wassén, A. M. (1948). *Arch. Biochem.* **18**, 361–370.

Bonnycastle, D. D., Bonnycastle, M. D., and Anderson, E. G. (1962). *Pharmacol. Exp. Ther.* **135**, 17–20.

Brady, R. O., Formica, J. V., and Koval, G. J. (1958). *J. Biol. Chem.* **233**, 1072–1076.

Bronaugh, R. L., and Erwin, V. G. (1973). *J. Neurochem.* **21**, 809–815.

Buchel, L. (1953). *Anesth. Analg.* **10**, 1–15.

Burbridge, T. N., Sutherland, V. C., Hine, C. H., and Simon, A. (1959). *J. Pharmacol. Exp. Ther.* **126**, 70–75.

Carlson, A., and Lindquist, M. (1973). *J. Pharm. Pharmacol.* **25**, 437–440.

Carpenter, D. O. (1970). *Comp. Biochem. Physiol.* **35**, 371–385.

Chance, B. (1947). *Acta Chem. Scand.* **1**, 236–267.

Chance, B., and Oshino, N. (1971). *Biochem. J.* **122**, 225–233.

Cherrick, G. R., and Leevy, C. N. (1965). *Biochim. Biophys. Acta* **107**, 29–37.

Corrodi, H., Fuxe, K., and Hokfelt, T. (1966). *J. Pharm. Pharmacol.* **18**, 821–823.

Cox, B. M., and Osman, O. H. (1970). *Br. J. Pharmacol.* **38**, 157–170.

Dalton, M. S., and Duncan, D. W. (1970). *Med. J. Aust.* **1**, 659–661.

Dalziel, K. (1958). *Acta Chem. Scand.* **12**, 459–464.

Davis, V. E., and Walsh, M. J. (1970). *Science* **167**, 1005–1007.

Davis, V. E., Brown, H., Huff, J. A., and Cashaw, J. L. (1967). *J. Lab. Clin. Med.* **69**, 787–799.

Deitrich, R. A. (1966). *Biochem. Pharmacol.* **15**, 1911–1922.

Dewan, J. G. (1943). *Q. J. Stud. Alcohol* **4**, 353–361.

Duritz, G., and Truitt, E. B., Jr. (1966). *Biochem. Pharmacol.* **15**, 711–721.

Erwin, V. G., and Deitrich, R. A. (1966). *J. Biol. Chem.* **241**, 3533–3539.

Feinstein, R. N., Braun, J. T., and Howard, J. B. (1967). *Arch. Biochem. Biophys.* **120**, 165–169.

Forsander, O. A. (1966). *Biochem. J.* **98**, 244–247.

Freund, G., and O'Hollaren, P. (1965). *J. Lipid Res.* **6**, 471–477.

Gatenbeck, S., and Ehrenberg, L. (1953). *Ark. Kemi* **5**, 333–340.

Glowinski, J., Kopin, I. J., and Axelrod, J. (1965). *J. Neurochem.* **12**, 25–30.

Gordon, E. R. (1967). *Can. J. Physiol. Pharmacol.* **45**, 915–918.

Greengard, P., McAfee, D. A., and Kebabian, J. W. (1972). *Adv. Cyclic Nucleotide Res.* **1**, 337–355.

170 ARUN K. RAWAT

Grenell, R. G. (1957). In "Alcoholism—Basic Aspects and Treatment" (H. P. Himwich, ed.), Publ. No. 47, pp. 7–17. Am. Assoc. Adv. Sci., Washington, D.C.
Gross, G. J., and Woodbury, D. M. (1972). J. Pharmacol. Exp. Ther. 181, 257–272.
Gupta, N. K., and Robinson, W. G. (1960). J. Biol. Chem. 235, 1609–1612.
Gupta, N. K., and Robinson, W. G. (1966). Biochim. Biophys. Acta 118, 431–434.
Gursey, D., and Olson, R. E. (1960). Proc. Soc. Exp. Biol. Med. 104, 280–281.
Hakkinen, H. M., and Kulonen, E. (1963). Nature (London) 198, 995.
Heim, F. (1950). Naunyn-Schmiedeberg's Arch. Exp. Pathol. Pharmakol. 210, 16–22.
Himwich, H. E., Nahum, L. H., Rakietin, N., Fazekas, J. F., DuBois, D., and Gilden, E. F. (1933). J. Am. Med. Assoc. 100, 651–654.
Hodgkin, A. L., and Keynes, R. D. (1955). J. Physiol. (London) 128, 28–60.
Hoffman, G. E., and Schulman, M. P. (1973). Pharmacologist 15, 160 (abstr.).
Hoffman, J. F. (1962). Circulation 26, 1201–1213.
Hokin, L. E. (1969). J. Gen. Physiol. 54, 527s–542s.
Holzer, H., and Schneider, S. (1955). Klin. Wochenschr. 33, 1006–1009.
Hornykiewicz, O. (1966). Pharmacol. Rev. 18, 925–964.
Hunt, W. A., and Majchrowicz, E. (1974). Brain Res. 72, 181–184.
Israel, M., and Kuriyama, K. (1971). Life Sci. 10, 591–599.
Israel, Y., Kalant, H., and Laufer, I. (1965). Biochem. Pharmacol. 14, 1803–1814.
Israel, Y., Kalant, H., and LeBlanc, A. E. (1966). Biochem. J. 100, 27–33.
Israel, Y., Carmichael, F. J., and Macdonald, J. A. (1973). Ann. N.Y. Acad. Sci. 215, 38–47.
Isselbacher, K. J., and Carter, E. A. (1970). Biochem. Biophys. Res. Commun. 39, 530–537.
Jarnefelt, J. (1961). Biochim. Biophys. Acta 48, 111–116.
Jofre de Breyer, I. J., Acevedo, C., and Torrelio, M. (1972). Arzneim.-Forsch. 22, 2140–2142.
Jones, K. L., and Smith, D. W. (1973). Lancet 2, 999–1001.
Jones, K. L., Smith, D. W., Ulleland, C. N., and Streissguth, A. P. (1973). Lancet 1, 1267–1271.
Jones, K. L., Smith, D. W., Streissguth, A. P., and Myrianthopoulos, N. C. (1974). Lancet 1, 1076–1078.
Kalant, H., Israel, Y., and Mahon, M. A. (1967). Can. J. Physiol. Pharmacol. 45, 172–176.
Katunuma, N., Okada, M., and Nishii, V. (1966). Adv. Enzyme Regul. 4, 317–335.
Keilin, D., and Hartree, E. F. (1936). Proc. R. Soc. London 119, 141–159.
Keilin, D., and Hartree, E. F. (1945). Biochem. J. 39, 294–301.
Kohn, L. D., and Jacoby, W. B. (1968). J. Biol. Chem. 243, 2494–2499.
Kopin, I. J. (1971). Fed. Proc., Fed. Am. Soc. Exp. Biol. 30, 904–907.
Kuriyama, K., and Israel, M. A. (1973). Biochem. Pharmacol. 22, 2919–2922.
Kuriyama, K., Sze, P. Y., and Rauscher, G. E. (1971). Life Sci. 10, 181–189.
Lee, Y. P., and Lardy, H. A. (1965). J. Biol. Chem. 240, 1427–1436.
Leloir, L. F., and Munoz, J. M. (1938). Biochem. J. 32, 299–307.
Lieber, C. S., and DeCarli, L. M. (1968). Science 162, 917–918.
Lindros, K. O., Vihma, R., and Fossander, O. A. (1972). Biochem. J. 126, 945–952.
Lubin, M., and Westerfeld, W. W. (1945). J. Biol. Chem. 161, 503–512.
Lundquist, F. (1960). Acta Physiol. Scand. 50, Suppl. 175, 97–99.
Lundquist, F., and Walthers, H. (1958). Acta Pharmacol. Toxicol. 14, 290–294.
Lundsgaard, E. (1938). C. R. Trav. Lab. Calsberg 22, 333–337.
Lutwak-Mann, C. (1938). Biochem. J. 32, 1364–1374.
McAfee, D. A., and Greengard, P. (1972). Science 178, 310–312.

McIlwain, H. (1961). *Biochem. J.* **78**, 24–32.
Majchrowicz, E. (1965). *Can. J. Biochem.* **43**, 1041–1051.
Mendelson, J. H. (1964). *Q. J. Stud. Alcohol* **25**, Suppl., 1–129.
Meyer, K. H. (1937). *Trans. Faraday Soc.* **33**, 1062–1068.
Mezey, E., and Tobon, F. (1971). *Gastroenterology* **61**, 707–715.
Moss, J. E., Smyth, R. D., Beck, H., and Martin, G. J. (1967). *Arch. Int. Pharma-codyn. Ther.* **168**, 235–238.
Murphy, D. L. (1972). *Am. J. Psychiatry* **129**, 141–148.
Muscholl, E., and Maitre, L. (1963). *Experientia* **19**, 658–659.
Mushahwar, I. K., and Koeppe, R. E. (1972). *Biochem. J.* **126**, 467–469.
Noble, E. P., and Tewari, S. (1973). *Ann. N.Y. Acad. Sci.* **215**, 333–345.
Noble, E. P., Parker, E., Alkana, R., Kohen, H., and Birch, H. (1973). *Fed. Proc., Fed. Am. Soc. Exp. Biol.* **32**, 724 (abstr.).
Orme-Johnson, W. H., and Ziegler, D. M. (1965). *Biochem. Biophys. Res. Commun.* **21**, 78–82.
Oshino, N., Oshino, R., and Chance, B. (1973). *Biochem. J.* **131**, 555–567.
Peng, T. C., Cooper, C. W., and Munson, P. L. (1972). *Endocrinology* **91**, 586–593.
Quastel, J. H. (1965). *Br. Med. Bull.* **21**, 49–56.
Raskin, N. H., and Sokoloff, L. (1968). *Science* **162**, 131–132.
Raskin, N. H., and Sokoloff, L. (1970). *J. Neurochem.* **17**, 1677–1687.
Raskin, N. H., and Sokoloff, L. (1972). *J. Neurochem.* **19**, 273–282.
Rawat, A. K. (1968). *Eur. J. Biochem.* **6**, 585–592.
Rawat, A. K. (1969a). *In* "Influence of Hormones and Other Factors on Hepatic Alcohol Metabolism" (A. K. Rawat, ed.), pp. 20–45. Kandrup & Wunch, Copenhagen.
Rawat, A. K. (1969b). *Eur. J. Biochem.* **9**, 93–100.
Rawat, A. K. (1970a). *Biochem. Pharmacol.* **19**, 2791–2728.
Rawat, A. K. (1970b). *Acta Chem. Scand.* **24**, 1163–1167.
Rawat, A. K. (1972). *Arch. Biochem. Biophys.* **151**, 93–101.
Rawat, A. K. (1973). *Adv. Exp. Med. Biol.* **35**, 145–166.
Rawat, A. K. (1974a). *Res. Commun. Chem. Pathol. Pharmacol.* **8**, 461–469.
Rawat, A. K. (1974b). *J. Neurochem.* **22**, 915–922.
Rawat, A. K. (1975a). *Adv. Exp. Med. Biol.* **56**, 165–177.
Rawat, A. K. (1975b). *Fed. Proc., Fed. Am. Soc. Exp. Biol.* **3**, 224 (abstr.).
Rawat, A. K. (1975c). *Res. Commun. Chem. Pathol. Pharmacol.* **12**, No. 4, 723–732.
Rawat, A. K. (1976a). *In* "The Role of Acetaldehyde in the Action of Ethanol," Satellite Symp. 6th Int. Congr. Pharmacol., 1975 (K. O. Lindros and C. J. P. Eriksson, eds.), pp. 159–176. *Finn. Found. Alcohol Stud.* Vol. 23.
Rawat, A. K. (1976b). *Ann. N. Y. Acad. Sci.* **273**, 175–187.
Rawat, A. K., and Kuriyama, K. (1972a). *Science* **176**, 1133–1135.
Rawat, A. K., and Kuriyama, K. (1972b). *Arch. Biochem. Biophys.* **152**, 44–52.
Rawat, A. K., and Lundquist, F. (1968). *Eur. J. Biochem.* **5**, 13–17.
Rawat, A. K., and Menahan, L. (1975). *Diabetes* **24**, 926–932.
Rawat, A. K., Kuriyama, K., and Mose, J. (1973). *J. Neurochem.* **20**, 23–33.
Recknagel, R. O., and Potter, R. V. (1951). *J. Biol. Chem.* **191**, 263–275.
Redetzki, H. M. (1967). *Q. J. Stud. Alcohol* **28**, 225–230.
Richter, D., and Crossland, J. (1949). *Am. J. Physiol.* **159**, 247–255.
Ridge, J. W. (1963). *Biochem. J.* **88**, 95–100.
Roach, M. K., Davis, D. L., Pennington, W., and Nordyke, E. (1973). *Life Sci.* **12**, 433–441.
Robbins, J. H. (1968). *Clin. Res.* **16**, 554.

Robinson, G. A., Butcher, R. W., and Sutherland, E. W. (1971). "Cyclic AMP." Academic Press, New York.

Ross, D. H., Medina, M. A., and Cardenas, H. L. (1974). *Science* **186**, 63–65.

Rothstein, A. (1968). *Annu. Rev. Physiol.* **530**, 15–72.

Rubin, R. P. (1970). *Pharmacol. Rev.* **22**, 389–428.

Sandor, S., and Amels, D. (1971). *Rev. Roum. Embryol. Cytol., Ser. Embryol.* **8**, 105–118.

Seeman, P. (1972). *Pharmacol. Rev.* **24**, 583–655.

Seeman, P., Chau, M., Goldberg, M., Sauks, T., and Sax, L. (1971). *Biochim. Biophys. Acta* **225**, 185–193.

Simpson, L. L. (1968). *J. Pharm. Pharmacol.* **20**, 889–910.

Skou, J. C. (1957). *Biochim. Biophys. Acta* **23**, 394–401.

Skou, J. C. (1958). *Biochim. Biophys. Acta* **30**, 625–629.

Smith, A. A., Hayashida, K., and Kim, Y. (1970). *J. Pharm. Pharmacol.* **22**, 644–645.

Smith, M. E., Newman, E. J., and Newman, H. W. (1957). *Proc. Soc. Exp. Biol. Med.* **95**, 541–543.

Sun, A. Y., and Somorajski, T. (1970). *J. Neurochem.* **17**, 1365–1372.

Sund, H., and Theorell, H. (1963). *In* "The Enzymes" (P. D. Boyer, H. Lardy, and K. Myrbäck, eds.), 2nd ed., Vol. 7, pp. 26–83. Academic Press, New York.

Sutherland, V. C., Burbridge, T. N., and Simon, A. (1958). *Fed. Proc., Fed. Am. Soc. Exp. Biol.* **17**, 413.

Swanson, P. D., and McIlwain, J. (1965). *J. Neurochem.* **12**, 877–891.

Sytinski, I. A., Guzikov, B. M., Gomanki, M. V., Eremin, V. P., and Konovalova, N. N. (1975). *J. Neurochem.* **25**, 43–48.

Tabakoff, B., and Erwin, V. G. (1970). *J. Biol. Chem.* **245**, 3262–3268.

Tague, L. L., and Shanbour, L. L. (1974). *Life Sci.* **14**, 1065–1073.

Theorell, H. (1967). *Harvey Lect.* **61**, 17–41.

Thieden, H. I. D., and Lundquist, F. (1967). *Biochem. J.* **102**, 177–180.

Thurman, R. G., Ley, H. G., and Scholz, R. (1972). *Eur. J. Biochem.* **25**, 420–450.

Thurman, R. G., Yonetani, T., Williamson, J. R., and Chance, B., eds. (1974). "Alcohol and Aldehyde Metabolizing Systems." Academic Press, New York.

Towne, J. C. (1964). *Nature (London)* **201**, 709–710.

Truitt, E. B., Jr., Bell, F. K., and Krantz, J. C., Jr. (1956). *Q. J. Stud. Alcohol* **17**, 594–600.

Tyce, G. M., Flock, E. V., Taylor, W. F., and Owens, C. A., Jr. (1970). *Proc. Soc. Exp. Biol. Med.* **134**, 40–44.

Ungar, G. (1966). *Fed. Proc., Fed. Am. Soc. Exp. Biol.* **25**, 207.

Veloso, D., Passonneau, J. P., and Veech, R. L. (1972). *J. Neurochem.* **19**, 2679–2686.

Victor, M., and Adams, R. D. (1953). *Res. Publ. Assoc. Res. Nerv. Ment. Dis.* **32**, 526–573.

Volicer, L., and Gold, B. I. (1973). *Life Sci.* **13**, 269–280.

Volicer, L., and Gold, B. I. (1975). *Adv. Exp. Med. Biol.* **56**, 211–237.

von Wartburg, J. P., Berli, W., and Aebei, H. (1961). *Helv. Med. Acta* **28**, 89–98.

Vorherr, H. (1974). *Postgrad. Med.* **56**, 97–104.

Wallgren, H. (1963). *J. Neurochem.* **10**, 349–362.

Wallgren, H. (1966). *Psychosom. Med.* **28**, 431–442.

Wallgren, H., and Kulonen, E. (1960). *Biochem. J.* **75**, 150–158.

Wallgren, H., Nikander, P., von Boguslawski, P., and Linkola, J. (1974). *Acta Physiol. Scand.* **91**, 83–93.

OCTOPAMINE AND SOME RELATED NONCATECHOLIC AMINES IN INVERTEBRATE NERVOUS SYSTEMS

By H. A. Robertson[1] and A. V. Juorio

Psychiatric Research Unit
University Hospital, Saskatoon, Saskatchewan, Canada

I. Introduction

In mammalian nervous tissue it is now reasonably well established that catecholamines (dopamine and noradrenaline) and the indole alkylamine, 5-hydroxytryptamine (5-HT, serotonin), serve as neurotransmitters. They are present in and synthesized by neurons, are released on stimulation, act on the postsynaptic membrane, and are inactivated (removed from the synaptic cleft)

[1] Present address: University Laboratory of Physiology, Parks Road, Oxford, OX1 3PT, England.

174   H. A. ROBERTSON AND A. V. JUORIO

by reuptake into the presynaptic terminal. These amines have long had a central position in theories of the etiology of psychiatric disorders. Dopamine, noradrenaline, and 5-HT have all, at one time or another, been suggested to be the transmitter involved in schizophrenia, one of the most common psychiatric disorders. Currently, dopamine appears to be the best neurotransmitter candidate for a role in schizophrenia. The relationship between phenothiazines and related antischizophrenic drugs and dopamine-receptor blockage has been well documented (see Snyder et al., 1974). Other hypotheses have postulated that depression is related to a deficiency in, and mania to an excess of, the activity of central monoaminergic neurons (see review by Weil-Malherbe, 1972).

In addition to these major monoamines, or classical neurotransmitters, whose role and importance is relatively well understood, there exists in the nervous tissue of all species examined to date a group of monoamines described variously as exotic amines, trace amines, or microamines. As we shall see, all these terms are in one way or another misleading, especially in reference to invertebrates. We propose, as an interim measure, to retain the term microamine, while keeping in mind that such a term is somewhat misleading, especially when the levels of the so-called microamines exceed those of the catecholamines and 5-HT.

Microamines have long been known to be pharmacologically active. Many of them were studied for physiological activity by Barger and Dale (1910). However, for many years these observations were of pharmacological interest only. Following technological advances, particularly the introduction of sensitive microassay procedures, it has become established that many of these amines are indeed present in mammalian nervous systems, albeit at exceedingly low concentrations. Among the endogenous microamines found in the mammalian brain are β-phenylethylamine, phenylethanolamine, m- and p-tyramine, octopamine (presumed to be the para isomer), and tryptamine. The structure of these and related compounds is shown in Fig. 1. Despite the very low concentrations of these microamines, they are interesting for several reasons: (1) They are heterogeneously distributed within the brain (Boulton, 1974, 1976a; Molinoff and Axelrod, 1972); (2) they are present in the same subcellular fraction and to about the same extent as catecholamines and 5-HT (Boulton and Baker, 1975; Molinoff and Axelrod, 1972); (3) they have a high turnover rate (Molinoff and Axelrod, 1972; Boulton and Wu, 1972; Wu and Boulton, 1974, 1975); (4) they release and/or replace catecholamines from storage sites and block reuptake (Burn and Rand, 1958; Burgen and Iversen, 1965; von Euler and Lishajko, 1968; (5) it has been claimed that they are excreted abnormally in the urine of patients with migraine (Sandler et al., 1974), Parkinson's disease (Boulton and Marjerrison, 1972), schizophrenia (Boulton, 1971), and depression (Fischer

a) Phenylethylamines

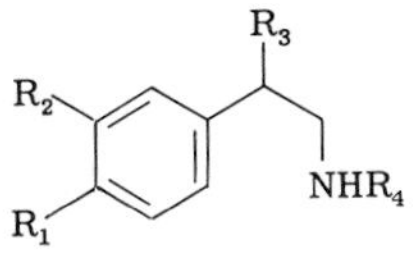

	R_1	R_2	R_3	R_4
β-Phenylethylamine	H	H	H	H
Phenylethanolamine	H	H	OH	H
p-Tyramine	OH	H	H	H
m-Tyramine	H	OH	H	H
p-Octopamine	OH	H	OH	H
m-Octopamine	H	OH	OH	H
p-Synephrine	OH	H	OH	CH_3
m-Synephrine	H	OH	OH	CH_3
Dopamine	OH	OH	H	H
Noradrenaline	OH	OH	OH	H
Adrenaline	OH	OH	OH	CH_3

b) Indolethylamines

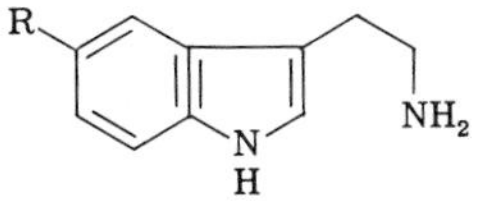

	R
Tryptamine	H
5-Hydroxytryptamine	OH

FIG. 1. Chemical structure of aryl alkylamines.

et al., 1972) ; (6) most interestingly, some are behaviorally active, mimicking the stereotypes of amphetamine (Faurbye, 1968; Saavedra *et al.*, 1970). It is clear that these microamines deserve further study. Unfortunately, their exceedingly low concentrations have hampered investigations. Phylogenetic distribution studies, however, have revealed that several of the more interesting microamines are present in the nervous tissues of some invertebrates in relatively high concentrations (see Table I for a summary of the phylogenetic distribution of monoamines in neural tissues).

In the past, invertebrate nervous systems have often been used as models in neurobiological investigations. The size of the neurons (up to 900 μm in some molluscs), the fact that many invertebrates possess identifiable neurons, and the ease of experimental manipulation make invertebrate preparations most amenable to study. These features, coupled with the high levels of microamines present, make invertebrate preparations the most suitable systems in which to investigate the role of these substances. Certain reservations must be kept in mind, however, with respect to the information obtained. First, we are interested in knowing how microamines are synthesized and how they are broken down and/or inactivated. It will be important to determine whether or not the enzymes and pathways of these processes are similar in invertebrates and vertebrates, and if certain chemical and physical manipulations affect the processes in a similar fashion. We expect many useful similarities to emerge from such studies, as it is well known that the cells are exceedingly conservative with respect to their biochemical organization. Second, we wish to identify those mechanisms that mediate the actions of microamines. Here again, we know from other systems that cells are rather conservative and that the mechanisms by which messages arriving at the cell surface are translated into a response are limited in number, involving cyclic nucleotides (cyclic adenosine- and guanosine-3',5'-monophosphate) and certain ions (Ca^{2+}, Na^+, and K^+). These appear to be the same in all organisms from bacteria to mammals (see Tomkins, 1975). Third, we are interested in knowing the function of microamines, and this is the crucial problem to consider in using invertebrates as models, for while we expect conservatism in metabolism and, to a lesser extent, in mechanisms of action, we do not necessarily expect it in the physiological use to which molecules are put. In the past, microamines have been regarded, in the mammalian nervous system, as metabolic accidents or minor by-products of more important biochemical pathways leading to catecholamines or 5-HT or, alternatively, at least in the case of octopamine, as cotransmitters of unknown function released simultaneously with a major transmitter, noradrenaline (Molinoff and Axelrod, 1972). Contrary to this situation, at least one microamine (octopamine) appears to fulfill a classical neurotransmitter role in invertebrates. The presence of various microamines in nervous tissues is now well

TABLE I

SUMMARY OF THE PHYLOGENETIC DISTRIBUTION OF MONOAMINES IN NEURAL TISSUES[a]

	PE	POA	TA	OA	DA	NA	A	TR	5-HT
Invertebrates									
Annelida	?	?	?	++++	++++	++++	?	?	+++
Mollusca	+	?	+++	++++	+++++	++	ND	+	+++++
Arthropoda	?	ND	+++	+++	++	+	?	ND	++++
Echinodermata	+	?	+	+++	+++	++++	ND	++++	ND
Vertebrates									
Fish	?	?	?	?	+++	++	+	?	+++
Amphibia	?	?	?	?	++	+++	++	?	++
Reptile	?	?	?	?	+++++	+++++	+++	?	++++
Bird	?	?	?	?	+++	++	++	++	++
Mammal	+	+	+	+	+++	+++	+++	++	++

[a] Amine concentrations in nanograms per gram. PE, Phenylethylamine; POA, phenylethanolamine; TA, p-tyramine; OA, octopamine (presumed para); DA, dopamine; NA, noradrenaline; A, adrenaline; TR, tryptamine; 5-HT, 5-hydroxytryptamine. ?, Unknown; ND, not detected; +, present <10; ++, >10 <100; +++, >100 <1000; ++++, >1000 <10,000; +++++ >10,000.

established. It remains to be determined whether or not they interact with receptors pre- and postsynaptically and, if so, exactly how, and whether or not they play an important role in nervous systems.

We should perhaps recall that advances in invertebrate neurobiology can actually precede and foretell advances in the mammalian field. 5-HT had already been suggested as a neurotransmitter in molluscs (Welsh, 1953) when it was discovered in the mammalian brain (Twarog and Page, 1953; Amin et al., 1954). Indeed, it was a bioassay using the clam heart that permitted its identification and quantitation in the mammalian brain.

In this article, while we refer to catecholamines and 5-HT for comparative purposes, our primary purpose is to consider the role of microamines in invertebrates. The literature on the classical transmitters in invertebrates has been reviewed by others (Gerschenfeld, 1973; Pitman, 1971; Murdock, 1971; Kerkut, 1973; Cottrell and Laverack, 1968; Welsh, 1972).

II. Analytical Procedures for Microamines

The fact that microamines all occur in mammalian nervous tissue in such minute amounts necessitated the development of sensitive methods for their analysis. This was fortunate because, although the levels of microamines found in invertebrate tissues are much higher, the amount of tissue available is usually much less. The current methods used for microamine assays are shown in Table II. To a considerable extent the choice of method depends on the background of the investigator and the equipment available. The most sensitive and specific methods available are radiochemical-enzymic assays and mass spectrometry. Mass spectrometry coupled with either thin-layer chromatography or gas chromatography is both sensitive and highly specific but requires expensive equipment and a high level of technical competence and sophistication. Radiochemical-enzymic assays require only a scintillation counter and are as sensitive as or more sensitive than mass spectrometry. These assays, however, are not always specific, and chromatographic confirmation of product identity is necessary.

A. RADIOCHEMICAL-ENZYMIC ASSAYS

A list of currently available radiochemical-enzymic procedures is shown in Table III. These assays all depend on the enzyme-catalyzed transfer of radioactively labeled methyl groups from a donor compound ([³H]- or [¹⁴C] S-adenosylmethionine) to the amine. The labeled, methylated product is isolated from the aqueous incubation mixture by extraction into an organic solvent. After removal of the organic solvent, the amount of radioactivity present is determined by liquid scintillation counting either directly or after

TABLE II
ANALYTICAL PROCEDURES FOR MICROAMINES

Procedure	Practical sensitivity	Advantages	Limitations
Enzymic-isotopic	^{14}C, 500–1000 pg; ^{3}H, 50–200 pg	Procedures developed for most biogenic amines; high sensitivity and reproducibility; possible to perform large numbers of samples; can be undertaken in most laboratories; requires minimum of equipment beyond scintillation counter	Not always specific; requires chromatographic identification of products
Mass spectrometric	100–500 pg	Highly sensitive and specific; can be adapted to most biogenic amines	Equipment (mass spectrometer) expensive; requires high degree of instrumental expertise; techniques not yet developed for all biogenic amines
Gas chromatographic	1–5 ng	Can be linked to mass spectrometer	Few methods available for biogenic amines
Fluorimetric	10–50 ng	Can be performed easily	Sensitivity and specificity limited
Labeled dansyl	500 pg	Fairly sensitive; potential of wide application	Specificity limited

chromatography, i.e., separation of the labeled products. The specificity of the method depends on the specificity of the enzyme used, solvent extraction, and chromatographic identification. Under the conditions employed, enzyme and cofactor being in excess, the substrate (amine) concentration is rate-limiting and the amount of radioactivity produced is directly proportional to the amine concentration. Figure 2 illustrates the biochemical basis of the octopamine assay as an example.

The procedure used in our laboratory for the simultaneous determination of octopamine and phenylethanolamine is illustrated in Fig. 3 [based on the method of Saavedra (1974a)]. To be able to assay β-phenylethylamine and tyramine, these amines must first be converted to their β-hydroxylated derivatives (phenylethanolamine and octopamine, respectively). The β-hydroxylated derivates are then quantitated after they are converted to their respective N-methyl derivatives (see Saavedra, 1974b).

To be sure that a single known substrate is being quantitated, it is essential that the identity of the product (i.e., the methylated amine) be

TABLE III

RADIOCHEMICAL-ENZYMIC ASSAYS FOR BIOGENIC AMINES[a]

Amine	Enzyme 1	Enzyme 2	Product	Sensitivity (pg)	References
Phenylethylamine	D-β-H	PNMT	N-Methylphenylethanolamine	200	Saavedra, 1974b
Phenylethanolamine	PNMT		N-Methylphenylethanolamine	100	Saavedra and Axelrod, 1973
Tyramine	D-β-H	PNMT	Synephrine	200	J. M. Saavedra, personal communication
Octopamine	PNMT		Synephrine	50	Saavedra, 1974a
Dopamine	COMT		3-Methoxytyramine	50–150	Cuello et al., 1973; Coyle
Noradrenaline	COMT		Normetanephrine	50–150	and Henry, 1973; Fry et
Adrenaline	COMT		Metanephrine	50–150	al., 1974
Tryptamine	Tryptamine-N-methyl transferase		N-Methyltryptamine	1000	Saavedra and Axelrod, 1972
5-Hydroxytryptamine	N-Acetyltransferase	HIOMT	Melatonin	50	Saavedra et al., 1973
Noradrenaline	PNMT		Adrenaline	25	Saelens et al., 1967; Henry et al., 1975

[a] COMT, Catechol-O-methyltransferase; D-β-H, dopamine-β-hydroxylase; HIOMT, hydroxyindole-O-methyltransferase; PNMT, phenylethanolamine-N-methyltransferase.

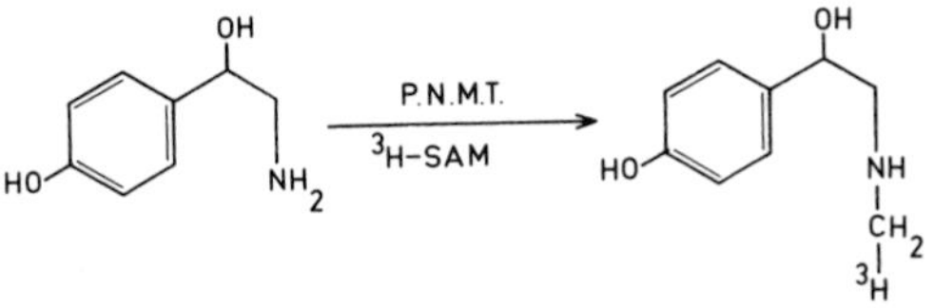

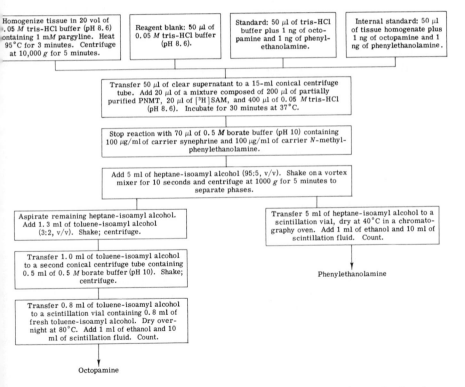

FIG. 2. Enzymic conversion of p-octopamine to labeled [^{3}H]p-synephrine by phenyl-ethanolamine-N-methyl transferase (PNMT). The cofactor is [^{3}H]S-adenosylmethionine ([^{3}H]SAM).

checked by chromatographic separation in three or more different solvent systems. It is also essential to include internal standards for every tissue sample analyzed. Internal standards are prepared by adding known amounts of biogenic amine to tissue samples. Unknown factors present in the tissue often exhibit inhibitory effects on methyltransferase activities.

Enzyme specificity, in some cases, is not yet known. For example, it has

FIG. 3. Procedure for simultaneous determination of octopamine and phenyl-ethanolamine.

tacitly been assumed that the octopamine located in extracts of nervous systems is the para isomer; this has never been checked, however. As both p- and m-tyramine are present in nervous tissue (Philips et al., 1974a, 1975), it is quite possible, perhaps even likely, that both positional isomers are present. p-Octopamine cannot be distinguished from m-octopamine by radiochemical-enzymic assay (H. A. Robertson, unpublished observations). However, an improved assay recently introduced now permits the simultaneous analysis of p-octopamine, m-octopamine, and phenylethanolamine (Danielson et al., 1976). In this procedure, p- and m-octopamine are first N-methylated with the enzyme phenylethanolamine-N-methyltransferase, using [^{3}H]-S-adenosylmethionine as a cofactor. The p- and m-synephrines are then converted to their dansyl derivatives and separated by thin layer chromatography in two different solvent systems. The zones containing p- and m-synephrine are eluted, and radioactivity is determined by liquid scintillation counting. Not only does this procedure allow the simultaneous determination of p- and m-octopamine and phenylethanolamine, but it increases the sensitivity and specificity of the assay. Furthermore, it is possible to quantitate p- and m-tyramine with this technique by first using the enzyme dopamine-β-hydroxylase to convert p- and m-tyramine to their respective β-hydroxylated derivatives.

A further point requiring clarification concerns the optical activity of naturally occurring octopamine (i.e., is it the D($-$)-isomer, the L($+$)-isomer, or a racemic mixture.

Despite the above-described disadvantages, radiochemical-enzymic methods remain the most convenient and inexpensive methods for the sensitive determination of many microamines.

B. MASS SPECTROMETRIC PROCEDURES

1. Thin-Layer Chromatography—Integrated Ion-Current Technique with a Direct Insertion Probe

Mass spectrometric–integrated ion-current technique with direct insertion probe (Jenkins and Majer, 1967) has been in use for several years for the analysis of metals and polycyclic hydrocarbons in pollution studies (Majer and Boulton, 1973), as well as for the estimation of polyamines (Seiler and Knodgen, 1973; Dolezalova et al., 1973) and monoamines (Durden et al., 1974) in animal tissue extracts. The analysis of amines in tissues by this technique is based on the formation of stable derivatives and chromatographic purification; any losses incurred in the overall procedure are compensated for by the use of deuterated internal standards (Durden et al., 1974). The protocol for the estimation of β-phenylethylamine, p-tyramine, m-tyramine, and tryptamine is outlined in Fig. 4. Complete details concerning the isola-

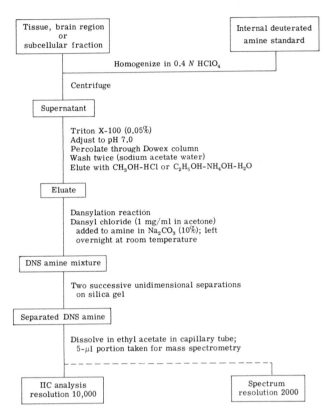

Fɪɢ. 4. Schematic procedure for the mass spectrometric estimation of aryl alkyl-amines. See text for more details.

tion, derivatization, and separation of amines susceptible to analysis by this procedure have been published (Philips *et al.,* 1974a,b, 1975; Durden *et al.,* 1973, 1974).

Tissues are homogenized in 0.1 N hydrochloric acid and deproteinized with perchloric acid (final concentration 0.4 N) or, alternatively, tissues are directly homogenized in 0.4 N perchloric acid. Deuterated internal standards are added in amounts equal to or greater than those expected to be present in the tissues, the amounts first being estimated by preliminary experiments. The tissue homogenate is mixed thoroughly, and then centrifuged at 12,000 g for 10 minutes (IEC B-20 centrifuge). The supernatant is decanted, and the nonionic detergent Triton X-100 (J. T. Baker Chemical Co., Phillipsburg, N.J.) is added (Boulton *et al.,* 1972), with stirring, to a final concentration of 0.05% (v/v). The solution is adjusted to pH 7 with 2 N sodium hydroxide and percolated through a column (1 cm in diameter and 6 cm long) of

Biorad AG 50W-X2 (H+) prepared according to the procedure of Kakimoto and Armstrong (1962). The column is washed successively with distilled water (10 ml), 0.1 M sodium acetate (20 ml), and distilled water (10 ml). The amine fraction is eluted from the resin with 15 ml of methanol–hydrochloric acid (73:27, v/v) in the case of phenylethylamine analyses, or 15 ml of ethanol–ammonium hydroxide–water (65:25:10, v/v) in the case of tyramine and tryptamine analyses. The extract is taken to dryness by rotary evaporation at 45°C. If the amount of tissue analyzed is small (less than 200 mg) the ion-exchange chromatographic separation step may be omitted. Tissues can be homogenized directly in saturated sodium carbonate solution. They are then frozen and thawed twice, and 2 vol of acetone is added. After centrifugation dansyl reagent is added directly to the supernatant (P. H. Wu, personal communication). The amines in the dried amine extract are dissolved in 1.0 ml of sodium carbonate (10%, w/v), and the dansyl derivatives prepared by adding 1.5–2.0 ml of dansyl reagent (Aldrich Chemical Co., Milwaukee, Wisc., 1 mg/ml acetone) to samples in which phenylethylamine is to be analyzed, or 3.5–4.5 ml of dansyl reagent to samples in which tyramines and tryptamine are to be analyzed. Following overnight reaction at room temperature, sodium carbonate is precipitated by the addition of 10 ml of acetone. The reaction mixture is centrifuged (500 g for 1 minute), and the clear supernatant transferred to a 50-ml, round-bottomed flask and evaporated to dryness at 45°C. The residue is dissolved in 4 ml of ethyl acetate, transferred to a test tube, and dried under a stream of nitrogen. It is then redissolved in 5 drops of ethyl acetate and transferred to a 20 × 20 cm glass plate coated with silica gel (Brinkmann Instruments Ltd., Rexdale, Ont.). The tube is rinsed once with 5 drops of ethyl acetate. Four tissue samples, as well as the appropriate dansyl amine standards, are applied to a single plate. To isolate dansyl phenylethylamine, the chromatogram is developed for approximately 2 hours in the solvent system chloroform–butyl acetate (4:1, v/v) and then removed from the chamber and sprayed with isopropanol–triethanolamine (4:1, v/v) to stabilize the fluorescence of the dansyl derivatives (Seiler and Wiechmann, 1966). The dansyl phenylethylamine zone is visualized in ultraviolet light (365 nm), outlined with a metal stylus, and scraped from the plate. Dansyl β-phenylethylamine is then eluted from the silica gel with two 2-ml portions of ethyl acetate; the extract is dried under a stream of nitrogen, redissolved in 5 drops of ethyl acetate, and reapplied to a second thin layer of silica gel. Following development of this chromatogram in the solvent system benzene–triethylamine (8:1, v/v) and spraying with isopropanol–triethanolamine, the dansyl phenylethylamine zone is again scraped from the plate, eluted, and separated a third time in the solvent system carbon tetrachloride–triethylamine (5:1, v/v). To isolate the dansyl tyramines and dansyl tryptamine, chromatograms containing the dansylated amine mixture are developed for 2 hours in the solvent system chloroform–butyl acetate (4:1, v/v). After spraying with isopropanol–triethanolamine, two zones are scraped from the plate, one containing dansyl tryptamine, and the other containing dansyl m- and p-tyramine. Dansyl tryptamine is eluted from the silica gel with two 2-ml portions of acetone–methanol (10:1, v/v). The extract is dried under nitrogen, redissolved in 5 drops of ethyl acetate, and applied to a second thin layer of silica gel. Final development is in the solvent system benzene–triethylamine (5:1, v/v). The dansyl tyramines are eluted from the silica gel with two 1-ml portions of benzene–acetone (10:1, v/v), and the extract is dried under nitrogen and redissolved in 5 drops of ethyl acetate. The meta and para isomers of dansyl tyramine are then separated on a second layer of silica gel in the solvent system benzene–triethylamine (12:1, v/v). Following the final chromatographic separation of each dansyl amine, the chromatogram is removed from the chamber and, without spraying with isopropanol–triethanolamine, the dansyl amines are prepared for mass spectrometric analysis as described previously (Philips et al., 1974a). Briefly, the dansyl amine zone is scraped from the plate and, with the use of a rotary vacuum pump, the silica gel powder is sucked into a constricted capillary tube containing a glass-fiber paper plug approximately 30 mm from one end. A second plug is placed in the tube to hold the powder in place. The dansyl amine is then eluted by drawing approximately 30 μl ethyl acetate through the powder by means of a 1-ml plastic disposable syringe adapted to fit the end of the capillary tube. The ends of the capillary tube are then sealed with Clay-Adams Seal Ease hematocrit sealing clay, and the tubes are refrigerated until mass spectrometric analysis. To analyze the sample, the end of the capillary is broken off, and an aliquot (5–10 μl) is withdrawn with a syringe and placed in a mass spectrometric direct insertion probe. Blanks are obtained by subjecting 0.4 N perchloric acid samples to an identical procedure, including the addition of deuterated amine, dansylation, chromatographic separation, and mass spectrometric analysis.

Integrated ion-current (IIC) profiles of the dansyl amines are recorded on an AEI MS902S mass spectrometer equipped with a direct insertion inlet and a Massmaster mass indicator. Profiles of dansyl phenylethylamine, dansyl tyramines, and dansyl tryptamine are obtained at ion source temperatures of 260 ± 10, 310 ± 5, and $260 \pm 5°$C, respectively, and at a resolution of 10,000. The procedure for quantitation of amines by the IIC technique has been described previously (Durden et al., 1973). The magnetic fields of the instrument are adjusted so that the m/e value of the molecule ion of the dansyl amine (354.1402 for β-phenylethylamine, 603.1861 for the tyramines, and 393.1511 for tryptamine) is focused in the low-mass position of the peak switching unit, while the m/e value due to the molecule ion of the dansyl deuterated amine (356.1527 for β-phenylethylamine, 605.1987 for the tyramines, and 395.1637 for tryptamine) is focused in the high-mass position. The peaks are located by means of the Massmaster and confirmed by comparison with ions arising from heptacosafluorotri-n-butylamine. An aliquot (5–10 μl) of the sample to be analyzed is withdrawn from the capillary tube, placed on the tip of the direct insertion probe, and evaporated to dryness on a small heater. With the instrument alternately focusing on the appropriate ionic species, the probe is inserted into the hot ion source, and the ion currents are recorded. The amount of amine in the sample is calculated from Eq. (1):

$$\text{Amine (nanograms/gram)} = \frac{A_1}{A_2 - x\% \, A_1} \times Y \qquad (1)$$

where A_1 and A_2 are the areas of the IIC profiles due to endogenous and deuterated dansyl amines, respectively, and Y is the amount, in nanograms, of the added internal standard (deuterated amine). The correction factor $x\%$ is characteristic of the amine analyzed. It is necessitated by the presence of a group of ion peaks due to the natural abundance of ^{13}C, ^{18}O, and ^{34}S isotopes, which are associated with the m/e value corresponding to the dansylated endogenous amine. They produce a composite peak which has a height $x\%$ that of the peak due to the molecule ion of the dansylated endogenous amine. At a resolution of 10,000, the composite peak is not separated from the molecule ion peak arising from the dansylated deuterated amine.

The identities of the dansyl amines isolated from tissues have previously been established by comparing the mass spectra to those of authentic dansylated amines (Durden et al., 1973; Philips et al., 1974a,b, 1975). Blank values range from 0.2 to 0.5 ng per sample for m-tyramine, p-tyramine, β-phenylethylamine, and tryptamine; the smallest amount of tissue amine estimated should contain at least twice the amount of amine in the blank.

The formation of derivatives, coupled with chromatographic separation followed by high-resolution mass spectrometry focusing on the molecule ions to be analyzed, provides a highly specific and sensitive analytical procedure. Disadvantages are that the method is somewhat time-consuming, depending on the procedure adopted (e.g., resin separation or direct dansylation) and the number of amines analyzed. The values found for brain β-phenylethylamine levels obtained by mass spectrometric (Durden et al., 1973), radiochemical (Saavedra, 1974b), gas chromatographic–mass spectrometric (Willner et al., 1974), and gas chromatographic (Martin and Baker, 1975) methods are in very good agreement, as has also been the case for phenylethanolamine (Saavedra and Axelrod, 1973; Willner et al., 1974) and p-tyramine (Philips et al., 1974b; J. M. Saavedra, personal communication). In contrast agreement has been not so good in the case of tryptamine.

With the use of radiochemical-enzymic methods (Saavedra and Axelrod, 1972), labeled dansyl techniques (Snodgrass and Horn, 1973), or fluorimetric methods (Sloan *et al.*, 1975) values estimated for the mammalian brain range from 20 to 80 ng/gm. Much lower values (0.05–0.5 ng/gm) were obtained after dansylation, separation by thin-layer chromatography, and quantification by the mass spectrometric integrated ion-current technique using internal standards labeled with a stable isotope (Philips *et al.*, 1974b; Boulton *et al.*, 1975b). No explanation has been found for this discrepancy; it may well be that a closely related tryptamine derivative, such as 5-methoxytryptamine, which has been identified in brain tissue (Björklund *et al.*, 1971) and found in relatively high concentrations [110 ng/gm in the hypothalamus (Green *et al.*, 1973)], reacts in a fashion similar to that of tryptamine, thus giving false high tryptamine levels in the brain.

2. Gas Chromatography–Mass Spectrometry

An alternative approach to mass spectrometric analysis of amines is provided by a combination of the techniques of gas chromatography and mass spectrometry (Holmstedt and Palmér, 1973). Briefly, in this method, amines are converted to suitable volatile derivatives. Quantitation is carried out by adding a deuterated internal standard at the beginning of the separation, or by adding supplements of the amine (or an analog). After separation on the gas column the amines are identified and quantitated by mass spectrometry. This column technique has been applied to the characterization of catecholamines and related β-hydroxyamines by their conversion to boronate derivatives (Anthony *et al.*, 1970), of indole alkylamines and aryl alkylamines by their conversion to pentafluoropropionate and heptafluorobutyrate derivatives (Cattabeni *et al.*, 1972; Karoum *et al.*, 1972; Willner *et al.*, 1974), and of aryl alkylamines by their conversion to isothiocyanate derivatives (Narasimhachmari and Vouros, 1972) and acetylcholine (Koslow *et al.*, 1974). Details of these techniques are given in recent reviews by Holmstedt and Palmér (1973) and Costa *et al.* (1975).

C. Gas Chromatographic Techniques

A gas chromatographic technique for β-phenylethylamine using electron capture for detection and quantification has been developed only recently (Martin and Baker, 1975). The amines are converted to N-acetyl derivatives in aqueous solution under mildly basic conditions using acetic anhydride. The N-acetyl derivatives are then purified by thin-layer chromatography on silica gel, eluted, and converted to pentafluoro derivatives with pentafluoropropionic anhydride. The resulting derivatives are introduced into a gas chromatograph. A sensitivity of 4 pg is claimed for β-phenylethylamine.

Sloan *et al.* (1975) used a gas chromatographic technique to confirm the presence of tryptamine as measured by a spectrofluorimetric method. Their procedure is described in Martin *et al.* (1974).

D. LABELED DANSYL TECHNIQUES

The labeled dansyl technique, using [³H]dansyl chloride, has been used to measure amines in nervous and other tissue. Briefly, amines are isolated from tissues by chemical extraction and reacted with [³H]dansyl chloride. The dansylated mixture is then subjected to two-dimensional thin-layer chromatography, the fluorescent spots are visualized under ultraviolet light and scraped into counting vials, and the amount of radioactivity is determined by liquid scintillation counting. The amine content is quantitated by comparison with known amounts of tryptamine added to the tissue extract. This method has been applied to tryptamine (Snodgrass and Horn, 1973; Osborne, 1974). Osborne (1974) has suggested that the [³H]dansyl technique lends itself well to the analysis of octopamine when the octopamine is converted to the acetylated derivative before dansylation. Such procedures may permit the analysis of other microamines, and possibly even catecholamines and 5-HT.

E. SPECTROPHOTOFLUORIMETRIC TECHNIQUES

Fluorimetric techniques were the first to be used in the investigation of *p*-tyramine and tryptamine in biological fluids (Sjoerdsma *et al.*, 1959). *p*-Tyramine yields a fluorescent derivative after condensation with 1-nitroso-2-naphthol; this reaction, coupled with ethyl acetate extraction, is the basis of the fluorimetric procedure for measuring this amine (Sjoerdsma *et al.*, 1959). In the absence of hydrolysis the assay measures unconjugated tyramine; however, related amines such as octopamine and synephrine, which are also present in urine (Kakimoto and Armstrong, 1962; Pisano *et al.*, 1961), exhibit only one-tenth the fluorescence of an equivalent amount of tyramine. A similar fluorimetric procedure was used for the determination of *p*-tyramine in nervous tissue (Spector *et al.*, 1963) but because of the lack of specificity of the method, values up to 3800 ng/gm were recorded in some regions of the mammalian brain. When tyramine was isolated by ion-exchange chromatography before condensation with 1-nitroso-2-naphthol, however, the mammalian brain levels obtained were less than 10 ng/gm (Gunne and Jonsson, 1965). This last estimate proved quite accurate, as the values obtained with mass spectrometric techniques indicated that *p*-tyramine exists in the mammalian brain in the range 0.4–2 ng/gm (Philips *et al.*, 1974a; Boulton *et al.*, 1975b).

Fluorimetric techniques have also been used for the determination of tryptamine in human urine (Sjoerdsma *et al.,* 1959); tryptamine is extracted in an organic solvent, and the native fluorescence produced at an alkaline pH is measured. An alternative technique is based on the fluorescence produced after condensation with formaldehyde to give a norharman derivative (Hess and Udenfriend, 1959); the sensitivity of this method is still low when applied to the brain and, in fact, tryptamine in tissues can be detected only after tryptophan administration or after inhibition of monoamine oxidase (MAO) (Hess *et al.,* 1959). More recently this method has been found to yield high tryptamine values for the mammalian brain, because of coextraction of brain tryptophan along with the tryptamine (Eccleston *et al.,* 1966). An additional ion-exchange chromatographic step has been added, which gives complete separation of these compounds; with this method, the sensitivity for tryptamine is about 80 ng (twice the blank), and tryptamine was detected in mammalian brain tissue only after L-tryptophan administration and MAO inhibition (Eccleston *et al.,* 1966). A similar method was used for the determination of tryptamine in the mammalian brain (Martin *et al.,* 1971; Sloan *et al.,* 1975).

III. Metabolism

A. BIOSYNTHESIS

In mammals, the amino acids phenylalanine, tyrosine, and tryptophan can be decarboxylated to form the biogenic amines β-phenylethylamine, tyramine, and tryptamine, respectively. However, the favored path (other than transamination) for metabolism of these amino acids in mammals is hydroxylation (Lovenberg *et al.,* 1962). Nevertheless, small amounts of β-phenylethylamine, *p*- and *m*-tyramine, and tryptamine are found in mammalian nervous tissue, as well as phenylethanolamine and octopamine, the products of β-hydroxylation of β-phenylethylamine and tyramine, respectively (Durden *et al.,* 1973; Philips *et al.,* 1974a; Saavedra and Axelrod, 1972; Axelrod and Saavedra, 1974). The exact route of biosynthesis of these microamines in mammals is still somewhat in doubt. In invertebrates the problem has been very little studied, although we may look to invertebrates for important clues to the biochemical pathways of biosynthesis. Unfortunately, to date, the biosynthesis of microamines has only been investigated in arthropods (in a crustacean, in the lobster, and in two insects, the cockroach and the locust) and in an annelid (*Hirudo medicinalis,* the leech). In both these phyla the synthesis appears to follow the proposed mammalian pattern shown in Fig. 5. In the leech, *H. medicinalis, in vitro* incubation of ganglia in [^{14}C]tyrosine

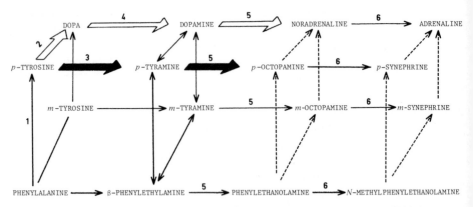

FIG. 5. Actual and potential metabolic interconversions between phenylalkylamines, phenolic amines, and catecholamines. Large solid arrows illustrate the proposed route of octopamine biosynthesis in invertebrates. Large open arrows indicate the biosynthetic pathway for noradrenaline (and adrenaline). Solid lines indicate demonstrated alternate pathways and interrupted lines other possible conversions. Identified enzymes as follows: 1, phenylalanine hydroxylase; 2, tyrosine hydroxylase; 3, tyrosine decarboxylase; 4, dopa decarboxylase; 5, dopamine-β-hydroxylase; 6, phenylethanolamine-N-methyltransferase. Modified after Boulton (1976b).

results in the production of ^{14}C-labeled dopamine, tyramine, and octopamine (Stuart *et al.*, 1974). It also appears that the rate of incorporation of [^{14}C]-tyrosine into octopamine is greater than that into dopamine. (This is also the case in insects.) The nervous system of another annelid, the earthworm, is known to contain more octopamine than dopamine (Robertson, 1975a). Similar *in vitro* incubations of lobster nervous system show incorporation of [^{14}C]tyrosine into dopamine, tyramine, octopamine, and possibly synephrine (Barker *et al.*, 1972). This study also reported the presence of tyrosine hydroxylase, dopamine-β-hydroxylase, and phenylethanolamine-N-methyltransferase in the lobster, but no MAO was detected. Dopamine-β-hydroxylase appears to be localized in octopamine-containing neurons (Wallace *et al.*, 1974). Recently, in our laboratory, we measured the endogenous levels of β-phenylethylamine, phenylethanolamine, and *p*-tyramine in the lobster; only *p*-tyramine appears to be present in significant amounts (up to 210 ng/gm) (A. V. Juorio, H. A. Robertson, and P. H. Wu, unpublished observation). Such a finding supports the biosynthetic route postulated by Barker *et al.* (1972).

There have been numerous studies on the biosynthesis and degradation of biogenic amines in the class Insecta, many of which have been concerned with the role of catecholamines as components in cuticle tanning (see the review by Murdock, 1971). It has been shown that insects possess a tyrosine decarboxylase and that tyramine may be an important intermediate in formation of the cuticular tanning agent N-acetyldopamine (Sekeris and Karlson, 1966). The pathway in hemocytes appears to involve tyrosine→tyramine → dopamine-N-acetyldopamine (Whitehead, 1969). As insect (cockroach) hemolymph contains the enzyme dopamine-β-hydroxylase which is capable of converting tyramine to octopamine, it is possible that octopamine is an intermediate in the biosynthesis of cuticular hardening agents such as 3,4-dihydroxybenzoic acid (protocatechuic acid) (Lake *et al.,* 1970).

The enzymes of biogenic amine metabolism in insect nervous tissue have not yet been investigated in detail, however. Robertson (1971) demonstrated that β-hydroxylation of [^{14}C]tyramine in cockroach ventral nerve cord occurs *in vitro* and, recently, two approaches to the problem have been exploited. First, the endogenous levels of putative precursors of octopamine in insect nervous tissue have been quantitated. The central nervous system (brain and ventral nerve cord, CNS) of the locust *Schistocerca gregaria* was found to contain relatively large amounts (74 ng/gm) of p-tyramine, but no m-tyramine, β-phenylethylamine, phenylethanolamine, or tryptamine (H. A. Robertson, S. R. Philips, P. H. Wu, and L. Dyck, unpublished observations). Second, brains and ventral nerve cords from the locust were incubated in [^{14}C]phenylalanine and [^{14}C]tyrosine *in vitro*. Catecholamines were isolated by adsorption on alumina followed by paper chromatography. Phenolic amines were isolated on a Dowex 50 (H$^+$ form) resin column and separated by subsequent paper chromatography. Incubation with [^{14}C]tyrosine resulted in the formation of both labeled tyramine and octopamine. No incorporation was found using [^{14}C]phenylalanine as substrate. In another series of experiments incorporation of [^{14}C]tyrosine into tyramine and dopamine was compared. The incorporation of label from [^{14}C]tyrosine was 10-fold higher into tyramine, compared with dopamine. This suggests that tyrosine decarboxylation is a more favored route than hydroxylation, at least in insects. Since the path from tyrosine to tyramine involves only one enzyme and that to dopamine two enzymes, the incorporation rates are not directly comparable. Nevertheless, when considered in light of the knowledge that the locust nervous system contains more octopamine than dopamine (Robertson, 1975b, 1976), it is of significance.

B. CATABOLISM

As well as possessing a system capable of producing and releasing a transmitter, it is necessary to have a mechanism by which the action of the transmitter can be terminated. In general, there are two mechanisms by which this can be achieved. Either the transmitter is broken down enzymically to yield inactive metabolites (as with acetylcholine) or, alternatively, it is removed from the synaptic cleft by reuptake into the presynaptic neurons and/or uptake into other tissues (as with noradrenaline) where it can then be reused or metabolized further. In the case of catecholamines and 5-HT, this latter metabolism usually involves mitochondrial MAO. Such also appears to be the case with respect to microamines, since they are known to be excellent substrates for MAO in mammalian systems; their tissue levels increase many times following MAO inhibition (Boulton, 1976b). In invertebrates, the inactivation of biogenic amines other than acetylcholine has received very little attention, and that of octopamine and other noncatecholic amines almost none. Nevertheless, certain indicators may be discerned concerning the possible means of catabolism of octopamine and other microamines.

1. Monoamine Oxidase

In contrast to the situation in mammalian systems MAO does not seem to be very important in invertebrates. An exception is octopus nervous tissue which contains both an active MAO (Blaschko and Hope, 1957) and the acid metabolites of dopamine and 5-HT (Juorio and Killick, 1972a). The administration of MAO inhibitors to the octopus results in large increases in the concentrations of β-phenylethylamine, p-tyramine, octopamine, dopamine, noradrenaline, tryptamine, and 5-HT (Juorio and Killick, 1972a; Juorio and Molinoff, 1974; Juorio and Philips, 1975, and unpublished observations). In contrast to this, there seems to be little MAO activity in gastropods (Juorio and Killick, 1972a; Wu and Juorio, 1975; Guthrie et al., 1975).

There is little MAO activity in arthropods (Boadle and Blaschko, 1968). MAO activity is present in cockroach and locust nervous tissue, where the activity is less than 0.1% of that in rat liver (H. A. Robertson, P. H. Wu, S. R. Philips, and L. Dyck, unpublished observations). Only cockroach Malpighian tubules (as reported earlier by Blaschko et al., 1961) exhibit significant MAO activity (i.e., about 10% of that in a rat liver homogenate). Octopamine, β-phenylethylamine, and tryptamine are all excellent substrates for insect MAO (H. A. Robertson, S. R. Philips, P. H. Wu, and L. Dyck, unpublished observations). In general, it seems that invertebrates employ mechanisms other than MAO to degrade monoamines.

2. N-Acetylation

There is good evidence, at least in insects, that N-acetylation is one of the methods for the inactivation of monoamines. N-Acetyltransferase activity in the fruit fly Drosophila melanogaster is at least 50 times that of MAO and more than 500 times that of catechol-O-methyltransferase (COMT) (Dewhurst et al., 1972). It is most interesting to note that tyramine is a better substrate for N-acetyltransferase than either dopamine or serotonin.

3. Conjugation

It has been shown recently that [^{14}C]noradrenaline is metabolized in cockroaches to protocatechuic acid glucoside (3-hydroxy-4-O-β-glucosylbenzoic acid) (Lake et al., 1975). Since noradrenaline is present in insects in only small amounts, this observation may be of little physiological significance. Octopamine, however, which is present in large amounts may, by analogy, be metabolized to 4-O-β-glucosylbenzoic acid.

4. Uptake

In mammals, uptake of noradrenaline is the major mechanism of inactivation, and it is assumed that uptake of dopamine and 5-HT is also of physiological importance in terminating the action of these amines (Iversen, 1974). It is possible that similar uptake mechanisms may be important for octopamine and other microamines in invertebrates, but this has not yet been studied. The only microamine uptake mechanism that has been investigated in invertebrates is octopamine uptake by the subesophageal ganglion of Helix pomatia (Osborne et al., 1975). It was demonstrated that octopamine and noradrenaline accumulate by a mechanism dependent on sodium ions and temperature. High tissue/medium ratios were obtained for 5-HT (30:1) and dopamine (18:1), while somewhat lower ratios were obtained for noradrenaline (4:1) and octopamine (5:1). Obviously, uptake is a mechanism capable of terminating neurotransmitter action in invertebrates and is certainly an area requiring further investigation.

In summary, current evidence suggests that the principal route of biosynthesis of octopamine in invertebrates is p-tyrosine $\rightarrow$ p-tyramine $\rightarrow$ p-octopamine. Evidence has been presented to substantiate the claim that some of the enzymes mediating this pathway are present in most of the higher invertebrates and tyramine, an intermediate in the sequence, has been identified and quantitated. Although conclusive proof for the scheme in Fig. 6 has not yet been provided, nor has the validity of the proposed pathway yet been tested by pharmacological manipulations, it appears to be the most likey at this time. Another question which remains to be answered is whether p-tyramine is merely a precursor of p-octopamine or whether it possesses a physiological role of its own in invertebrates.

The mechanism by which octopamine and microamines are removed from the site of action and/or degraded into inactive metabolites is unclear. MAO, while playing a role in some species, is absent in others, and thus alternate mechanisms of monoamine inactivation must be sought. Several possibilities deserve earnest attention. These include N-acetylation, uptake, and conjugation.

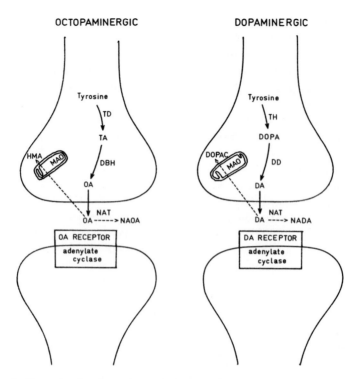

FIG. 6. Generalized schematic model comparing proposed octopaminergic and catecholaminergic neurons from invertebrate nervous systems. Possible inactivation mechanisms are shown as dashed lines. DA, Dopamine; DBH, dopamine-β-hydroxylase; DD, dopa decarboxylase; DOPAC, dihydroxyphenylacetic acid; HMA, p-hydroxymandelic acid; MAO, monoamine oxidase, NAT, N-acetyltransferase; NADA, N-acetyldopamine; NAOA, N-acetyloctopamine; OA, octopamine; TD, tyrosine decarboxylase; TH, tyrosine hydroxylase.

IV. Octopamine in Invertebrate Nervous Systems

So far as invertebrates are concerned, octopamine appears to be the most interesting and, thus far, the best described and best understood of the newly discovered microamines. Octopamine was first identified in the posterior salivary gland of *Octopus vulgaris* by Erspamer (1948, 1952). The demonstration that octopamine is present in mammalian organs and urine during inhibition of MAO systems and normally present in human urine (Kakimoto and Armstrong, 1962) indicated that octopamine may be important in its own right and not merely a metabolic accident and/or false transmitter. Following the development of a sensitive radiochemical-enzymic assay by Molinoff and Axelrod (1969), it became possible to quantitate octopamine and demonstrate its presence in all sympathetically innervated organs in mammals. The simultaneous fall in both octopamine and noradrenaline concentration after sympathectomy of rat salivary glands suggested that octopamine is present in noradrenergic nerves (Molinoff and Axelrod, 1972). Other studies had shown that both [³H]octopamine (resulting from the incubation of tissues with [³H]tyramine) and endogenous octopamine can be released from cat splenic nerve together with noradrenaline (Kopin et al., 1964; Molinoff and Axelrod, 1972). Molinoff and Axelrod (1972) thus suggested that octopamine, since it appeared to be stored in and released from noradrenergic nerves, may conveniently be termed a cotransmitter. Recent work, however, has contradicted some of these earlier results, and it now appears that, at least in rat salivary gland, octopamine is not present in noradrenergic nerves (Coyle et al., 1974; Wooten et al., 1975). Similarly, treatments designed to destroy central noradrenergic nerves in mouse brain or to deplete nerves of their transmitter substances have little or no effect on the levels of octopamine (Harmar and Horn, 1975).

Much recent work on octopamine has centered on its possible role as a primary transmitter at synapses in invertebrates, and there have been suggestions of octopaminergic neurotransmission. No doubt such findings and claims will accelerate the search for a role for octopamine in the vertebrate, especially the mammalian, nervous system.

A. PHYLOGENETIC DISTRIBUTION

Octopamine derives its name from the fact that it was first discovered in the octopus, an invertebrate. Nevertheless, only recently has this compound been definitely associated with the nervous system in invertebrates, as opposed to nonneural tissue such as octopus salivary gland (Juorio and Molinoff, 1971, 1974). The phylogenetic distribution of octopamine and other biogenic amines is shown in Table IV. Octopamine occurs in large amounts in the nervous systems of species representing the phylum Arthropoda (including the classes Insecta (Robertson and Steele, 1974; Robertson, 1975b, 1976) and Crustacea (Barker et al., 1972; Wallace et al., 1974; Evans et al., 1975). Recent work in our laboratory has shown that octopamine is present in large amounts in the annelid Lumbricus (Robertson, 1975a). While the amounts of octopamine present in invertebrates vary considerably, in general the levels have been found to be several orders of magnitude higher than in mammals. In cephalopods, the large amounts of octopamine present seem to reflect, at least in part, increased levels of other amines. For example, in the superior buccal lobes of Octopus brain, octopamine content is 4.6 μg/gm, but this region also contains 16.7 μg/gm of noradrenaline (Juorio

TABLE IV

THE QUANTITATIVE DISTRIBUTION OF AMINES IN SOME REPRESENTATIVE INVERTEBRATE SPECIES[a,b]

Phylum and Species	Tissue	TA	OA	DA	NA	5-HT
Echinodermata						
Class Asteroidea						
Pycnopodia helianthoides (sunflower starfish)	Arm nerve	2.5[1]	260[1]	6,000[1]	2,130[1]	<40[1]
	Tube feet	<1.1[1]	160[1]	370[1]	80[1]	<20[1]
	Stomach	21[1]	53[1]			
Annelida						
Class Oligochaeta						
Lumbricus terrestris (earthworm)	Cerebral ganglia		7,390[2]			
	Subpharyngeal ganglia		8,110[2]			
	Ventral nerve cord		5,340[2]	1,970[3]	1,390[3]	10.4[4]
	Gut (gizzard)		1,060[2]			
	Muscle		<33[2]			
Arthropoda						
Class Insecta						
Periplaneta americana (American cockroach)	Supraesophageal ganglion		3,450; 4,250[5]	2,350[6]	370[6]	
	Subesophageal ganglion and thoracic nerve cord		940[5]			
	Abdominal nerve cord		1,010[5]			
Schistocerca gregaria (desert locust)	Supraesophageal ganglia		2,430[7]	870[7]	110[7]	
	Optic lobes		3,910[7]	660[7]		
	Brain minus optic lobes		860[7]	770[7]		
	Whole CNS	74[8]	1,820[7]			
	Salivary gland		<23[9]	330[12]		
	Fat body		<18[9]			
	CNS		500[9]			
Melanoplus sanguinipes (prairie locust)						790; 1,470[11]
Manduca sexta (tobacco hornworm moth)	Thoracic ganglia		300[9]			

Photuris versicolor (firefly)					
Lantern		125[10]			15[15,c]
Class Crustacea					
Homarus americanus (lobster)					
Supraesophageal ganglion	210[13]	226[13]			<20[15]
Subesophageal ganglion and thoracic nerve cord	150[13]				
Abdominal nerve cord	160[13]				
Subesophageal ganglion		117[14]			
Thoracic 1		74[14]			
Thoracic 2, 3		117[14]			
Thoracic 4, 5		140[14]			
Abdominal 1		109[14]			
Abdominal 2 to 5		55[14]			
Abdominal 6		73[14]			
Peripheral nerve bundle		11[14]			
Thoracic connective		379[14]			
Abdominal connective		41[14]			
Muscle		<2[14]			
CNS			200[14]		
Mollusca					
Class Gastropoda					
Helix aspersa (garden snail)					
Circumesophageal ganglia	24[16]	127[18] 0.75 μg/gm protein[19]	5,160[17]	70[17,19]	5,100[17]
Heart	19[16]	0[18] 1.32 μg/gm protein[19]	<40[17]		7,240[17]
Aplysia californica (ref. 17 *A. limacina*) (sea hare)					
Abdominal ganglia		35[28]	1,850[27]		
Cerebral ganglia		283[28]	2,610[27]		2,500[27]
Buccal ganglia		130[28]	800[27]		
Pedal ganglia		161[28]	5,020[17]	<85[17]	8,430[17]
Pleural ganglia		31[28]	760[17]	<85[17]	

(Continued)

TABLE IV (Continued)

Phylum and Species	Tissue	TA	OA	DA	NA	5-HT
Class Cephalopoda, order Dibranchia, suborder Octopoda Octopus vulgaris (Mediterranean octopus)						
	Circumesophageal ganglia		1,200[20]	11,900[20]	4,400[20]	3,700[20]
	Supraesophageal ganglia					
	Vertical lobe		720[20]	2,050[24]	3,620[24]	4,700[23]
	Superior frontal lobe		530[20]	4,480[24]	4,290[24]	
	Inferior buccal lobe		1,140[20]	1,570[24]	700[24]	
	Superior buccal lobe		4,610[20]	10,000[24]	16,700[24]	7,270[26]
	Posterior buccal lobe		2,050[20]	7,100[24]	2,600[24]	
	Basal lobe system		1,460[20]	4,600[24]	4,960[24]	
	Optic lobes		1,310[20]	15,000[24]	4,530[24]	4,990[20]
	Optic tract		1,330[20]	2,790[24]	2,600[24]	
	Subesophageal ganglia					
	Anterior region		1,000[20]	5,730[24]	1,770[24]	
	Median region		700[20]	1,630[24]	1,590[24]	
	Posterior region		570[20]	2,990[24]	1,520[24]	
	Other tissues					
	Stellate ganglia		210[20]	840[24]	<70[24]	
	Gastric ganglia		340[20]	5,600[24]	4,040[24]	
	Lens		80[20]				
	Retina		50[20]	320[25]	<50[25]	360[25]
	Branchial heart		250[20]	<30[25]	<30[25]	<40[25]
	Systemic heart		30[20]	<30[25]	<30[25]	<40[25]
	Cephalic aorta		20[20]				
	Cecum		2[20]	<30[25]	<30[25]	<40[25]
	Stomach		30[20]	<30[25]	<30[25]	<40[25]
	Crop		100[20]	90[25]	270[25]	<40[25]
	Esophagus		80[20]	260[25]	850[25]	<40[25]
	Anterior salivary gland		60[20]	<10[25]	<10[25]	<30[25]
	Posterior salivary gland		1,310,000[20]	3,070[25]	5,780[25]	455,000[25]

Species and tissue	OA	DA	NA	TA
Octopus dofleini martini (Pacific octopus)				
Mantle skin	130[22]	<30[25]	<30[25]	<30[25]
Superior buccal lobe	170[22]	670[22]	5,460[23]	4,660[23]
Optic lobes	525[22]	820[22]		
Inferior buccal lobe	4[22]	8,900[22]		
Posterior salivary gland	4,900[23]	14,300[23]	4,800[23]	34,200[23]
Octopus macropus				
Optic lobes	1,770[23]	10,900[23]		
Eledone moschata				
Optic lobes	2,210[20]	19,200[21]	5,240[21]	7,490[21]
Posterior salivary gland	182,000[20]	21,100[21]	9,210[21]	7,000[21]
Class Cephalopoda, order Dibranchia, suborder Decapoda				
Sepia officinalis (cuttlefish)				
Vertical lobe	20[20]	590[23]	930[23]	
Optic lobes	220[20]	6,940[21]	3,200[21]	2,520[21]
Stellate ganglia	10[20]	890[25]	1,490[25]	<70[25]
Posterior salivary gland	90[20]	510[23]	590[23]	
Loligo vulgaris (squid)				
Vertical lobe	180[20]	5,040[21]	2,830[21]	860[21]
Optic lobes	430[20]	70[23]	170[23]	
Stellate ganglia	40[20]	120[25]		
Preganglionic nerve	10[20]			
Fin and stellate nerve	20[20]			
Posterior salivary gland	20[20]		1,890[25]	
Systemic heart	20[20]			<40[25]

[a] Amine concentrations given in nanograms per gram of fresh tissue unless otherwise noted. TA, p-tyramine; OA, octopamine; DA, dopamine; NA, noradrenaline.

[b] Superscript numbers indicate references: (1) A. V. Juorio and H. A. Robertson, unpublished observations, 1975; (2) Robertson, 1975a; (3) Gardner and Cashin, 1975; (4) Welsh and Moorhead, 1960; (5) Robertson and Steele, 1974; (6) Frontali and Häggendal, 1969; (7) Robertson, 1976; (8) Robertson, 1975a; (9) H. A. Robertson, unpublished observations; (10) Robertson, 1975d; (11) Klemm and Axelsson, 1973; (12) Robertson, 1975c; (13) A. V. Juorio, H. A. Robertson, and P. H. Wu, unpublished observations, 1975; (14) Barker et al., 1972; (15) Welsh and Moorhead, 1960; (16) Wu and Juorio, 1975; (17) Juorio and Killick, 1972a; (18) H. A. Robertson, unpublished observations, 1975; (19) Walker et al., 1972; (20) Juorio and Molinoff, 1974; (21) Juorio and Killick, 1972a; (22) Juorio and Philips, 1975; (23) Juorio and Killick, 1973; (24) Juorio, 1971; (25) Juorio and Killick, 1973; (26) Barlow et al., 1974; (27) Carpenter et al., 1971; (28) Saavedra et al., 1974a.

[c] Nerve cord.

and Molinoff, 1974). In contrast to this situation, the brain of the locust
S. gregaria contains 2.5 µg/gm of octopamine and only 0.1 µg/gm of noradrenaline (Robertson, 1976). The brain of the cockroach (*Periplaneta
americana*) contains about 4 µg/gm of octopamine (Robertson and
Steele, 1974) and 0.4 µg/gm of noradrenaline (Frontali and Häggendal, 1969), and lobster (*Homarus*) brain contains 229 ng/gm of octopamine
and no detectable noradrenaline (Barker *et al.*, 1972). In arthropods, it is
clearly of great significance that high levels of octopamine are found only
in conjunction with very low levels of noradrenaline or in its absence. Likewise, octopamine but no noradrenaline is found in the ganglia of the marine
gastropod *Aplysia;* dopamine, however, is present (Carpenter *et al.*, 1971;
Juorio and Killick, 1972a; Saavedra *et al.*, 1974a). In the earthworm, *Lumbricus,* the only annelid well studied, octopamine (5 µg/gm in the ventral
nerve cord) is present in much higher concentrations than dopamine (1.97
µg/gm) or noradrenaline (1.39 µg/gm) (Gardner and Cashin, 1975). Is
there a phylogenetic pattern here? It would be nice to be able to present a
story of two discrete systems in higher invertebrates composed of two different types of neurons, an octopaminergic neuron and a dopaminergic
neuron. The octopaminergic neuron probably would contain a tyrosine decarboxylase and tyramine-β-hydroxylase (which may be identical to the enzyme known as dopamine-β-hydroxylase). The dopaminergic neuron would
be characterized by the enzymes tyrosine hydroxylase and dopadecarboxylase.
The evidence for the existence of such discrete systems is compelling in the
case of arthropods (Barker *et al.*, 1972; Wallace *et al.*, 1974; Robertson and
Steele, 1974; Robertson, 1975b, 1976) and the gastropod mollusc *Aplysia*
(Saavedra *et al.*, 1974a). However, in the case of some higher invertebrates
there is evidence indicating large amounts of noradrenaline in addition to
dopamine and octopamine, and so presumably a noradrenergic neuron type,
possessing tyrosine hydroxylase, dopa decarboxylase, and dopamine-β-hydroxylase, must also be present in these animals. Examples include cephalo-
pod molluscs (see Juorio and Molinoff, 1974) and the annelid *Lumbricus
terrestris* (Gardner and Cashin, 1975; Robertson, 1975a). Even in insects,
a small amount of noradrenaline is present in the CNS (Klemm and Axelsson, 1973; Robertson, 1975, 1976). It is possible that dopamine released
from dopaminergic neurons is taken up by a nonspecific mechanism into
octopaminergic neurons and there converted to noradrenaline.

In addition to being a putative central transmitter there is evidence to
suggest that octopamine is a peripheral transmitter in higher invertebrates.
In arthropods (insects and crustaceans) there is some evidence suggesting a
role in neuromuscular transmission. This is not to say that octopamine is the
neuromuscular transmitter, but rather that it may possess a modulating influence on nerve–muscle interaction (see Evans *et al.*, 1975; Hoyle, 1975).

Similarly, there is substantial circumstantial evidence to suggest that octo-pamine is the principal transmitter in the firefly lantern (Carlson, 1969; Robertson, 1975d; Robertson and Carlson, 1976a). In annelids, it is possible that octopamine acts as a transmitter in the gut (Robertson, 1975a). In the mollusc *Aplysia,* octopamine-containing neurons (Saavedra *et al.,* 1974a) project to gill and siphon muscles (Kupfermann *et al.,* 1974). It is not known, however, whether these octopamine-containing neurons in *Aplysia* actually release octopamine at their neuromuscular contacts. These neurons contain more than one transmitter (Brownstein *et al.,* 1974).

In summary, octopamine is widely distributed in all higher invertebrates and is present in amounts comparable to or in excess of those of catechol-amines. There is evidence for specific octopaminergic and dopaminergic neu-rons in arthropods and in some molluscs. Some other molluscs (the gastropod snail *Helix aspersa,* and cephalopods), and annelids, may possess noradren-ergic neurons as well. It is also possible that octopamine serves as a trans-mitter in some peripheral tissues.

B. Cellular Localization

To establish whether or not a substance is a transmitter, several criteria must be fulfilled (see Phillis, 1970). One of these criteria is that the sus-pected transmitter substance exist within the neuron. There are now several procedures by which this can be demonstrated, such as (1) fluorescence light microscopy (for catecholamines and 5-HT), (2) electron microscope visualization after special fixation techniques, (3) autoradiography at the light and electron microscope levels, (4) immunohistochemistry, and (5) microdissection of neurons followed by analysis of contents.

Fluorescence microscopy is not an option for *p*-octopamine, since the Falck–Hillarp technique depends on a reaction that does not occur with this amine (Fuxe and Jonsson, 1973). At the electron microscope level, we can-not as yet assign any characteristics to octopamine-containing neurons, al-though several systems in which octopamine may be the putative transmitter have been described. The ultrastructure of the nerve endings of the pre-sumed octopamine neurons in the second roots of the lobster thoracic ganglia has been examined by Evans *et al.* (1975). These nerve endings are full of granules ($\simeq$100 nm in diameter) of varying electron density. Another sys-tem that has been examined by electron microscopy, and which only recently has been proposed to be octopaminergic (Robertson, 1975d; Robertson and Carlson, 1976a), is the firefly lantern. Its ultrastructure has been described by Smith (1963) and by Peterson (1970). There appear to be few if any discernible similarities between the supposed octopaminergic neurons of the lobster and the firefly, except perhaps that they both contain numerous elongated dense-core vesicles. Autoradiography at the light and electron microscope levels has not yet been attempted on systems suspected to be octopaminergic. The fact that octopamine possesses a reactive amino group, which presumably binds to glutaraldehyde (Bloom, 1970), suggests that this approach should be successful.

Immunofluorescent histochemical mapping has not yet been attempted. However, since most of the species in which putative octopaminergic systems occur do not contain noradrenaline, the enzyme dopamine-β-hydroxylase can be utilized as a specific marker for these neurons just as it has for noradrenergic systems in mammals (see Hartman et al., 1972).

Microdissection techniques have been applied successfully in the isolation of specific octopamine-containing neurons. This work was much facilitated by the fact that the neurons of many invertebrates are not only large but also identifiable from individual to individual. Thus Saavedra et al., (1974a) dissected and isolated individual identified neurons from various ganglia of Aplysia californica and measured their octopamine content. These cells are large and, most important, have no synapses. All known synaptic contacts in molluscs are axoaxonic (Tauc, 1967). The possibility that the octopamine identified as being present in such cells is present in the adhering nerve terminals from other cells can therefore be discounted. Certain neurons were found to contain octopamine, but not dopamine or noradrenaline. Although dopamine is present in Aplysia ganglia (Saavedra et al., 1974a), it is not present in the octopamine-containing neurons. However, what is anomalous about Aplysiaa neurons is that they contain several putative transmitters (Brownstein et al., 1974). For example, cell L-7 from the abdominal ganglion contains octopamine, but also measurable amounts of 5-HT, histamine, acetylcholine, glutamate, and glutamine, all of which are putative transmitters in Aplysia, since there are specific postsynaptic receptors for all these substances in this species (Brownstein et al., 1974). A possible explanation of this apparent violation of Dale's principle (that a neuron makes and releases only one transmitter) may lie in the specificity of transport systems. For example, in Aplysia, while both serotonergic and cholinergic neurons can convert 5-hydroxytryptophan (5-HTP) to 5-HT, only in the serotonergic neurons is 5-HT stored and transported down the axon (Goldman and Schwartz, 1974). By analogy then, octopaminergic cells may thus contain other transmitter substances which, because they are not transported, cannot be released or, alternatively, cells containing octopamine may not be able to transport it to the nerve terminals.

Another instance in which microdissection has been possible is the isolation of the octopamine-containing cells in the second root of the thoracic ganglia of the lobster. This is possible because the neurons lie outside the CNS and can be visualized by the neutral red vital staining technique (Wallace et al., 1974). The cells exhibit dopamine-β-hydroxylase activity, and it appears likely that octopamine is present in the cells rather than in nerve terminals impinging on them. The input to these cells appears to be cholinergic (Wallace *et al.*, 1974). Although the neutral red technique was useful in visualizing the above cells, it is a fact that this vital stain is also taken up by other monoaminergic cells in the CNS of several species including the snail *H. aspersa*, the earthworm *L. terrestris*, the leech *H. medicinalis*, and the lobster *Homarus americanus* (Stuart *et al.*, 1974), and in several species of insects (H. A. Robertson, unpublished observations).

C. SUBCELLULAR LOCALIZATION

Although microdissection and analysis of neuronal perikarya provide good evidence that octopamine is present in a cell body, they do not provide conclusive evidence that a particular substance is a transmitter. As several putative transmitters may coexist in a single neuron, it is necessary to demonstrate in addition that the substance is present in the nerve ending and is released on stimulation. The localization of most putative neurotransmitters in synaptosomes (pinched-off nerve endings) has been demonstrated. Octopamine was shown by Juorio and Molinoff (1974) to be located in a synaptosome fraction isolated from an homogenate of octopus brain after density gradient centrifugation. Dopamine and noradrenaline were also present in the same regions of the gradient as octopamine (see Fig. 7). The presence of octopamine in granule-containing synaptosomes from octopus brain, together with the fact that reserpine depletes these granules, supports the contention that octopamine is stored in reserpine-sensitive storage granules. A problem remaining to be solved is whether octopamine exists in the same nerve endings as noradrenaline or whether there are specific octopaminergic nerve endings. Reserpine produces a long-lasting reduction in the concentration of certain amines in mammalian nerves, and it is generally accepted that this drug impairs the transport of amines into storage granules (Carlsson *et al.*, 1963). The administration of reserpine to the octopus in comparatively low doses produced a marked and long-lasting reduction in the concentration of amines measured in the optic lobes (Table V). Relatively high doses of reserpine (60 mg/kg) have been shown to deplete octopamine levels in locust brain (Robertson, 1975b, 1976). Similar high doses of reserpine were required to deplete catecholamine stores in insects (Frontali, 1968). These biochemical and morphological findings strongly suggest that, in octopus ganglia, octopamine, noradrenaline, and dopamine are stored in granules sensitive to reserpine treatment; the same may be true for insects.

The large size and accessibility of identified neurons in some invertebrates provides a splendid example of a system in which a combination of physiological, anatomical, and biochemical techniques can be focused on a single neuron. An indication of the range of feasible experiments is demon-

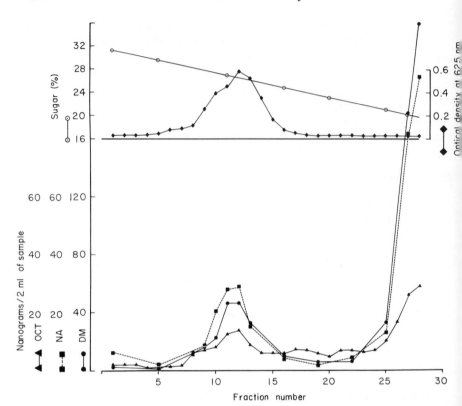

FIG. 7. Subcellular fractionation of *O. vulgaris* circumesophageal ganglia. Tissue weighing 396 mg was obtained from one animal. The tissue was homogenized in 4.8 ml of a 1:1 mixture of 13% glucose solution and saline. A 3-ml portion was then layered onto 52 ml of a sugar–salt gradient containing 205 mM sodium chloride, 4 mM potassium chloride, 5 mM calcium chloride, and 50 μg/ml of pargyline. The sugar concentration in the gradient extended from a minimum value of 7.5% to a maximum of 35%. The gradient was then centrifuged for 90 minutes at 106,900 g_{max}. The open circles in the upper diagram represent the sugar content, as determined by refractometry, and the dots light scattering as measured at 625 nm. In the lower diagram the amine (octopamine, noradrenaline, and dopamine) concentration is expressed in nanograms per 2 ml of sample. This figure has been redrawn from data listed by A. V. Juorio and P. B. Molinoff (1974) and from unpublished results.

strated by the work performed using a giant neuron in the cerebral ganglion of the snail *H. pomatia*. This cell was identified as serotonergic on the basis of anatomical and bioassay techniques (Cottrell and Osborne, 1970). With this knowledge, Pentreath and Cottrell (1974) injected, iontophoretically, [³H]5-HT or it precursor [³H]5-HTP directly into the identified neuron. Then, using autoradiographic techniques on serial sections, the entire axonal projection was mapped. These studies showed for the first time that pre-synaptic nerve terminals of a specific individual neuron of known trans-mitter type can be studied in direct relation to the cell body. In future studies, it may be possible to inject labeled precursor into the cell body and to demonstrate release of labeled transmitter at the target organ. Techniques similar to those described, applied to known octopaminergic neurons such as those found in insects, crustaceans, and molluscs may be expected to augment greatly our knowledge of these neurons and their functions.

D. PHYSIOLOGICAL ROLES FOR OCTOPAMINE

In view of the large concentrations of octopamine existing in inverte-brates it is not surprising that most of the speculation with respect to its potential physiological role is centered on these animals. It seems likely, at least in some species, that octopamine is synthesized in specific octopaminergic neurons and that it may function as a neurotransmitter.

1. Arthropoda

The earliest suggestion that octopamine may function as a transmitter was made by Carlson (1968a,b), who investigated the pharmacology of the firefly lantern. It has been known since the work of Kastle and McDermott (1910) that adrenaline induces luminescence when injected into fireflies. Carlson (1968a,b) tested a large number of adrenergic drugs on an *in vitro* preparation of firefly lantern and found synephrine and octopamine to be many times more potent than dopamine or any other adrenergic compound. The idea that a monophenolic amine could be the transmitter was challenged by Murdock (1971), who argued that octopamine had not been identified in insects, while dopamine was at least present in insects and functioned as a peripheral neurotransmitter (see Robertson, 1974, 1975c). Following the development of a suitable assay procedure, octopamine was found to be present in insects and at concentration levels exceeding those of catechol-amines (Robertson and Steele, 1974). It has recently been shown that the firefly lantern contains octopamine (Robertson, 1975d; Robertson and Carl-son, 1976a). Carlson (1972) compared the action of the endogenous trans-mitter on the firefly lantern with that of synephrine. The transmitter and synephrine both act directly on the lantern with similar latencies. Neither transmitter nor synephrine show enhanced activity in the presence of MAO inhibitors. Both are blocked by chlorpromazine, an α-blocking drug. The only difference found was that luminescence induced by the transmitter was more rapidly extinguished than that induced by synephrine. As the analytical data now point to octopamine rather than synephrine as the transmitter, the extinction rates of octopamine and of the native transmitter should be compared. With respect to the lack of effect of MAO inhibitors, it has recently been shown that insect nervous tissue contains very little MAO activity and that other mechanisms of inactivation such as reuptake and N-acetylation must be considered the means of inactivating monoamine transmitters in insects (H. A. Robertson, S. R. Philips, P. H. Wu, and L. Dyck, unpublished observations).

Another early suggestion that octopamine possesses a role of its own in insects involved the discovery that octopamine and related amines (synephrine, tyramine) exhibited a powerful stimulatory effect on the enzyme glycogen phosphorylase in the ventral nerve cord of the cockroach P. americana (Robertson and Steele, 1970, 1972). Octopamine, but not dopamine, noradrenaline, or adrenaline, produced significant decreases in nerve cord glycogen levels and increases in phosphorylase activity (Robertson and Steele, 1973). The effects of octopamine were mimicked by cyclic adenosine-3',5'-monophosphate (cAMP) and by the phosphodiesterase inhibitor caffeine (Robertson and Steele, 1972). Phosphorylase activation, as shown by Steele (1963), was also produced by a factor from the corpus cardiacum (an organ analogous to the mammalian posterior pituitary), but this factor was shown to be a peptide and not octopamine (Robertson and Steele, 1973). Subsequent studies by Nathanson and Greengard (1973) demonstrated a specific octopamine-sensitive adenylate cyclase in the nerve cord of the cockroach, as well as specific dopamine- and 5-HT-sensitive adenylate cyclases. The function of octopamine-induced phosphorylase activation and the resulting glycogenolysis is still unknown. Insect ganglia contain large stores of glycogen as an energy source, possibly because the insect nervous system is avascular (Wigglesworth, 1960; Treherne, 1966). It is possible that, in addition to being a transmitter, octopamine plays a role in carbohydrate metabolism in the insect nervous system by regulating the breakdown of glycogen to glucose. However, there is no evidence for the direct activation of insect nerve cord phosphorylase by octopamine or even by cAMP, and it is possible that both octopamine and cAMP activate only ATP-requiring processes in the cell, which lead to conditions favoring increased carbohydrate metabolism and phosphorylase activation.

The role of octopamine in Crustacea has been investigated by Kravitz and his colleagues. In the lobster (Homarus), discrete octopamine-containing cells are present in the second roots of the subesophageal and thoracic ganglia (Wallace et al., 1974). The location of these cells outside the CNS, their probable cholinergic input, and their position and number indicated to Wallace et al. (1974) that perhaps this is a primitive analog of the mammalian sympathetic nervous system. Evans et al. (1975) injected the dye Procion yellow into the octopamine neurons in order to trace their processes. They saw that fine processes of the cells branched extensively in the vicinity of the cells. Electron micrographs indicated granule-filled endings which appeared not to be associated with any particular target, suggesting a neurosecretory role (i.e., that the octopamine is released into the hemolymph rather than at a specific target organ).

Experiments using high-potassium lobster saline to depolarize the nerves after preloading with either [^{3}H]tyrosine or [^{3}H]tyramine revealed a calcium-dependent release of [^{3}H]octopamine (Evans et al., 1975). It was suggested that lobster muscle may be the site of action of octopamine, and the effects of octopamine on the opener muscle of lobster walking legs were examined. Octopamine (10 μM) produced a long-lasting contraction of the walking-leg opener muscle. It is of relevance that both nerve and muscle from the lobster contain an octopamine-sensitive adenylate cyclase (Sullivan and Barker, 1975). The physiological significance of these observations is still unknown. A similar system of octopaminergic neurons has been reported recently in insects. Large nerve cell bodies found in the midlines of the dorsal surface of cockroach and locust (S. gregaria) thoracic ganglia appear to be homologous to the octopaminergic cells of the second roots of the subesophageal and thoracic ganglia. These cells, described by Hoyle et al. (1974) as dorsal unpaired median (or DUM) cells, give off a single median axon which makes a T branch and provides symmetrical left and right efferent axons to the major skeletal leg muscles. The final branches of this neuron parallel the fast axon (which probably releases glutamate, the transmitter at the insect neuromuscular junction). All the fibers in the muscle are innervated by the fast axon, but only a few receive terminals of the dorsal neuron which has neurosecretory-type endings (Hoyle et al., 1974). Stimulation of these DUM cells leads to long-term inhibition of the slow intrinsic rhythm of contraction of the leg muscle, and this inhibition is mimicked by the infusion of saline containing monoamines into the leg of the locust. Again, like the firefly lantern, the muscle is most sensitive to octopamine and is much less sensitive to dopamine and noradrenaline (Hoyle, 1975). DUM cells do not show fluorescence after the Falck-Hillarp treatment (Hoyle, 1975), and when ganglia, somata of DUM cells, and leg nerves were incubated in the presence of [^{3}H]tyrosine, labeled tyramine and octopamine were formed. Small amounts of endogenous octopamine (90 ng/gm) are present in the leg muscle of S. gregaria (H. A. Robertson, unpublished observations).

2. Mollusca

Evidence supporting a physiological role for octopamine is well documented in molluscs, the phylum in which it was first identified. Numerous features make the molluscs a popular group for experimentation. Cephalopods are the most advanced (behaviorally) of the invertebrates and possess large brains (by invertebrate standards) (Young, 1971). The nervous system of gastropod molluscs is ideal for neurochemical and neurophysiological investigation, because of the large and distinct neurons, many of which can be identified on the basis of position, size, and color.

a. *Gastropoda*. From an experimental point of view, the most important feature of the gastropod nervous system is that individual neurons can be identified from one animal to the next. This means that many identical neurons from several preparations can be collected for chemical analysis, that physiological techniques can be standardized, and that experimental manipulations can be performed at the level of the individual neuron. Most important, it allows ready correlation among results from different experimental approaches to the same problem. For example, it is reported that the motor neuron L-7 from the abdominal ganglion of *Aplysia* mediates an excitatory response at the gill and mantle shelf (Kupfermann *et al.*, 1974). This can immediately be correlated with biochemical information showing that L-7 contains large amounts of octopamine (Saavedra *et al.*, 1974a). The large size of *Aplysia* neurons makes it possible to microdissect and analyze single neurons. The intracellular location of octopamine in individual identified neurons of *Aplysia* has been demonstrated (Saavedra *et al.*, 1974a), and Carpenter and Gaubatz (1974) have recorded intracellularly from *Aplysia* neurons and found specific receptors for octopamine, dopamine, and phenylethanolamine. Octopamine caused either a depolarizing sodium conductance or a hyperpolarizing potassium conductance. Octopamine receptors were generally found on cells other than those possessing dopamine or phenylethanolamine receptors, but a few cells possessed all three receptors. Octopamine receptors were also sensitive to noradrenaline, but to a lesser extent. Since noradrenaline is not present in *Aplysia* (Saavedra *et al.*, 1974a), this is of no functional significance, but the cells also respond weakly to phenylethanolamine which is present (Carpenter and Gaubatz, 1974). Further evidence for a neurotransmitter role for octopamine in *Aplysia* comes from the work of Levitan and Barondes (1974), who showed octopamine- and 5-HT-stimulated phosphorylation of a specific protein (MW $\sim$120,000) in the abdominal ganglion. This stimulatory effect of octopamine was inhibited by phentolamine and mimicked by dibutyryl cAMP. The changes produced in the ganglia persist for hours after removal of octopamine. These investigators suggested that neurotransmitters (such as octopamine) produce relatively long-lasting changes in phosphoprotein in postsynaptic cells. It is, however, impossible to determine the site of the change in protein phosphorylation in this system. In mammalian systems, catecholamines have been shown to stimulate adenylate cyclase (hence to increase cAMP levels) both in postsynaptic neurons (Siggins *et al.*, 1973) and in glioblastoma (Gilman and Nirenberg, 1971). The ease with which the nervous system of molluscs such as *Aplysia* can be manipulated both electrophysiologically and biochemically suggests that this system may be useful in working out the role of neurotransmitters in the long-term changes in synaptic function associated with learning.

Octopamine and 5-HT both produced increases in cAMP in abdominal ganglia, and the octopamine- and 5-HT-induced increases were blocked by phentolamine and methysergide, respectively (Levitan *et al.*, 1974). Unfortunately, no attempt was made to block octopamine with methysergide or 5-HT with phentolamine to determine if specific receptors are involved in this process.

The evidence that octopamine is a neurotransmitter in *Aplysia* may be summarized as follows. (1) It is present in individual identified neurons that do not contain dopamine or noradrenaline; (2) octopamine receptors are found on a few neurons and only in the neuropile, where functional synapses occur; (3) the receptors have a marked sensitivity for octopamine and do not respond to the only endogenous catecholamine, dopamine; and (4) *Aplysia* ganglia contain an octopamine-sensitive adenylate cyclase, and such adenylate cyclases have been suggested to be receptors in octopaminergic, dopaminergic, and serotonergic neurotransmission (Greengard *et al.*, 1973).

In another gastropod, *H. aspersa*, octopamine has been shown to exert specific action on individual neurons. Walker *et al.* (1972) first identified octopamine in the CNS of gastropods and demonstrated that it, like dopamine and noradrenaline, was a potent inhibitor of the spontaneous firing of neurons. The activity of cells was inhibited by dopamine, noradrenaline, and octopamine, and the membrane potential was hyperpolarized. However, the potency of octopamine as compared to dopamine was from equipotent to 100 times less potent. Octopamine was at least 10 times more potent than noradrenaline. Several arguments have been advanced to support the concept of the presence of distinct octopamine receptors. Cells desensitized by repeated application of octopamine still responded to standard doses of noradrenaline. Low doses of ergotamine blocked the action of dopamine and noradrenaline, but not octopamine. Dibenzyline blocked all three compounds, but propanolol failed to antagonize their actions. Cocaine ($10 \ \mu g/ml$) inhibited the action of 50 pmoles of octopamine. These investigators argue that the blocking of octopamine action by cocaine is evidence for indirect action. Walker *et al.* (1972) also claimed to have identified octopamine ($1.32 \ \mu g/gm$ protein) in the heart of *H. aspersa*. However, it has not been possible, using a more sensitive assay, to confirm this (A. V. Juorio, H. A. Robertson, and P. H. Wu, unpublished observations). No octopamine was present in the heart of *Helix* in November; it is possible that the level of octopamine in *Helix* heart, like that of 5-HT, fluctuates seasonally (see Cardot, 1971; Juorio and Killick, 1972a).

b. Cephalopoda. While octopamine exists in relatively high concentrations in octopus ganglia (Juorio and Molinoff, 1974), there is not as yet any conclusive evidence to support the claim that it is a neurotransmitter in this animal. A possible explanation for this may be that, because the octopus possesses large numbers (about 1.6×10^8 cells, Young, 1963) of comparatively small neurons (20- to 80-μm body diameter; Osborne, 1974), the single-cell dissection technique and electrode implantation are more difficult than in gastropods (cell body diameter up to 800 μm, Osborne, 1974). The giant nerve system of squid stellate ganglia (preganglionic, fin, and stellate nerves) has long axons (diameter, 700–900 μm, Osborne, 1974) but contains only 10–20 ng/gm of octopamine (Juorio and Molinoff, 1974). This appears to rule out the possibility that octopamine acts as a transmitter in these regions. The presence of large amounts of octopamine (and also 5-HT and *p*-tyramine) in the posterior salivary glands of cephalopods may indicate physiological significance, especially since octopamine and possibly 5-HT and *p*-tyramine are transmitters in crustaceans. It is now well established that crabs are rapidly killed by octopus saliva (Lo Bianco, 1898). The fact that a crab-killing glycoprotein has been isolated from the posterior salivary gland of some cephalopods (Guiretti, 1960) suggests that octopamine, and other amines secreted by the glands of these animals, may have a function other than directly killing the prey, for example, improving toxin absorption or prolonging its effects (Juorio and Killick, 1973).

3. Annelida and Other Invertebrates

Octopamine is present in large amounts in the CNS of the earthworm *L. terrestris,* and it is also found in the gut (gizzard); such findings raise the possibility that it is both a central and peripheral transmitter in annelids (Robertson, 1975a). Octopamine is also synthesized from [^{14}C]tyrosine by isolated ganglia from the leech *H. medicinalis* (Stuart *et al.,* 1974). No information with respect to the physiological role of octopamine is available for annelids or any other lower invertebrate.

In summary, it may be stated that there appears to be good evidence to support the concept that octopamine acts as a transmitter in higher invertebrate phyla. In all higher invertebrates, the levels of the amine are relatively high and, in some groups, such as gastropod molluscs and insects, there is evidence in support of the existence of octopaminergic neurons terminating on octopaminergic receptors which may be identical to, or associated with, a specific octopamine-sensitive adenylate cyclase.

In addition to its potential role as a central transmitter, there is some evidence, from several groups, to support the view that octopamine operates as a transmitter at peripheral effector organs including somatic muscle (in molluscs, insects, and crustaceans), gut muscle (in annelids), and the firefly lantern. In both the CNS and the periphery, the mechanism of action of octopamine seems to involve an octopamine-sensitive adenylate cyclase. Whether or not specific octopamine receptors are present in the above tissues has not been investigated, except in a few instances, and the relationship between the receptor and the adenylate cyclase system, even in well-studied systems, remains unclear. Despite these limitations, our knowledge of octopamine has moved from a consideration of whether or not it is a transmitter to that of considering its physiological role as a transmitter. It is evident that octopamine plays some role in neuromuscular physiology in arthropods (insects and crustaceans) and possibly in molluscus and annelids as well, and this must be considered exciting, since it may lead to advances in our knowledge of how the nervous system maintains the integrity of muscle. That octopamine may also play a role in the regulation of carbohydrate metabolism in invertebrate nervous systems is also evident. Perhaps its role in the invertebrate nervous system is to maintain neurons in a state of readiness by regulating cAMP levels, which in turn woud be seen as changes in phosphorylase activation, protein synthesis, membrane permeability, or any of the myriad other parameters of cell physiology affected by cyclic nucleotide levels. Indeed, the role of octopamine in invertebrate muscle may also be interpreted in a similar vein.

V. Other Microamines

A. β-PHENYLETHYLAMINE AND PHENYLETHANOLAMINE

The presence of β-phenylethylamine in mammalian tissues has been suspected since the amine was detected in brain tissue following the administration of its precursor amino acid both in the presence and absence of a MAO inhibitor (Nakajima et al., 1964; Edwards and Blau, 1973). As a result of the recent development of specific and sensitive mass spectrometric (Durden et al. 1973), mass fragmentographic (Willner et al., 1974), enzymic-isotopic assay (Saavedra, 1974b), and gas chromatographic (Martin and Baker, 1975) techniques, the β-phenylethylamine concentration in rat brain has been found to be between 1.5 and 1.8 ng/gm. The values found in the circumesophageal ganglia of the snail were about 7 ng/gm, and even lower values were observed in *Octopus dofleini* optic lobes (A. V. Juorio and S. R. Philips, unpublished observations) and in insect nervous tissue (H. A. Robertson and S. R. Philips, unpublished observations) (see Table VII).

Since phenylethanolamine-N-methyltransferase, the enzyme responsible for the transformation of β-phenylethylamine into phenylethanolamine, is present in mammalian brain (Axelrod, 1962), it is not surprising to find that this amine is also present in this tissue; concentrations for rat brain range from 4 to 7 ng/gm (Saavedra and Axelrod, 1973; Willner et al., 1974). Very little is known about the presence of phenylethanolamine in invertebrate ganglia. It appears that phenylethanolamine is present in Aplysia neurons (J. M. Saavedra, M. J. Brownstein, and J. Axelrod, unpublished, cited by Carpenter and Gaubatz, 1974). Recent attempts to identify phenylethanolamine in the optic lobes of O. dofleini have shown that, if it is present, even after pargyline treatment its levels are below the limits of sensitivity of the method (A. V. Juorio and S. R. Philips, unpublished observations).

B. p- AND m-TYRAMINE

p-Tyramine is a constituent of normal urine, and daily excretion in humans is about 200–500 μg/liter (Levine et al., 1962); the amount excreted increases severalfold after treatment with MAO inhibitors (Sjoerdsma et al., 1959). p-Tyramine has also been implicated in some pathological conditions. After oral administration it has been reported to produce migraine attacks in patients who suffer from migraine (Hanington, 1967) and, following ingestion, it is excreted in conjugated form in significantly smaller quantities in migraine patients than in normals (Youdim et al., 1971); urinary excretion of unconjugated tyramine is abnormal in patients suffering from Parkinson's disease (Boulton et al., 1967; Boulton and Marjerrison, 1972; Smith and Kellow, 1969; Marjerrison et al., 1971) and schizophrenia (Boulton et al., 1971; Boulton, 1971). These findings suggested that p-tyramine exists endogenously in tissues, but only after the development of a specific and sensitive mass spectrometric technique was a value of 2 ng/gm found for rat brain (Philips et al., 1974a).

Chromogenic reactions after solvent extraction have indicated that high concentrations of p-tyramine are present in the posterior salivary gland of the octopus (Henze, 1913; Erspamer, 1948). This gland also contains octopamine, dopamine, noradrenaline, and 5-HT (Table IV), and unequal concentrations of these amines have been found in the various lobes of octopus ganglia (Table IV), thus indicating that relatively high concentrations of p-tyramine may also be present. Mass spectrometric analysis of chromatographically purified dansyl-p-tyramine from the optic lobes of Octopus dofleini martini indicated that the molecular ion possesses a m/e ratio identical to that obtained for exogenously added p-tyramine (Juorio and Philips, 1975), and the concentration of p-tyramine in the optic lobes was about 170 ng/gm. Similar values were observed for the superior buccal lobe, in contrast to the inferior buccal lobe, in which p-tyramine levels were very low and close to the limit of sensitivity of the method (Table IV). The administration of a MAO inhibitor (100 mg/kg pargyline hydrochloride injected 3 hours before death) produced more than a fivefold increase in the concen-

TABLE V

THE CONTENT OF AMINES IN THE OPTIC LOBES OF *O. vulgaris* AT VARIOUS TIMES
AFTER THE ADMINISTRATION OF THE MAO INHIBITOR PARGYLINE (100 mg/kg)[a]

Duration of treatment	TA	OA	DA	NA	5-HT
Untreated	174[3,b]	1,310[2] 525[4,b]	17,400[1]	4,960[1]	5,160[1]
3 hours	853[3,b,c]	2,020[2,c] 1,490[4,b,c]	27,000[1,c]	8,240[1,c]	6,400[1,c]
10 hours		2,620[2,c]	2,200[1]	6,780[1,c]	6,180[1,c]
36 hours		1,880[2]	22,400[1]	6,100[1]	5,430[1,c]

[a] Concentrations given in nanograms per gram of fresh tissue. TA, *p*-Tyramine; OA, octopamine; DA, dopamine; NA, noradrenaline; 5-HT, 5-hydroxytryptamine. Superscript numbers indicate references: (1) Juorio and Killick, 1972a; (2) Juorio and Molinoff, 1974; (3) Juorio and Philips, 1974; (4) A. V. Juorio, unpublished observations.

[b] *Octopus dofleini martini.*

[c] Statistically different from controls.

tration of *p*-tyramine in the optic lobes and superior buccal lobes, and more marked increases were observed for the inferior buccal lobe (Juorio and Philips, 1975, Table V).

There is no available information on the effect of reserpine administration on the levels of *p*-tyramine in nervous tissues of gastropod molluscs and arthropods, nevertheless some species of these groups are known to be reserpine-resistant, requiring 30–60 mg/kg to give clear-cut amine reductions (Dahl *et al.,* 1966; Juorio and Killick, 1972b; Robertson, 1975b, 1976), and similar high doses are expected to be necessary in the case of *p*-tyramine. In contrast, the octopus responds to reserpine administration in a way similar to higher vertebrates; relatively low doses (1–4 mg/kg) produce substantial reductions in the concentrations of dopamine, noradrenaline, and 5-HT, and also *p*-tyramine and octopamine (Table V). Recent experiments have shown that reserpine treatment (0.4–10 mg/kg) markedly reduces rat caudate nucleus *p*-tyramine levels (Boulton *et al.,* 1975a).

C. TRYPTAMINE

Tryptamine also has been found in human urine (Rodnight, 1956), and in mammalian brain after the administration of its amino acid precursor and MAO inhibitors (Eccleston *et al.,* 1966). More recently, the presence of tryptamine in bovine brain and in rat brain has been reported (Martin *et al.,* 1971; Saavedra and Axelrod, 1972; Philips *et al.,* 1974b; Snodgrass and

TABLE VI

THE CONTENT OF AMINES IN THE OPTIC LOBES OF *O. vulgaris* AT VARIOUS TIMES
AFTER THE ADMINISTRATION OF A SINGLE DOSE OF RESERPINE (4 mg/kg)[a]

Duration of treatment	TA	OA	DA	NA	5-HT
Untreated	174[3,b]	1,131[2] 525[4,b]	17,400[1] 8,900[3,b]	4,960[1]	5,160[1]
6 hours		680[2]	8,580[1,c]	5,590[1]	1,700[1,c]
12 hours		290[2,c]	4,750[1,c]	2,960[1,c]	1,740[1,c]
24 hours		140[2,c]	1,770[1,c]	1,520[1,c]	<30[1,c]
48–72 hours	40[3,b,c]	51[4,b]	780[1,c] 476[4,b,c]	320[1,c]	
6 days		60[2,c]	2,340[1,c]	330[1,c]	260[1,c]
16 days		110[2,c]	2,420[1,c]	940[1,c]	1,130[1,c]

[a] Amine concentrations are given in nanograms per gram of fresh tissue. TA, *p*-Tyramine; OA, octopamine; DA, dopamine; NA, noradrenaline; 5-HT, 5-hydroxytryptamine. Superscript numbers indicate references: (1) Juorio and Killick, 1972b; (2) Juorio and Molinoff, 1974; (3) Juorio and Philips, 1975; (4) A. V. Juorio, unpublished observations.
[b] *Octopus dofleini martini*.
[c] Statistically different from controls.

TABLE VII

CONCENTRATIONS OF β-PHENYLETHYLAMINE, *m*-TYRAMINE AND TRYPTAMINE
IN NERVOUS TISSUES[a]

	β-Phenylethylamine	*m*-Tyramine	Tryptamine
Invertebrates			
Octopus dofleini martini (octopus), optic lobes	2.9[1]	0.6[1]	<0.5[1]
Helix aspersa (snail), ganglia	6.6[2]		3.6[2]
Schistocerca gregaria (locust), whole nervous system	<2.0[7]	<2.0[7]	<2.0[7]
Pycnopodia helianthoides (starfish), arm nerve	3.9[3]		1250[3]
Vertebrate			
Rattus norvegicus (rat), brain	1.8[4]	0.30[6]	0.5[5]
Oryctolagus cuniculus (rabbit), brain	0.44[6]	0.16[6]	0.05[6]

[a] Concentrations are given in nanograms per gram of fresh tissue. Superscript numbers indicate references: (1) A. V. Juorio and S. R. Philips, unpublished observations; (2) Wu and Juorio, 1975; (3) A. V. Juorio and H. A. Robertson, unpublished observations; (4) Durden *et al.*, 1973; (5) Philips *et al.*, 1974b; (6) Boulton *et al.*, 1975b; (7) H. A. Robertson, S. R. Philips, P. H. Wu, and L. Dyck, unpublished observations.

Horn, 1973; Sloan *et al.*, 1975) ; concentrations are generally low, though the results obtained by radiochemical or spectrofluorimetric methods are higher than those obtained by mass spectrometric techniques (for the rat brain 20–80 ng/gm versus 0.1 ng/gm; see Section II).

The levels of tryptamine in the nervous tissues of the invertebrates so far investigated are, with one notable exception, generally low (Table VIII). Among molluscs, the highest concentration was found in snail ganglia (about 4 ng/gm). Octopus ganglia contain <0.5 ng/gm; the tryptamine levels in *O. dofleini martini* optic lobes are greatly increased after MAO inhibition (A. V. Juorio and S. R. Philips, unpublished observations). However, after a similar treatment, no changes were observed in snail circumesophageal ganglia (Wu and Juorio, 1975). In arthropod nervous tissue the concentration of tryptamine is below the limits of sensitivity of the methods (Table VII). Most interestingly, the only species so far examined that has high levels of tryptamine in its nervous system is the echinoderm *Pycnopodia helianthiodes* (Table VII). There is very little 5-HT in the nervous system of this starfish; perhaps tryptamine rather than 5-HT is the important indole alkylamine in echinoderms.

VI. Some Phylogenetic Considerations

As we have seen, it appears that octopamine is an important transmitter in several invertebrate phyla, but that it is found only in small amounts in the mammalian nervous system and that its role is somewhat in doubt. Therefore it is important that we consider the relationship between these two situations as a means by which we may better understand the development, both phylogenetic and ontogenetic, of nervous systems. Several features of transmitters are important in this discussion. Transmitters appear before nervous systems both phylogenetically and ontogenetically. Catecholamines are present and may have physiological significance even in single-cell organisms (Protozoa) (see Welsh, 1972). Similarly, in development, transmitters generally appear before the nervous system begins to function and may be involved in the actual organization of embryological development; thus, as well as functioning as mediators of fast chemical transmission of nerve impulses, transmitters may act as intercellular messengers for the relatively slow communication of developmental information in the embryo (see review by MacMahon, 1974).

The probable relationships of the major phyla of the animal kingdom are shown in Fig. 8. We notice that there is a pattern. The invertebrate phyla described by the embryological term protostomia (meaning "first mouth," i.e., the blastopore forms the mouth) have high octopamine levels and little

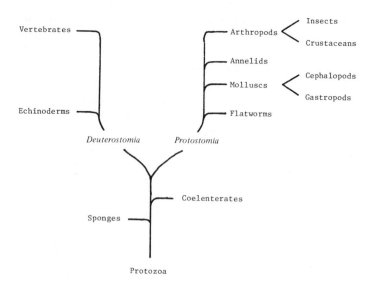

Fig. 8. Probable relationships of the major phyla of the animal kingdom.

if any noradrenaline (cephalopods are an exception, as usual). The phyla described by the embryological term deuterostomia ("second mouth," i.e., the mouth develops from a second invagination, not from the blastopore) have low octopamine levels and generally high noradrenaline levels. It has been suggested that this reflects a fundamental biochemical dichotomy between protostomia and deuterostomia. If we were to predict from this model, we would say that echinoderms (the starfish and sea urchin family) have noradrenaline and relatively little octopamine. We have recently shown that this is at least partially true. Noradrenaline levels in nerves from the starfish *P. helianthiodes* greatly exceed octopamine levels (A. V. Juorio and H. A. Robertson, unpublished observations). It is worth mentioning the exceptions. Cephalopods have high levels of noradrenaline, as well as high levels of octopamine. Cephalopods are also atypical among invertebrates in that they have a low CNS dopamine/noradrenaline ratio of 3:1 as compared to the more usual ratio of at least 10:1 (Kerkut, 1973), and high MAO activity (Blaschko and Hawkins, 1952). Table VIII shows the ratio of octopamine to noradrenaline in various invertebrate brains. For comparison, the levels of octopamine in the developing and adult rat brain are also included. It can be seen that in all protostomia, with the exception of cephalopods, the octopamine/noradrenaline ratio is greater than unity, while in deuterostomia (and in cephalopods) the ratio is less than unity.

The terms protostomia and deuterostomia are embryological ones, and it is interesting and perhaps significant that, in mammalian (rat) brain

TABLE VIII

THE OCTOPAMINE/NORADRENALINE RATIO IN NERVOUS TISSUES[a]

Species	Class	Tissue	Ratio OA/NA
Periplaneta americana (cockroach)	Insecta	Brain	10.4
Schistocerca gregaria (desert locust)	Insecta	Brain	22.1
Homarus americanus (lobster)	Crustacea	Brain	>10
Lumbricus terrestris (earthworm)	Oligochaeta	Ventral nerve cord	3.8
Helix aspersa (garden snail)	Gastropoda	Brain	1.8
Octopus vulgaris (Mediterranean octopus)	Cephalopoda	Brain	0.3
Octopus dofleini martini (Pacific octopus)	Cephalopoda	Optic lobes	0.1
Sepia officinalis (cuttlefish)	Cephalopoda	Optic lobes	<0.1
Loligo vulgaris (squid)	Cephalopoda	Optic lobes	0.2
Pycnopodia helianthoides (starfish)	Asteroidea	Arm nerve	0.1
Rattus norvegicus (rat)	Mammalia	Brain, day 15 gestation	1.56[b]
		Brain, day 16 gestation	1.85[b]
		Brain, day 17 gestation	0.39[b]
		Brain, day 22 gestation (birth)	0.04[b]
		Brain, adult	0.01[b]

[a] OA, Octopamine; NA, noradrenaline.
[b] Saavedra *et al.* (1974b).

development, octopamine levels fall from a high of 30 ng/gm at day 16 of gestation to 6.24 ng/gm at birth, while the noradrenaline content climbs from 16.4 ng/gm at day 16 to 156 ng/gm at birth (Coyle and Henry, 1973; Saavedra *et al.*, 1974b). It is tempting, but highly speculative, to refer here to the "biogenetic law" of Haeckel, which proposes that ontogeny tends to recapitulate phylogeny. Perhaps the high octopamine levels in developing rat brain only reflect "biochemical noise" in the developing noradrenergic system, but they may also reflect a real physiological role for octopamine in the embryonic nervous system.

The phylogenetic distribution of the other microamines shows little evidence of any pattern. Not surprisingly, p-tyramine is highest in species with high concentration levels of octopamine, namely, the lobster, locust, and octopus (Table IV). β-Phenylethylamine and m-tyramine are relatively uniformly distributed in the species examined (Table VII). The most anomalous observation is the very high level of tryptamine in the nervous tissue of the starfish. In all other species examined, the highest tissue concentration found was 3.6 ng/gm in the snail (Table VII). By contrast, in starfish arm nerve, a tissue concentration of 1250 ng/gm was observed (Table VII).

VII. Conclusions

Six years ago, when the presence of endogenous octopamine in nervous tissue was first reported (Molinoff and Axelrod, 1969), it would have been difficult to imagine that this amine would be established as such a strong transmitter candidate so rapidly. Octopamine has, in one invertebrate species or another, fulfilled six of the seven criteria for identification of chemical transmitters listed by Phillis (1970).

1. Octopamine is present in all nervous systems investigated to date, and it has been shown to be localized in neurons in several instances.

2. The necessary enzymic mechanisms for the manufacture of octopamine are present in a variety of groups including insects, crustaceans, and mammals.

3. The presence of precursors and intermediates, in this case tyramine, has been demonstrated in insects, gastropods, cephalopods, and mammals.

4. During stimulation of nerves containing octopamine, it is released and can be detected in extracellular fluid collected from the preparation. This has been shown only in the octopaminergic cells in the lobster (Evans et al., 1975).

5. When applied to the postsynaptic structure, octopamine mimics the effects of a synaptically released transmitter. This has been shown in crustaceans (Evans et al., 1975) and in insects (Hoyle, 1975).

6. Pharmacological agents interact with both the synaptically released transmitter and octopamine in an identical manner. This has been shown to some extent in the firefly lantern.

7. A means by which octopamine is inactivated has not yet been demonstrated in any species. Octopamine is a substrate for MAO, in insects at least (H. A. Robertson, P. H. Wu, S. R. Philips, and L. Dyck, unpublished observations), and may be a substrate for N-acetyltransferase (Dewhurst et al., 1972); in the octopus the administration of a MAO inhibitor produced a significant increase in optic lobe octopamine concentration (Juorio and Molinoff, 1974); the physiological means of inactivation and/or removal from the synapse, however, remain unknown.

Several other features of octopamine fall outside the formal criteria. For example, it is now recognized that the membrane-bound enzyme adenylate cyclase and its product cAMP are somehow involved in neurotransmission (Greengard et al., 1973). It is significant, then, that octopamine-sensitive adenylate cyclases have been found in nervous tissue from insects (Nathanson and Greengard, 1973), molluscs (Levitan *et al.*, 1974), and crustaceans (Sullivan and Barker, 1975). Similarly, octopamine has been shown to be the most potent agonist at some receptors on neurons in *Aplysia* ganglia (Carpenter and Gaubatz, 1974), but it is not yet known whether these neurons receive an octopaminergic input.

Octopamine thus fulfills many criteria for a neurotransmitter, and the gaps in our knowledge, for example, of the mechanism of inactivation of octopamine, are more the result of a complete absence of studies in this area rather than a lack of understanding. Unfortunately, all criteria have not yet been satisfied in any one preparation. The principal reason for this is that, until recently, an appropriate preparation was not available. Several putative octopaminergic systems have now been described. These include the firefly lantern (Carlson, 1968a,b; Robertson, 1975d; Robertson and Carlson, 1976), the DUM neurons innervating the extensor tibia muscle in the locust (Hoyle, 1975; Hoyle and Barker, 1975), and the nerve–gill muscle preparation from *Aplysia* (Kupfermann *et al.*, 1974; Saavedra *et al.*, 1974a). It can be expected that in the near future studies on these and other invertebrate systems will lead to substantiation, beyond reasonable doubt, of the neurotransmitter role of octopamine in invertebrates.

Among the other microamines, there is little evidence for a role in invertebrates. p-Tyramine is detected in relatively high concentrations in the ganglia of crustaceans, insects, and molluscs (cephalopods and gastropods). It is stored by a reserpine-sensitive mechanism and is a substrate for MAO. There is no evidence, however, for a tyraminergic receptor, for intraneuronal localization, or for release after stimulation. In at least one instance, it has been shown that p-tyramine does not activate adenylate cyclase (Nathanson and Greengard, 1973). It is tempting to assume that p-tyramine is merely a precursor of octopamine. However, p-tyramine is present in concentrations as high as octopamine in at least one species (the lobster), and it is possible that it may have a role of its own.

The status of β-phenylethylamine and tryptamine in invertebrates is even less well established than that of p-tyramine, and we must assume on the basis of present information that these amines are present only in very small amounts in the nervous systems of vertebrates and invertebrates alike. Further investigation of the neurochemistry of invertebrates may be expected to turn up exceptions, such as the finding that tryptamine values are high in the starfish, and so open up new areas for neurobiological research.

ACKNOWLEDGMENTS

The authors wish to express their gratitude to Dr. A. A. Boulton for encouragement and critical reading of the manuscript. We are grateful to Dr. S. R. Philips for details of the mass spectrographic analysis. H. A. Robertson is a fellow of the MRC of Canada. A. V. Juorio thanks the Psychiatric Services Branch, Province of Saskatchewan, and the MRC of Canada for financial support.

References

Amin, A. H., Crawford, T. B. B., and Gaddum, J. H. (1954). *J. Physiol.* (*London*) **126**, 596.

Anthony, G. M., Brooks, C. J. W., and Middleditch, B. S. (1970). *J. Pharm. Pharmacol.* **22**, 205.

Axelrod, J. (1962). *J. Biol. Chem.* **237**, 1657.

Axelrod, J., and Saavedra, J. M. (1974). *Ciba Found. Symp.* **22**, 51.

Barger, G., and Dale, H. H. (1910). *J. Physiol.* (*London*) **41**, 19.

Barker, D. L., Molinoff, P. B., and Kravitz, E. A. (1972). *Nature* (*London*), *New Biol.* **236**, 61.

Barlow, J. J., Juorio, A. V., and Martin, R. (1974). *J. Comp. Physiol.* **89**, 105.

Björklund, A., Falck, B., and Stenevi, V. (1971). *Brain Res.* **32**, 266.

Blaschko, H., and Hawkins, J. (1952). *J. Physiol.* (*London*) **118**, 88.

Blaschko, H., and Hope, D. B. (1957). *Arch. Biochem. Biophys.* **69**, 10.

Blaschko, H., and Levine, W. G. (1966). *Handbk. Exp. Pharmakol.* **19**, 212.

Blaschko, H., Colhoun, E. H., and Frontali, N. (1961). *J. Physiol.* (*London*) **156**, 28P.

Bloom, F. E. (1970). *Int. Rev. Neurobiol.* **13**, 27.

Boadle, M. C., and Blaschko, H. (1968). *Comp. Biochem. Physiol.* **25**, 129.

Boulton, A. A. (1971). *Nature* (*London*) **231**, 22.

Boulton, A. A. (1974). *Lancet* **2**, 7871.

Boulton, A. A. (1976a). *Adv. Biochem. Psychopharmacol.* (in press).

Boulton, A. A. (1976b). *In* "Trace Amines in the Brain" (E. Usdin and M. Sandler, eds.). Dekker, New York (in press).

Boulton, A. A., and Baker, G. B. (1975). *J. Neurochem.* **25**, 477.

Boulton, A. A., and Majer, J. R. (1970). *J. Chromatogr.* **48**, 322.

Boulton, A. A., and Marjerrison, G. L. (1972). *Nature* (*London*) **236**, 76.

Boulton, A. A. and Wu, P. H. (1972). *Can. J. Biochem.* **50**, 261.

Boulton, A. A., Pollit, R. J., Majer, J. R. (1967). *Nature* (*London*) **215**, 132.

Boulton, A. A., Marjerrison, G. L., and Majer, J. R. (1971). *J. Acad. Med. Sci.* (*USSR*) **5**, 68.

Boulton, A. A., Wu, P. H., and Philips, S. R. (1972). *Can. J. Biochem.* **50**, 1210.

Boulton, A. A., Juorio, A. V., Philips, S. R., and Wu, P. H. (1975a). *Br. J. Pharmacol.* **55**, 296P.

Boultin, A. A., Juorio, A. V., Philips, S. R., and Wu, P. H. (1975b). *Brain Res.* **96**, 212.

Brownstein, M. J., Saavedra, J. M., Axelrod, J., Zeman, G. H., and Carpenter, D. O. (1974). *Proc. Natl. Acad. Sci. U.S.A.* **71**, 4662.

Burgen, A. S. V., and Iversen, L. L. (1965). *Br. J. Pharmacol. Chemother.* **25**, 34.

Burn, J. H., and Rand, M. J. (1958). *J. Physiol.* (*London*) **144**, 314.

Cardot, J. (1971). *C. R. Seances Soc. Biol. Ses Fil.* **165**, 338.

Carlson, A. D. (1968a). *J. Exp. Biol.* **48**, 381.

Carlson, A. D. (1968b). *J. Exp. Biol.* **49**, 195.

Carlson, A. D. (1969). *Adv. Insect Physiol.* **6**, 51.

Carlson, A. D. (1972). *J. Exp. Biol.* **57**, 737.

Carlsson, A., Hillarp, N.-A., and Waldeck, B. (1963). *Acta Physiol. Scand.* **59**, Suppl. 215, 1

Carpenter, D., Breese, G., Schanberg, S., and Kopin, I. (1971). *Int. J. Neurosci.* **2**, 49.

Carpenter, D. O., and Gaubatz, G. L. (1974). *Nature (London)* **252**, 483.

Cattabeni, F., Koslow, S. H., and Costa, E. (1972). *Science* **178**, 166.

Costa, E., Koslow, S. H., and LeFebre, H. F. (1975). *Handb. Psychopharmacol.* **1**, 1.

Cottrell, G. A., and Laverack, M. S. (1968). *Annu. Rev. Pharmacol.* **8**, 273.

Cottrell, G. A., and Osborne, N. N. (1970). *Nature (London)* **225**, 470.

Coyle, J. T., and Henry, D. (1973). *J. Neurochem.* **21**, 61.

Coyle, J. T., Wooten, G. F., and Axelrod, J. (1974). *J. Neurochem.* **22**, 923.

Cuello, A. C., Hiley, R., and Iversen, L. L. (1973). *J. Neurochem.* **21**, 1337.

Dahl, E., Falck, B., Mecklenburg, C. V., Myhrberg, H., and Rosengren, E. (1966). *Z. Zellforsch. Mikrosk. Anat.* **71**, 489.

Danielson, T. J., Boulton, A. A., and Robertson, H. A. (1976). In preparation.

Dewhurst, S. A., Croker, S. G., Ikeda, K., and McCaman, R. E. (1972). *Comp. Biochem. Physiol. B* **43**, 975.

Dolezalova, H., Giacobini, E., Seiler, N., and Schneider, H. H. (1973). *Brain Res.* **55**, 242.

Durden, D. A., Philips, S. R., and Boulton, A. A. (1973). *Can. J. Biochem.* **51**, 995.

Durden, D. A., Davis, B. A., and Boulton, A. A. (1974). *Biomed. Mass Spectrom.* **1**, 83.

Eccleston, D., Ashcroft, G. W., Crawford, T. B. B., and Loose, R. (1966). *J. Neurochem.* **13**, 93.

Edwards, D. J., and Blau, K. (1973). *Biochem. J.* **132**, 95.

Erspamer, V. (1948). *Acta Pharmacol. Toxicol.* **4**, 224.

Erspamer, V. (1952). *Nature (London)* **169**, 375.

Evans, P. D., Talamo, B. R., and Kravitz, E. A. (1975). *Brain Res.* **90**, 340.

Faurbye, A. (1968). *Compr. Psychiatry* **9**, 155.

Fischer, E., Spatz, H., Heller, B., and Reggiani, H. (1972). *Experientia* **28**, 307.

Frontali, N. (1968). *J. Insect Physiol.* **14**, 881.

Frontali, N., and Häggendal, J. (1969). *Brain Res.* **14**, 540.

Fry, J. P., House, C. R., and Sharman, D. F. (1974). *Br. J. Pharmacol.* **51**, 116P.

Fuxe, K., and Jonsson, G. (1973). *J. Histochem. Cytochem.* **21**, 293.

Gardner, C. R., and Cashin, C. H. (1975). *Neuropharmacology* **14**, 493.

Gerschenfeld, H. M. (1973). *Physiol. Rev.* **53**, 1.

Gilman, A. G., and Nirenberg, M. (1971). *Proc. Natl. Acad. Sci. U.S.A.* **68**, 2165.

Goldman, J. E., and Schwartz, J. H. (1974). *J. Physiol. (London)* **242**, 61.

Green, A. R., Koslow, S. H., and Costa, E. (1973). *Brain Res.* **51**, 371.

Greengard, P., Nathanson, J. A., and Kebabian, J. W. (1973). In "Frontiers in Catecholamine Research" (E. Usdin and S. Snyder, eds.), p. 377. Pergamon, Oxford.

Guiretti, F. (1960). *Ann. N.Y. Acad. Sci.* **90**, 726.

Gunne, L-M., and Ponsson, J. (1965). *Acta Physiol. Scand.* **64**, 434.

Guthrie, P. B., Neuhoff, V., and Osborne, N. N. (1975). *Experientia* **31**, 775.

Hanington, E. (1967). *Br. Med. J.* **2**, 550.

Harmar, A. J., and Horn, A. S. (1975). *Abstr., Int. Meet. Int. Soc. Neurochem., 5th,* p. 440.

Hartman, B. K., Zide, D., and Udenfriend, S. (1972). *Proc. Natl. Acad. Sci. U.S.A.* **69**, 2722.

222   H. A. ROBERTSON AND A. V. JUORIO

Henry, D. P., Starman, B. J., Johnson, D. G., and Williams, R. H. (1975). *Life Sci.* **16**, 375.

Henze, M. (1913). *Hoppe-Seyler's Z. Physiol. Chem.* **87**, 51.

Hess, S. M., and Udenfriend, S. (1959). *J. Pharmacol. Exp. Ther.* **127**, 175.

Hess, S. M., Redfield, B. G., and Udenfriend, S. (1959). *J. Pharmacol. Exp. Ther.* **127**, 178.

Holmstedt, B., and Palmér, L. (1973). *Adv. Biochem. Psychopharmacol.* **7**, 1.

Hoyle, G. (1975). *J. Exp. Zool.* **193**, 425.

Hoyle, G., and Barker, D. (1975). *J. Exp. Zool.* **193**, 433.

Hoyle, G., Dagan, D., Moberly, B., and Colquhoun, W. (1974). *J. Exp. Zool.* **187**, 159.

Iversen, L. L. (1974). *Biochem. Pharmacol.* **23**, 1927.

Jenkins, A. E., and Majer, J. R. (1967). *Talanta* **14**, 777.

Juorio, A. V. (1971). *J. Physiol. (London)* **216**, 213.

Juorio, A. V., and Killick, S. W. (1972a). *Comp. Gen. Pharmacol.* **3**, 283.

Juorio, A. V., and Killick, S. W. (1972b). *Int. J. Neurosci.* **4**, 195.

Juorio, A. V., and Killick, S. W. (1973). *Comp. Biochem. Physiol.* **44A**, 1059.

Juorio, A. V., and Molinoff, P. B. (1971). *Br. J. Pharmacol.* **43**, 438P.

Juorio, A. V., and Molinoff, P. B. (1974). *J. Neurochem.* **22**, 271.

Juorio, A. V., and Philips, S. R. (1975). *Brain Res.* **83**, 180.

Kakimoto, Y., and Armstrong, M. D. (1962). *J. Biol. Chem.* **237**, 422.

Karoum, F., Cattabeni, F., Costa, E., Ruthven, C. R. J., and Sandler, M. (1972). *Anal. Biochem.* **47**, 550.

Kastle, J. H., and McDermott, F. A. (1910). *Am. J. Physiol.* **27**, 122.

Kerkut, G. A. (1973). *Br. Med. Bull.* **29**, 100.

Klemm, N., and Axelsson, S. (1973). *Brain Res.* **57**, 289.

Kopin, I. J., Fischer, J. E., Musacchio, J. M., and Horst, W. D. (1964). *Proc. Natl. Acad. Sci. U.S.A.* **52**, 716.

Koslow, S. H., Racagni, G., and Costa, E. (1974). *Neuropharmacology* **13**, 1123.

Kupfermann, I., Carew, T. J., and Kandel, E. R. (1974). *J. Neurophysiol.* **37**, 996.

Lake, C. R., Mills, R. R., and Brunet, P. C. J. (1970). *Biochim. Biophys. Acta* **215**, 226.

Lake, C. R., Mills, R. R., and Koeppe, J. K. (1975). *Insect Biochem.* **5**, 223.

Levine, R., Oates, J. A., Vendsalu, A., and Sjoerdsma, A. (1962). *J. Clin Endocrinol. Metab.* **22**, 1242.

Levitan, I. B., and Barondes, S. H. (1974). *Proc. Natl. Acad. Sci. U.S.A.* **71**, 1145.

Levitan, I. B., Madsen, C. J., and Barondes, S. H. (1974). *J. Neurobiol.* **5**, 511.

Lo Bianco, S. (1898). *Mitt. Zool. Stn. Neapel* **13**, 448.

Lovenberg, W., Weissbach, H., and Udenfriend, S. (1962). *J. Biol. Chem.* **237**, 89.

MacMahon, D. (1974). *Science* **185**, 1012.

Majer, J. R., and Boulton, A. A. (1973). *Methods Biochem. Anal.* **21**, 467.

Marjerrison, G. L., Boulton, A. A., and Rajput, A. (1971). *Int. J. Clin. Pharmacol.* **4**, 263.

Martin, I. L., and Baker, G. B. (1975). *Abstr. Int. Meet. Int. Soc. Neurochem., 5th,* p. 540.

Martin, W. R., Sloan, J. W., and Christian, S. T. (1971). *Fed. Proc., Fed. Am. Soc. Exp. Biol.* **30**, 271.

Martin, W. R., Sloan, J. W., Buchwald, W. R., and Bridges, S. R. (1974). *Psychopharmacologia* **37**, 189.

Molinoff, P. B., and Axelrod, J. (1969). *Science* **164**, 428.

Molinoff, P. B., and Axelrod, J. (1972). *J. Neurochem.* **19**, 157.

Murdock, L. L. (1971). *Comp. Gen. Pharmacol.* **2**, 254.

Nakajima, T., Kakimoto, Y., and Sano, I. (1964). *J. Pharmacol. Exp. Ther.* **143**, 319.

Narasimhachari, N., and Vouros, P. (1972). *Anal. Biochem.* **45**, 154.

Nathanson, J. A., and Greengard, P. (1973). *Science* **180**, 308.

Osborne, N. N. (1974). "Microchemical Analysis of Nervous Tissue." Pergamon, Oxford.

Osborne, N. N., Hiripi, L., and Neuhoff, V. (1975). *Biochem. Pharmacol.* **24**, 2141.

Pentreath, V. W., and Cottrell, G. A. (1974). *Nature (London)* **250**, 655.

Peterson, M. K. (1970). *J. Morphol.* **131**, 103.

Philips, S. R., Durden, D. A., and Boulton, A. A. (1974a). *Can. J. Biochem.* **52**, 366.

Philips, S. R., Durden, D. A., and Boulton, A. A. (1947b). *Can. J. Biochem.* **52**, 447.

Philips, S. R., Davis, D. A., and Boulton, A. A. (1975). *Can. J. Biochem.* **53**, 65.

Phillis, J. W. (1970). "The Pharmacology of Synapses." Pergamon, Oxford.

Pisano, J. J., Oates, J. A., Karmen, A., Sjoerdsma, A., and Udenfriend, S. (1961). *J. Biol. Chem.* **236**, 898.

Pitman, R. M. (1971). *Comp. Gen. Pharmacol.* **2**, 347.

Robertson, H. A. (1971). M.Sc. Thesis, University of Western Ontario.

Robertson, H. A. (1974). *Cell Tissue Res.* **148**, 237.

Robertson, H. A. (1975a). *Experientia* **31**, 1006.

Robertson, H. A. (1975b). *Abstr., Int. Meet. Int. Soc. Neurochem., 5th,* p. 8.

Robertson, H. A. (1975c). *J. Exp. Biol.* **63**, 413.

Robertson, H. A. (1975d). *Proc. Can. Fed. Biol. Soc.* **18**, 66.

Robertson, H. A. (1976). *Experientia* **32**, 522.

Robertson, H. A., and Carlson, A. D. (1976). *J. Exp. Zool.* **195**, 159.

Robertson, H. A., and Steele, J. E. (1970). *Proc. Can. Fed. Biol. Soc.* **13**, 137.

Robertson, H. A., and Steele, J. E. (1972). *J. Neurochem.* **19**, 1603.

Robertson, H. A., and Steele, J. E. (1973). *Insect Biochem.* **3**, 53.

Robertson, H. A., and Steele, J. E. (1974). *J. Physiol. (London)* **237**, 34P.

Rodnight, R. (1956). *Biochem. J.* **64**, 621.

Saavedra, J. M. (1974a). *Anal. Biochem.* **59**, 628.

Saavedra, J. M. (1974b). *J. Neurochem.* **22**, 211.

Saavedra, J. M., and Axelrod, J. (1972). *J. Pharmacol. Exp. Ther.* **182**, 363.

Saavedra, J. M., and Axelrod, J. (1973). *Proc. Natl. Acad. U.S.A.* **70**, 769.

Saavedra, J. M., Heller, B., and Fischer, E. (1970). *Nature (London)* **226**, 868.

Saavedra, J. M., Brownstein, M., and Axelrod, J. (1973). *J. Pharmacol. Exp. Ther.* **186**, 508.

Saavedra, J. M., Brownstein, M. J., Carpenter, D. O., and Axelrod, J. (1974a). *Science* **185**, 364.

Saavedra, J. M., Coyle, J. T., and Axelrod, J. (1974b). *J. Neurochem.* **23**, 511.

Saelens, J. K., Schoen, M. S., and Kovacsics, G. B. (1967). *Biochem. Pharmacol.* **16**, 1043.

Sandler, M., Youdim, M. B. H., and Hanington, E. (1974). *Nature (London)* **250**, 335.

Seiler, N., and Knodgen, B. (1973). *Org. Mass Spectrom.* **7**, 97.

Seiler, N., and Wiechmann, M. (1966). *Z. Anal. Chem.* **220**, 109.

Sekeris, C. E., and Karlson, P. (1966). *Pharmacol. Rev.* **18**, 89.

Siggins, G. R., Battenberg, E. F., Hoffer, B. J., Bloom, F. E., and Steiner, A. R. (1973). *Science* **179**, 585.

Sjoerdsma, A., Lovenberg, W., Oates, J. A., Crout, J. R., and Udenfriend, S. (1959). *Science* **130**, 225.

Sloan, J. W., Martin, W. R., Clements, T. H., Buchwald, W. F., and Bridges, S. R. (1975). *J. Neurochem.* **24**, 523.

Smith, D. S. (1963). *J. Cell Biol.* **16**, 323.

Smith, I., and Kellow, A. H. (1969). *Nature (London)* **221**, 1261.

Snodgrass, S. R., and Horn, A. S. (1973). *J. Neurochem.* **21**, 687.

Snyder, S. H., Banerjee, S. P., Yamamura, H. I., and Greenberg, D. (1974). *Science* **184**, 1243.

Spector, S., Melmon, K., Lovenberg, W., and Sjoerdsma, A. (1963). *J. Pharmacol. Exp. Ther.* **140**, 229.

Steele, J. E. (1963). *Gen. Comp. Endocrinol.* **3**, 46.

Stuart, A. E., Hudspeth, A. J., and Hall, Z. W. (1974). *Cell Tissue Res.* **153**, 55.

Sullivan, R. E., and Barker, D. L. (1975). *5th Annu. Meet. Soc. Neurosci.* p. 394.

Tauc, L. (1967). *Physiol. Rev.* **47**, 521.

Tomkins, G. M. (1975). *Science* **189**, 760.

Treherne, J. E. (1966). "The Neurochemistry of Arthropods." Cambridge Univ. Press, London and New York.

Twarog, B. M., and Page, I. H. (1953). *Am. J. Physiol.* **175**, 157.

von Euler, U. S., and Lishajko, F. (1968). *Acta Physiol. Scand.* **73**, 78.

Walker, R. J., Ramage, A. G., and Woodruff, G. N. (1972). *Experientia* **28**, 1173.

Wallace, B. G., Talamo, B. R., Evans, P. P., and Kravitz, E. A. (1974). *Brain Res.* **74**, 349.

Weil-Malherbe, H. (1972). *Handb. Neurochem.* **7**, 371.

Welsh, J. H. (1953). *Naunyn-Schmiedeberg's Arch. Exp. Pathol. Pharmakol.* **219**, 23.

Welsh, J. H. (1972). *Handb. Exp. Pharmakol.* **33**, 79.

Welsh, J. H., and Moorhead, M. (1960). *J. Neurochem.* **6**, 146.

Whitehead, D. L. (1969). *Nature (London)* **224**, 721.

Wigglesworth, V. B. (1960). *J. Exp. Biol.* **37**, 500.

Willner, J., LeFevre, H. F., and Costa, E. (1974). *J. Neurochem.* **23**, 857.

Wooten, G. F., Jacobowiz, D. M., Saavedra, J. M., and Axelrod, J. (1975). *J. Neurochem.* **24**, 1107.

Wu, P. H., and Boulton, A. A. (1974). *Can. J. Biochem.* **52**, 374.

Wu, P. H., and Boulton, A. A. (1975). *Can. J. Biochem.* **53**, 42.

Wu, P. H., and Juorio, A. V. (1975). *Abstr., Int. Meet. Int. Soc. Neurochem., 5th,* p. 79.

Youdim, M. B. H., Carter, S. B., Sandler, M., Hanington, E., and Wilkinson, M. (1971). *Nature (London)* **230**, 127.

Young, J. Z. (1963). *Proc. Zool. Soc. London* **140**, 229.

Young, J. Z. (1971). "The Anatomy of the Nervous System of *Octopus vulgaris*." Oxford Univ. Press (Clarendon), London and New York.

APOMORPHINE: CHEMISTRY, PHARMACOLOGY, BIOCHEMISTRY

By F. C. Colpaert, W. F. M. Van Bever, and J. E. M. F. Leysen

Department of Pharmacology, Janssen Pharmaceutica Research Laboratories, Beerse, Belgium

I. Introduction: Major Clinical Data

The literature covered by this review is limited in several ways. First, only articles dealing with intrinsic chemical, pharmacological, or biochemical properties of apomorphine were included, and reports on research in which apomorphine was merely used as an investigational tool have not been incorporated. Second, only papers available before December 1, 1975 were considered. Also, in view of the extremely large amount of information on apomorphine, it seems inevitable that a number of relevant articles have been overlooked, and we apologize for such unintentional omissions.

Since it was discovered to be a powerful stereotypogenic compound (Harnack, 1874), apomorphine (APO) has gained much interest in the field of neuropsychopharmacological research. The early finding that bulbocapnine (3,4-methylenedioxy-6-apomorphine), which itself produces behavioral symptoms reminiscent of Parkinson's disease in monkeys, antagonizes APO-induced stereotyped behavior (Brücke, 1935), led to the clinical discovery (Schwab et al., 1951; Vernier and Unna, 1951) that APO alleviates Parkinson's disease in humans. However, the emetic effects of APO (Isaacs and MacArthur, 1954) have severely limited its therapeutic use, though subemetic APO doses may still be useful in the treatment of Parkinson's disease (Castaigne et al., 1971; Cotzias et al., 1967, 1970; Struppler and von Uexküll, 1953; Vernier, 1952; von Uexküll, 1953) and of Huntington's chorea (Tolosa and Sparber, 1974; see, however, Lal et al., 1973). Apart from these beneficial effects, single injections of subemetic APO doses (0.5–1.0 mg) in humans produce dizziness, faintness, and sleepiness, as well as hypotension and bradycardia (Cotzias et al., 1970; Schwab et al., 1951). In individuals with a latent disposition to depression, chronic (12–14 days) APO (0.5–1.0 mg, three times daily) administration may exert a reserpine-like (Bunney and Davis, 1965) depressogenic effect (Tesařová, 1972). This finding may be related to the proposed use (Dent, 1955; Ziegler and Schneider, 1974) of APO in behavioral therapy for drug addiction, as suggested by animal studies (Garcia et al., 1966) showing that APO can be effectively applied as an aversive stimulus.

II. Chemistry: Structure and Activity

APO is a tertiary base with the empirical formula $C_{17}H_{17}NO_2$. Its molecular skeleton consists of four fused six-membered rings, giving the molecule a semirigid structure. Its molecular skeleton is that of an aporphine alkaloid; owing to the catechol moiety in ring D, it oxidizes rapidly and becomes green on exposure to air and in solution.

Levorotatory APO (II) was synthesized, more than a century ago, by treatment of naturally occurring levorotatory morphine (I) with mineral acids (Matthiessen and Wright, 1870) or with zinc chloride (Mayer, 1871). Milder acids, such as phosphoric acid or oxalic acid, afford better yields (Small *et al.*, 1940). This acid-catalyzed conversion of I into II consists

I, (-)-morphine   II, (-)-apomorphine   III, aporphine

of dehydration followed by skeletal rearrangement, whereby four of the five asymmetric centers of morphine are destroyed while the nine-carbon atom, corresponding to the 6a-carbon atom of APO, retains its configuration.

In 1902 the chemical structure of APO was elucidated by Pshorr *et al.* (1902; Pshorr, 1907), and in 1955 its absolute configuration was proven to be 6aR via stereoselective degradation (Corrodi and Hardegger, 1955). The conformation of the crystal structure has been described by Giesecke (1973).

More recent interest in the study of APO and its congeners was triggered by the report of Ernst (1965), who drew attention to the structural similarities between APO and dopamine (DA), as shown in structure III. This section is consequently limited to a brief survey of the most recent developments in the field. Although no complete set of comparable data is available, an attempt is made to discuss the structure–activity relationships of APO and its congeners in terms of their ability to induce stereotyped behavior in rodents and of their emetic activity in dogs.

A. (6aR)- AND (6aS)-APO

Dopaminergic and emetic activity reside mainly in the (6aR)-levorotatory enantiomer of APO. (—)-Apomorphine is about twice as potent as the corresponding racemic mixture (Schoenfeld *et al.*, 1975; Neumeyer *et al.*, 1973) while the (6aS)-enantiomer is virtually inactive (Saari and King, 1973). This stereoselectivity is also valid for other APO derivatives (Atkinson *et al.*, 1975; Schoenfeld *et al.*, 1975).

B. MODIFICATION OF THE *N*-METHYL GROUP OF APO

Several reports on the *N*-alkyl derivatives of APO are available (Atkinson *et al.*, 1975; Hensiak *et al.*, 1965; Koch *et al.*, 1968; Neumeyer *et al.*, 1973;

Schoenfeld *et al.*, 1975). Norapomorphine is very weakly active (more than 300 times less potent than APO with respect to the induction of stereotyped behavior). The corresponding *N*-ethyl- and *N*-*n*-propylnorapomorphines, respectively 48 and 24 times more potent than APO with respect to emesis in dogs, are by far the most potent *N*-alkyl derivatives of norapomorphine. However, the *N*-*n*-propyl compound is superior to the *N*-ethyl derivative with respect to the induction of stereotyped behavior in rodents. *n*-Butyl-norapomorphine is much less active than APO, in contrast to the very similar *N*-(2-chloro-*n*-butyl) compound which is equipotent with APO as an emetic. *N*-allyl- and *N*-cyclopropylmethylnorapomorphine are, respectively, two and six times more potent as emetics, while *N*-propargyl-, *N*-phenylmethyl-, and *N*-phenylethylnorapomorphine are far less active than APO. It is worthwhile to note that, within the above-mentioned series, emetic potency does not correlate with ability to induce stereotyped behavior.

C. Modification of the Catechol Moiety of APO

APO can be acetylated to diacetylapomorphine without loss of potency (Cannon *et al.*, 1963). However, etherification leads invariably to less active or inactive compounds. 11-Hydroxy-10-methoxyaporphine (apocodeine) and 10,11-methylenedioxyaporphine are about four times less potent than APO in inducing stereotyped gnawing in rats, while 10,11-dimethoxyaporphine is inactive (Lal *et al.*, 1972a; Neumeyer *et al.*, 1973; Saari *et al.*, 1974).

Monohydroxy derivatives of aporphine are inactive. However, when the *N*-methyl group of 10- or 11-hydroxyaporphine is replaced by a *N*-*n*-propyl substituent, some activity is retained; these compounds are nevertheless still considerably less potent than APO (Neumeyer *et al.*, 1974; Saari *et al.*, 1974; Schoenfeld *et al.*, 1975). Introduction of the dihydroxy substitution pattern in other parts of the molecule, or introduction of the monohydroxy group in still other parts of the molecule, or, finally, introduction of additional hydroxy functions greatly diminishes or completely abolishes the activity of the parent molecule. Thus 9,10-dihydroxyaporphine (isoapomorphine) (Neumeyer *et al.*, 1973; Saari *et al.*, 1974), 9-hydroxyaporphine (Saari *et al.*, 1974), 1,2-dihydroxyaporphine, 1,2-dimethoxyaporphine (nuciferine) (Neumeyer *et al.*, 1973), 2,11-dihydroxy-10-methoxyaporphine (morphothebaine), 2,10,11-trihydroxyaporphine, 1,2,10,11-tetrahydroxyaporphine (Lal *et al.*, 1972a), and 1,2,9,10-tetrahydroxyaporphine (Neumeyer *et al.*, 1973) all are very weakly active or completely inactive compounds. Finally, oxidation of the catechol moiety of APO to the corresponding 5,6-dihydro-6-methyl-4*H*-dibenzo-[*d,e,g*] quinoline-10,11-dione, also results in an inactive compound (Lal *et al.*, 1972a).

It can be concluded that the 10,11-dihydroxy substitution pattern of

APO is an absolute requirement for optimal activity. It should be noted that APO contains the DA structural moiety in an *anti* disposition, as shown in IV and VI, while inactive 1,2-dihydroxyaporphine contains the DA moiety in a gauche disposition (V and VII). This is in agreement with the observation that the *anti* disposition (VI) of the catechol ring and of the amino group of DA are the biologically active ones (Horn, 1974; Rekker *et al.*, 1972).

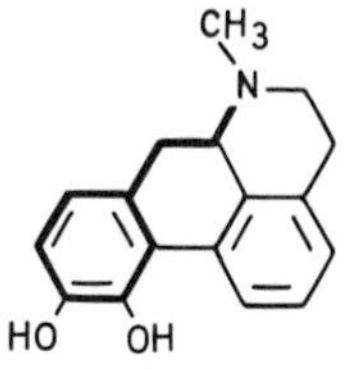

IV

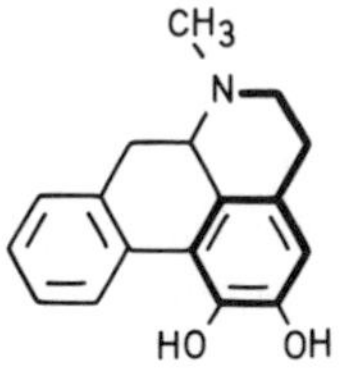

V

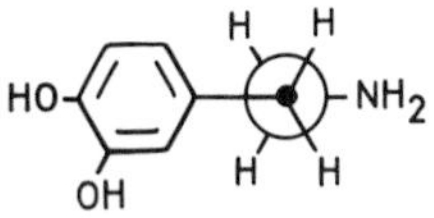

VI , anti

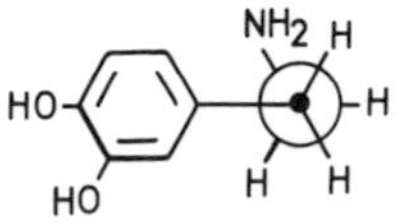

VII , gauche

D. MODIFICATIONS REPRESENTING A SIMPLIFICATION
   OF THE APO SKELETON

Hofmann and Emde degradation of APO and nuciferine, leading to opening of the B ring and resulting in the corresponding dihydrophenanthrene congeners (VIII, IX, and XI) of APO and nuciferine, as well as

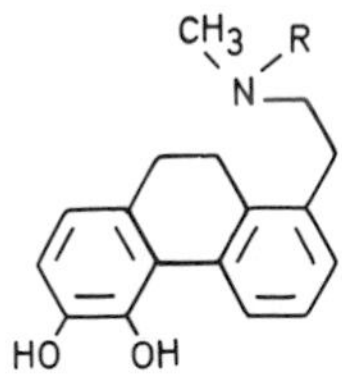

VIII   R = Me
        or R = Et

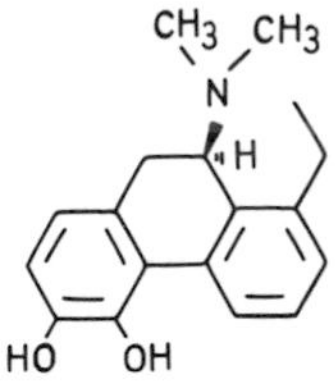

IX

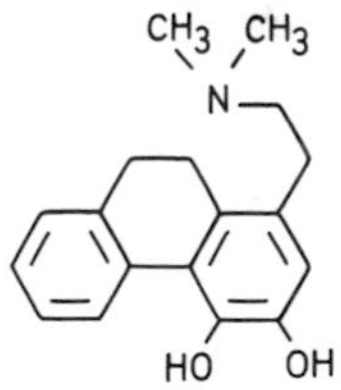

X

the conformational aspects of these dihydrophenanthrene derivatives, have been described in a series of reports by Cannon *et al.* (1973, 1975a,b). This type of structural modification always leads to far less active or to inactive compounds. The corresponding phenanthrene derivatives are completely

XI   XII

devoid of activity. The surprisingly very low level of activity of XI has been explained in terms of conformational changes (Cannon *et al.*, 1975a). The great impact of conformational changes on activity is further exemplified by the seven-membered B-ring analog (XII) of APO, which is completely devoid of dopaminergic activity (Berney *et al.*, 1975).

XIII   XIV   XV

The derivatives of 2-amino-4,5-dihydroxyindan (XIII) (Cannon *et al.*, 1972b) and of 2-amino-5,6-dihydroxy-1,2,3,4-tetrahydronaphthalene (XIV) (Cannon *et al.*, 1972b; McDermed *et al.*, 1975) can be considered a group of compounds without the A and B rings of APO, as shown in structure XV. In XIII and XIV, R_1 and R_2 represent small alkyl groups (methyl, ethyl, or *n*-propyl). Indan derivatives (XIII) are less potent than corresponding tetrahydronaphthalene derivatives (XIV). Primary amines of types XIII and XIV are very weakly active or inactive; secondary amines are less active than tertiary amines, while cyclic tertiary amines of type XIV are inactive. The most interesting compounds are the dimethylamino, diethylamino, and di-*n*-propylamino derivatives of XIV, which are, respectively, 2, 54, and 46 times more potent than APO as emetics in dogs and, respectively, 2.5 times more, 6 times less, and 17 times more potent than APO as dopaminergic agonists in rats. The 2-di-*n*-butylamino derivative of XIV is much less active than the 2-di-*n*-propyl compound. It should be noted that these results are very similar to those observed for the series of *N*-methyl, *N*-ethyl, *N*-*n*-propyl, and *N*-*n*-butyl derivatives of norapomorphine, and that emetic activity and dopaminergic activity again do not correlate.

The *N*-methyl and *N*-*n*-propyl derivatives of 2-(3,4-dihydroxyphenyl-methylpiperidine (XVI) and of 1-(2,3-dihydroxyphenylmethyl)-1,2,3,4-

XVI   R = Me   XVII   R = Me
   or R = N-prop   or   R = N-prop

tetrahydroisoquinoline (XVII) can be considered as analogs of APO lacking, respectively, the C and A rings and the C ring of APO. Compounds XVI and XVII were found to be devoid of dopaminergic activity (Ginos *et al.*, 1975).

E. Conclusions

From the above it can be concluded that the 10,11-dihydroxy substitution pattern (catechol) and the D ring in *anti* disposition with respect to the tertiary amine (IV) are essential for optimal activity. Small conformational changes influencing the *anti* disposition drastically reduce the activity of APO. Since 9,10-dihydroxyaporphine (isoapomorphine) is practically inactive, it is also concluded that the angle between the plane of the D ring and the plane formed by C_7, C_{6a}, and the nitrogen atom is another important conformational parameter. Finally, the N-methyl group itself is not optimal and can be replaced by a N-ethyl substituent or, most advantageously, by a N-n-propyl group.

III. Pharmacology

A. Emesis and the Gastrointestinal Tract

The induction of emesis by APO constitutes one of the best documented effects of the drug and has been demonstrated in cats (Mitchell, 1950), dogs (Boyd and Boyd, 1953), and humans (Isaacs and MacArthur, 1954); monkeys appear to be resistant to this effect of APO (Brizzee *et al.*, 1955; Peng and Wang, 1962; Shintomi and Yamamura, 1975). Although pigeons have also been reported (Koster, 1957; Weissman, 1975) to peck or to vomit after APO administration, there is still some doubt (Burkman, 1973) about the nature of this response. Some tachyphylaxis to the emetic effect of APO may develop in dogs (Boyd *et al.*, 1955; Dresse and Niemegeers, 1961;

Niemegeers, 1971). The emetic effect of APO is generally considered (Wang and Borison, 1950, 1952; Bhargava *et al.*, 1961; Share *et al.*, 1965; Peng, 1963) to be due to APO's action on the chemoreceptor trigger zone of the fourth ventricle (the area postrema, Borison, 1974). Neuroleptics (Janssen and Niemegeers, 1959), narcotic analgesics (Shemano *et al.*, 1961), and a limited number of pharmacologically heterogeneous compounds (Niemegeers, 1960, 1971) may attenuate APO-induced vomiting, and antagonism to APO-induced emesis in dogs is currently used in predicting clinical dosages of neuroleptic drugs (Janssen *et al.*, 1965b, Niemegeers, 1971).

It has been observed (Cannon, 1898) that APO reduces gastric motility and, at subemetic doses not producing nausea, delays gastric emptying in humans (Ramsbottom and Hunt, 1970). Recent studies (Abrahamsson *et al.*, 1971, 1973) suggest that APO-induced relaxation of the proximal part of the stomach is mediated through vagal relaxatory fibers (Martinson, 1965) which, along with splanchnic adrenergic fibers (Jansson and Martinson, 1966), exert an inhibitory influence on gastric motility. Such an inhibitory phase occurs early in the vomiting act (Cannon, 1898). This effect of APO is interesting in view of the possibility that DA, rather than merely being a precursor of adrenaline and noradrenaline at peripheral sites (Axelrod and Weinshilboum, 1972), also constitutes a neurotransmitter in the autonomic nervous system including, in particular, the gastrointestinal tract (Christensen *et al.*, 1975). DA is present in gastrointestinal mucosa of the stomach (Håkanson, 1970) and of other parts of the gastrointestinal tract (Håkanson and Owman, 1967; Håkanson *et al.*, 1970). The DA receptor-blocking agent metoclopramide (Borenstein and Bles, 1965) produces peristalsis and dilation of the pylorus and duodenum (Justin-Besançon, 1964), thus opposing the action of APO. These effects of metoclopramide are antagonized by atropine (Jacoby and Brodie, 1967), and it has been suggested (Thorner, 1975) that DA modulates cholinergic function at this site and, as such, acts as a transmitter in its own right. However, no convincing evidence is thus far available to substantiate the possible role of DA as a peripheral transmitter substance.

B. BODY TEMPERATURE

In rabbits, systemic (Hill and Horita, 1972; Quock and Horita, 1974; Roszell and Horita, 1975) or intraventricular injection (Quock *et al.*, 1975) of APO produces an hyperthermic response which is effectively antagonized by haloperidol and pimozide.

In mice, hypothermia is produced by systemic (Barnett *et al.*, 1972; Puech *et al.*, 1974) or intraventricular application (Lapin and Samsonova, 1968) of APO; this effect is antagonized by haloperidol and pimozide (Fuxe and Sjöqvist, 1972) and abolished by electrolytic lesions aimed at destroying the caudate nucleus (Glick and Marsanico, 1974).

In rats, systemic (Scheel-Krüger and Hasselager, 1974; Schelkunov and Strabrovsky, 1971) or intraventricular injection (Kruk and Brittain, 1972) of APO likewise produces hypothermia which is antagonized by pimozide (Kruk, 1972). Electrolytic lesions of the midbrain raphe nuclei attenuate the hypothermic response to APO in rats (Grabowska, 1974), and it has been suggested (Grabowska et al., 1973a) that indirect serotonergic stimulation may be involved in this response.

C. Blood Pressure

APO lowers blood pressure in humans (Cotzias et al., 1970; Konzett and Strieder, 1969), dogs (Antonaccio and Robson, 1974), rabbits (Hills and Horita, 1972), cats (Barnett and Fiore, 1971; Lecomte and Dresse, 1962), and rats (Finch and Haeusler, 1973; Lecomte and Dresse, 1962), and lowers heart frequency in the same species (Barnett and Fiore, 1971; Fadhel, 1967; Finch and Haeusler, 1973; Konzett and Strieder, 1969; Lecomte and Dresse, 1962). At relatively high doses, APO may also increase blood pressure in cats and dogs (Barnett and Fiore, 1971; Fadhel, 1967), and this effect has been ascribed (e.g., Patil et al., 1973) to its adrenergic activity. Vagal stimulation (Fadhel, 1967; Finch and Haeusler, 1973) and central DA receptor stimulation (Antonaccio and Robson, 1974; Barnett and Fiore, 1971) have been proposed as possible central mechanisms by which APO exerts its hypotensive effect. However, interference with orthosympathetic innervation at the level of the ganglia (Willems, 1973; Willems and Bogaert, 1975) or the peripheral nerve endings (Enero and Langer, 1975; Long et al., 1975), and direct renal vasodilation (Goldberg, 1972; Setler et al., 1975), may also be involved. These orthosympathetic interferences seem to be based on interaction with a specific DA receptor (Enero and Langer, 1975; Goldberg, 1972, 1975; Long et al., 1975; Setler et al., 1975; Willems, 1973).

D. Hormone Release

It has been reported (Lal et al., 1972b; Nilsson, 1975) that APO raises the serum level of human growth hormone, and the use of APO as a provocative agent to assess the adequacy of human growth hormone secretion has been recommended.

APO also decreases the plasma prolactin concentration in ovariectomized female rats treated with estrogens (Horowski et al., 1975), as well as in intact male rats (Brown et al., 1975). These and other (Nilsson et al., 1975) findings corroborate the hypothesis (Macleod and Lehmeyer, 1974; Kamberi *et al.*, 1970; Hökfelt and Fuxe, 1972) that dopaminergic tuberoinfundibular neurons are involved in the regulation of pituitary hormone secretion. Drugs decreasing dopaminergic neurotransmission conversely raise the serum level of prolactin (e.g., Meites and Clemens, 1972), and it has been postulated (Fuxe *et al.*, 1975) that the ability of the DA receptor-blocking neuroleptic, pimozide (Janssen *et al.*, 1968), to increase DA turnover in the median eminence is due to a drug-induced increase in prolactin secretion.

E. EEG Changes

It has been reported that APO produces increased desynchronization of EEG activity in rats (Votava and Dyntarova, 1968); the duration of APO-induced desynchronization is reduced by haloperidol (Kadzielawa, 1974). These observations may be related to the behavioral findings that APO enhances the susceptibility of rats to environmental stimuli generating behavioral arousal (Janssen *et al.*, 1962) and that APO produces a loss of habituation (Carlsson, 1972).

F. Convulsions

APO increases the lethal effects of pentylenetetrazol in rats and mice and potentiates convulsions in rats induced by the latter drug (Soroko and McKenzie, 1970). In rats, but not in mice, APO possesses some anticonvulsant activity in that it protects against maximal electroshock seizures (McKenzie and Soroko, 1972).

G. Metabolism

According to the work by Kaul *et al.* (1961a,b,c; Kaul and Conway, 1971), glucuronide formation appears to constitute the major metabolic pathway for APO in rodents and accounts for 70–80% of the amount of APO administered. Methylation of the drug by catechol-*O*-methyltransferase (COMT) may be the second major pathway (Cannon *et al.*, 1972a; McKenzie and White, 1973; Missala *et al.*, 1973; White and McKenzie, 1971).

Since monoamine oxidase (MAO) inhibitors fail to potentiate the stereotypogenic action of APO (Ernst, 1967), and as there is no evidence that APO can possibly be a substrate for MAO, it is unlikely that *in vivo* deamination significantly contributes to inactivation of the drug (see also Di Chiara *et al.*, 1974).

IV. Neuropsychopharmacology

A. STEREOTYPED BEHAVIOR

It was originally reported (Amsler, 1923) that systemic APO administration produced chewing (*Zwangsnagen*) and excitation in rats and guinea pigs. The first more detailed account of APO-induced behavioral effects in rats (Janssen *et al.,* 1960) revealed that the intravenous injection of APO (dose range, 0.08–40 mg/kg) induced intense and repetitive (stereotyped) sniffing, licking, agitation, chewing, and increased reactivity to environmental stimuli which in normal rats would be relatively ineffective in generating behavioral arousal (see also Janssen *et al.,* 1962). These effects are clearly dose-related as regards incidence, intensity, and duration. At high doses (2.5–40 mg/kg) exophthalmia, straub, tremors, convulsions, and salivation are also observed (Janssen *et al.,* 1960). However, the characteristics of APO-induced stereotyped behavior (APO SB) vary according to the different stages of the rat's ontogeny (Lal and Sourkes, 1973); also, the duration and distinctiveness of APO SB decrease with repeated administration of the drug (Divac, 1972; Costentin *et al.,* 1975).

Although most studies on APO-induced behavioral effects have been made in rats, the stereotypogenic action of the drug has been documented in various animal species including mice (Puech *et al.,* 1974; Ther and Schramm, 1962), guinea pigs (Frommel *et al.,* 1965), pigeons (Burkman, 1960; Dhawan and Saxena, 1960; Dhawan *et al.,* 1961; Koster, 1957), cats (Cools, 1971; Mitchell, 1950), rabbits (Hill and Horita, 1972; Muacevic *et al.,* 1965), dogs (Koster, 1957; Nymark, 1972; Rotrosen *et al.,* 1972b; Willner *et al.,* 1970), and monkeys (Brizzee *et al.,* 1955; Peng and Wang, 1962; Shintomi and Yamamura, 1975). In most of these species, the APO- (or amphetamine-) induced SB is typically "purposeless" (Emele *et al.,* 1961) and, for this reason, seems to be related to schizophrenic behavior in humans (Randrup and Munkvad, 1967).

The well-known assumption that APO's stereotypogenic effects critically depend on *the integrity of the basal ganglia* was originally proposed by Amsler (1923); this investigator found that striatal lesions, but not decortication, abolished APO SB in rats. The subsequent work by Ernst and Smelik (Ernst, 1962, 1965; Ernst and Smelik, 1966; Smelik and Ernst, 1966) further supported this assumption in that it was shown (Ernst and Smelik, 1966) that implantation of crystalline 3,4-dihydroxyphenylalanine (dopa) or APO in the dorsal part of the caudate nucleus and the globus pallidus of rats resulted in a "gnawing compulsion" syndrome; implantations in other brain areas (i.e., the ventral part of the caudate nucleus, subthalamic structures, substantia nigra) were reported to be ineffective.

The thus established fact that APO can mimic some behavioral effects of the DA precursor (Blaschko, 1939), dopa, generated the idea (Ernst and Smelik, 1966) that APO exerts these effects through *direct activation of central DA receptors.* This was further substantiated by the finding (Ernst, 1967) that neither the dopa decarboxylase inhibitor, α-methyldopa (which depletes catecholamines and serotonin: Dengler and Reichel, 1958; Hess *et al.,* 1961; Sourkes, 1954), nor the tyrosine hydroxylase inhibitor, α-methyltyrosine (which inhibits catecholamine biosynthesis: Spector *et al.,* 1965), affected the APO-induced gnawing compulsion. However, the conclusiveness of the latter results was later challenged by the possibility that the doses used in these experiments were not appropriate (Srimal and Dhawan, 1970).

It was also shown (Smelik and Ernst, 1966) that application of the cholinesterase inhibitor, physostigmine, in the substantia nigra likewise resulted in a gnawing compulsion; caudate and pallidal applications were reported not to do so. This supported the hypothesis that cholinergic nerve fibers end synaptically on dopaminergic nigra cells; accumulation of acetylcholine by physostigmine would then activate the dopaminergic nigrostriatal fibers and thus cause an accumulation of DA at striatal nerve endings (Smelik and Ernst, 1966). This hypothesis on the functional significance of the dopaminergic nigrostriatal system was felt (Ernst, 1969) to be entirely consistent with the observation that electrical stimulation of the substantia nigra produces an increased release of DA (Andén *et al.,* 1964; Brodal, 1963; McLennan, 1965; Portig and Vogt, 1968, 1969; Vogt, 1969), as well as unit responses (Connor, 1968, 1970; Frigyesi and Purpura, 1967) in the caudate nucleus.

B. Brain Areas Involved in APO SB

The assumption that APO exerts its stereotypogenic action through a (direct) DA mimicking effect at central DA receptor sites (Ernst and Smelik, 1966; Ernst, 1967) has prompted research efforts to concentrate on those brain areas in which dopaminergic nerve endings have been demonstrated. According to recent studies on the organization of ascending catecholamine pathways in rat brain (Ungerstedt, 1971a; Lindvall and Björklund, 1974), the following areas are implicated; (1) the nigrostriatal DA system, (2) the mesolimbic DA system, and (3) the tuberoinfundibular DA system. In addition, evidence has accumulated (Berger *et al.,* 1974; Hökfelt *et al.,* 1974a,b; Lindvall *et al.,* 1974; Thierry *et al.,* 1974) to include (4) cortical dopaminergic innervation (Thierry *et al.,* 1973) as well.

Research on the site of action involved in APO SB has benefited considerably from some earlier work on the sites involved in amphetamine SB. The latter had been shown to depend critically on catecholamines (Scheel-Krüger and Randrup, 1967; Taylor and Snyder, 1971; Tseng and Loh, 1974; Weinstok and Speiser, 1974; Weissman et al., 1966), and studies using brain lesion techniques revealed the caudate–putamen complex (Fog et al., 1970) and the globus pallidus (Naylor and Olley, 1972) to play a prominent role in amphetamine SB.

At the outset of this discussion, however, it should be pointed out that the relevance of some of the techniques commonly used to study behavioral functions of the brain is limited, for one thing, by the intrinsic effects of such techniques. Thus, for example, electrolytic lesions of striatal (Fog and Pakkenberg, 1971) or nigral tissue (Baum et al., 1971; Costall et al., 1971; Simpson and Iversen, 1971) themselves produce a form of SB that is not (Fog and Pakkenberg, 1971), or only at very large doses (Costall et al., 1972), antagonized by the otherwise extremely effective neuroleptic, halo-peridol (Janssen, 1967). Similar comments apply both to the use of 6-hy-droxydopamine (6-OHDA) to produce degeneration of catecholamine path-ways (Kostrzewa and Jacobowitz, 1974) and to the implantation of can-nulas to inject drugs directly into the brain (Routtenberg, 1972; see, however, Singer and Montgomery, 1973).

6-OHDA-induced degeneration of the nigrostriatal ascending system, then, results in enhanced sensitivity (denervation supersensitivity) to APO-induced rotational behavior (Ungerstedt, 1971b), as well as to other behaviorally stimulating effects of APO (Jalfre and Haefely, 1971; Unger-stedt, 1971c). This contrasts to the finding (Baum et al., 1971; Costall et al., 1972) that bilateral electrolytic lesions of the substantia nigra severely im-pair the occurrence of APO SB. According to the latter result, the integrity of the substantia nigra pars compacta (A9, Dahlström and Fuxe, 1964) is critical to APO SB, whereas it is not to amphetamine SB (Costall et al., 1972).

These seemingly contradictory findings established by different lesion techniques may be reconsidered in view of the possibility (Baum et al., 1971; Iversen, 1971) that the electrolytic lesions were insufficient to disrupt the nigrostriatal pathway entirely. Over 90% depletion of striatal DA indeed is required to impair amphetamine-induced behavioral responses effectively (Creese and Iversen, 1972); only nearly total striatal DA depletion resulting from either neonatal 6-OHDA treatment (Creese and Iversen, 1973) or acute 6-OHDA injection into the substantia nigra (Creese and Iversen, 1972, 1975) is completely effective in this respect. In contrast to its effects on amphetamine-induced behavioral responses, 6-OHDA injection into the sub-stantia nigra increases behavioral responses to APO (Creese and Iversen, 1975).

These differential effects of electrolytic (Baum et al., 1971; Costall et al., 1972) and 6-OHDA-induced (Creese and Iversen, 1975) damage to the substantia nigra on APO SB draw attention to some rather poorly investigated factors which may conceivably contribute to this result. Thus, for example, the conclusions reached by Costall et al. (1972) are based on a score system which attributes quantitatively different scores to morphologically distinct behavioral items. Such an approach may actually confound different effects, as Baum et al. (1971, 1972) have shown that electrolytic lesions similar to those described by Costall et al. (1972) produced a marked qualitative modification of APO SB rather than merely reducing it quantitatively.

Drug studies may likewise reveal this phenomenon; specific DA receptor-blocking neuroleptics such as haloperidol (Janssen, 1967), pimozide (Janssen et al., 1968), penfluridol (Janssen et al., 1970), and clopimozide (Janssen et al., 1975) have been found (Colpaert et al., 1976a) to antagonize APO-induced chewing and agitation, to potentiate licking and rearing, and to exert a biphasic effect on sniffing. Combined reserpine and α-methyl-p-tyrosine treatment also differentially affects various components of APO SB (Costall and Naylor, 1973a, 1975; Cox and Tha, 1973; see, however, Andén et al., 1967). The effects of neuroleptic drugs on amphetamine SB have similarly been described (Kjellberg and Randrup, 1974; Munkvad and Randrup, 1966; Randrup and Munkvad, 1965) in terms of (partial) restoration of normal activity, rather than in terms of mere inhibition of abnormal behavior (i.e., SB). One therefore inevitably arrives at the conclusion that different APO SB components are differentially affected by the same electrolytic nigral lesions (Costall et al., 1975). Conversely, bilateral electrolytic lesions of the substantia nigra involving to a varying degree the pars compacta and the pars reticulata differentially affect APO SB (Baum et al., 1972) and striatal DA and serotonin contents (Baum et al., 1972; Faull and Laverty, 1969; Goldstein et al., 1969; Sourkes and Poirier, 1968; Ungerstedt, 1971a).

Regardless of this behavioral differentiation, then, extensive lesions of the caudate–putamen complex have been reported either to leave APO SB unaffected (Costall and Naylor, 1973a; Divac, 1972; McKenzie, 1972) or to potentiate some of its components (Kelly et al., 1975; Wolfarth, 1974). In contrast, amphetamine SB is abolished by lesions destroying over 30% of the neostriatal tissue (Fog et al., 1970).

Lesions of the globus pallidus, which also contains DA fibers originating in the A9 area (Broch and Marsden, 1972; Hornykiewicz, 1966), markedly reduce or abolish APO SB (Costall and Naylor, 1973b; Wolfarth, 1974), as do lesions of the nucleus amygdaloideus lateralis (Costall and Naylor, 1972) and centralis (Costall and Naylor, 1973a, 1974a).

Bilateral intracaudate APO injection does not result in SB (Costall and

Naylor, 1974b); DA application at the same site may likewise fail to affect general motor function (Bondareff *et al.,* 1970; Costall *et al.,* 1974; Hull *et al.,* 1967). However, these negative findings may possibly be attributed to methodological problems, as intracaudate or intrapallidal DA injection, given at a sufficiently high dose, may nevertheless produce characteristic rotational behavior (Costall and Naylor, 1974c).

Lesions at various mesolimbic sites of dopaminergic innervation have been reported to produce less conflicting results. During either the acute (Costall and Naylor, 1973b; McKenzie 1971b, 1972) or the chronic stage (Costall and Naylor, 1973b) of lesions in the tuberculum olfactorium, APO SB is markedly reduced or even abolished (the sniffing component). APO injection into the tuberculum olfactorium effectively induces SB (McKenzie, 1971b). Lesions of the nucleus accumbens septi have been found either to abolish APO-induced sniffing (Costall and Naylor, 1973b) or to exert no effect at all (McKenzie, 1972). Finally, lesions of the stria terminalis, for the purpose of assessing the possible involvement of the nucleus interstitialis striae terminalis, were reported not to affect APO SB (Costall and Naylor, 1973b).

From these studies related to the brain locus of APO SB it can be concluded that, in contrast to the original idea of a specific and exclusive role of striatal tissue (Ernst, 1967), both the nigrostriatal and mesolimbic DA systems are involved in this effect. However, there are some inconsistencies among lesion studies using different or similar lesion techniques, as well as among studies using local intracranial application of drugs in liquid or solid form. It is further indicated that adequate analysis of this locus of action requires detailed differentiation, both qualitatively and quantitatively, of the distinct behavioral effects of APO (Costall and Naylor, 1973c, 1975; Costall *et al.,* 1975); specification of the type of effect with regard to locus also seems warranted (Bieger *et al.,* 1972). Finally, the possible role of other brain areas containing DA nerve terminals, such as the cortical DA system, has thus far not, or only poorly, been investigated.

C. Drugs Affecting APO SB

The finding (Janssen *et al.,* 1960) that neuroleptic drugs, and also narcotic analgesics, effectively antagonize APO SB in rats constitutes a major argument for the now generally accepted hypothesis that the antipsychotic activity of neuroleptics is primarily based on their ability to block DA receptors (Van Rossum, 1966). Subsequent research (Janssen *et al.,* 1965a, 1967) has essentially duplicated this finding, and no other drugs seem to be able to block APO SB effectively. Under particular experimental conditions, reserpine (Fekete *et al.,* 1970), α-methyl-L-tyrosine (Pedersen, 1968), and the serotonin precursor 5-hydroxytryptophan (Weiner et al., 1975) may attenuate APO SB. However, other workers have found the two former drugs either to be ineffective (Ernst, 1967; Rotrosen et al., 1972a; Andén et al., 1967) or to potentiate APO SB (Ther and Schramm, 1962; Goetz and Klawans, 1974; Rotrosen et al., 1972b; Costall and Naylor, 1973a). At least some of these discrepancies can be explained by the differences in APO doses used in these studies (see discussion in Weiner et al., 1975).

Tricyclic antidepressants, pethidine, and phenobarbital, as well as several anticholinergic and antihistaminic drugs, have been found (Ther and Schramm, 1962; Pedersen, 1967, 1968) to potentiate APO SB in mice. It is interesting to note that the anticholinergic potentiation of APO SB is more effectively counteracted by physostigmine than by spiramide (Scheel-Krüger, 1970); this finding is relevant in view of the hypothesis (Klawans, 1968) that the normal function of the corpus striatum depends on a DA-acetylcholine balance.

Various MAO inhibitors have been reported to potentiate APO SB in mice (Fekete et al., 1970) and rats (Maj et al., 1972); this contrasts to earlier results (Ernst, 1967) indicating that these drugs fail to affect APO SB.

Methysergide and lysergic acid diethylamide potentiate APO SB in rats (Grabowska and Michaluk, 1974) and guinea pigs (Weiner et al., 1975), thus evidencing a serotonergic modulatory influence on APO SB. The fact that the COMT inhibitors, pyrogallol, tropolone, and 8-hydroxyquinoline, potentiate APO SB (McKenzie and White, 1973) corroborates the finding (White and McKenzie, 1971) that O-methylation is a major metabolic pathway for APO.

Finally, the central DA receptors presumably involved in the behavioral effects of APO are subject to rapid changes in sensitivity to APO (Costentin et al., 1975), and drugs increasing receptor sensitivity may thereby potentiate APO SB (Asper et al., 1973; Gianutsos et al., 1975; Gudelsky et al., 1975; Nahorski, 1975; Sayers et al., 1975; Tarsy and Baldessarini, 1973, 1974; Vonvoigtlander et al., 1975; Yarbrough, 1975).

D. Locomotor Activity

In rats and mice, APO may either increase (Frommel, 1965; Thomas, 1970; Maj et al., 1972) or decrease (Puech et al., 1974; Kulkarni and Dandiya, 1975) locomotor activity, the direction of the effect depending on the dose and the time interval after APO injection (Sahakian and Robbins, 1975).

The locomotor stimulant effect of APO in rats partially depends on social experience (Sahakian et al., 1975) and can be potentiated by food deprivation (Sahakian and Robbins, 1975). It has been suggested (Sahakian *et al.*, 1975) that APO-induced locomotor stimulant effects are pharmacologically distinct from APO SB. Intraventricular 6-OHDA injections (Nahorski, 1975), presumably destroying catecholamine-containing nerve terminals (Uretsky and Iversen, 1970; Breese and Traylor, 1970), or lesions of the midbrain raphe nuclei (Grabowska, 1974), potentiate this locomotor stimulant effect, and serotonergic systems (Grabowska, 1974; Grabowska and Michaluk, 1974) as well as an interaction between dopaminergic and noradrenergic mechanisms (Sahakian and Robbins, 1975) may be involved in this effect.

It is relevant to note here that a serotonergic involvement has also been proposed in APO SB (Costall *et al.*, 1975; Jacobs, 1974; Weiner *et al.*, 1975; see, however, Rotrosen *et al.*, 1972b); whether such involvement actually bears on the same behavioral effect (assessed as either locomotion or SB) is not clear from the available data.

E. AGGRESSION

APO is known to induce intraspecies aggression in rats (Schneider, 1968; Senault, 1968; Van Rossum, 1970) and monkeys (Peng and Wang, 1962); interspecies aggression is unaffected by the drug (Senault, 1970). External stimulation of different modalities such as auditive (Senault, 1970) or noxious (McKenzie, 1971a) enhance the rat's susceptibility to this effect which, per se, is more clearly evident in adult and male rats than in young and female animals (Senault, 1970; McKenzie, 1971a). Also, social isolation increases the aggressive response to APO (Senault, 1971), but this result is confounded by the fact that such isolation itself may enhance aggression (Bevan *et al.*, 1951).

In a competitive situation for food (Lindzey *et al.*, 1961), APO increases the number of victories in male (Terada and Masur, 1973) and female rats (Masur and Benedito, 1974a,b), irrespective of whether the animals are genetically winners or losers (Masur *et al.*, 1975). APO also potentiates narcotic withdrawal-produced aggression in rats (Puri and Lal, 1973), and the latter type of aggression has been claimed (Lal *et al.*, 1971) to be similar to APO-induced aggressive behavior.

The morphological distinction between fighting behavior and biting responses has led to the hypothesis (Patni and Dandiya, 1974) that APO-induced aggressive behavior is not exclusively due to direct stimulation of a single DA receptor (Lal *et al.*, 1971). Patni and Dandiya (1974) indeed argued that the APO-induced biting response must result from the activation of some central nervous system receptor for which APO must have a higher affinity than DA.

F. Sexual Behavior

It has been shown (Butcher *et al.*, 1969) that, in male rats, APO can restore sexual behavior abolished by tetrabenazine; APO itself decreases intromission frequency, increases postejaculatory latency, and does not affect ejaculatory latency. The effect of APO on male sexual behavior is antagonized by haloperidol (Tagliamonte *et al.*, 1974), and a dopaminergic (Butcher *et al.*, 1969; Everitt *et al.*, 1974; Malmnas, 1973) and possibly a serotonergic mechanism (Tagliamonte *et al.*, 1974) may be involved in male, and also in female (Hamburger-Bar and Rigter, 1975), sexual behavior.

G. Conditioned Behavior

APO can increase as well as decrease conditioned responding in rats (Butcher, 1968) and pigeons (Weismann, 1966), and can overcome the inhibition of conditioned behavior induced by haloperidol (Davies *et al.*, 1973) or tetrabenazine (Butcher and Andén, 1969). Conversely, APO-induced decreased responding for food can be partially restored by haloperidol (Colpaert *et al.*, 1975). The intrinsic effects of APO can be demonstrated using operant procedures involving either positive (Broekkamp and Van Rossum, 1974; De Oliviera and Graeff, 1972; Kadzielawa, 1974; Liebman and Butcher, 1973, 1974; St.-Laurent *et al.*, 1973; Wauquier and Niemegeers, 1973; Weissman, 1966) or negative (Butcher, 1968) reinforcement, though they may be differentially featured according to the nature of the reinforcement applied. For example, after APO the response rate in a Sidman avoidance situation bears no systematic relationship to the dose (Butcher, 1968), whereas it does so when electrical stimulation of the medial forebrain bundle (at the level of the lateral hypothalamus) is used as a reward (Wauquier and Niemegeers, 1973). Also, APO-produced response stimulation as revealed under the latter experimental conditions is related to the control response rates in individual rats (Wauquier and Niemegeers, 1973), whereas this does not seem to be the case in the avoidance procedure (Butcher, 1968).

Interpretation of data on the effects of APO on operant behavior is generally inspired by the role of DA in the extrapyramidal motor system (Hornykiewicz, 1973; Klawans, 1968) which partly consists of the basal ganglia. The latter group of brain structures is commonly thought to subserve subcortical sensory-motor integratory functions, and it has been proposed accordingly that APO's response stimulatory effect is due to mere facilitation of motor output (Wauquier and Niemegeers, 1973). Such facilitation may result either in stereotyped execution of the learned response and thus cause response increase (Butcher, 1968), or in the increased occurrence of competing alternative (unlearned) responses and thus cause response decrease (Colpaert et al., 1975).

An alternative hypothesis is based on the role of biogenic amines in memory formation (Dismukes and Rake, 1972; Kety, 1970); such interference may readily account for the differences that exist (Davies et al., 1974) between APO's effects on the acquisition of a new response and the performance of a learned one.

H. The Concept of Direct DA Receptor Stimulation in the Caudate–Putamen Complex

The early studies by Ernst (Ernst and Smelik, 1966; Ernst, 1967) have critically contributed to the widely accepted (Hornykiewicz, 1972) concept of a direct receptor stimulation at central DA receptor sites by APO, and the use of APO as a tool in neuropsychopharmacological research is largely based on this concept. From the above, however, it follows that the present status of knowledge casts some doubt on this concept. As for the direct nature of the presumed effect of APO on DA receptors, some data (Costall and Naylor, 1973a,b; Cox and Tha, 1973) have been presented which suggest that a presynaptic event is also critically involved in APO SB. Thus, for example, electrolytic lesions of the substantia nigra attenuate APO SB (Baum et al., 1972; Costall et al., 1972), suggesting that direct DA receptor activation at striatal sites does not constitute a sufficient condition to make APO elicit SB.

Other evidence has accumulated which argues for primary or secondary involvement of neurotransmitter substances other than DA (e.g., serotonin and noradrenaline) in APO SB (Costall et al., 1975; Taylor and Snyder, 1971; Weiner et al., 1975), increased locomotor activity (Maj et al., 1972; Grabowska, 1974), and aggression (Terada and Masur, 1973). Some investigators (Patni and Dandiya, 1974; Kulkarni and Dandiya, 1975) have proposed a separate central receptor for which APO may have a higher affinity than DA itself; this proposal may be appreciated in terms of a model with two DA receptors (Cools, 1973; Struyker-Boudier, 1975).

It also has been substantiated (see, for example, Costall and Naylor, 1973b; Costall et al., 1975) that, not only the caudate–putamen complex, but also numerous brain structures pertaining to the nigrostriatal as well as to the mesolimbic DA systems, are involved in various aspects or components of APO SB, and the possible role of still other DA-innervated structures remains to be determined. Perusal of the literature in this area further reveals that an adequate interpretation of data requires detailed knowledge and appropriate application of the techniques used in such studies. Thus, apart from the necessity, as discussed above, to differentiate between distinct components of APO SB, appreciation of whether the proposed involvement of serotonin in APO SB (Costall *et al.,* 1975; Weiner *et al.,* 1975) basically pertains to the same behavioral effect which, alternatively, would have been measured as locomotor activity (Grabowska, 1974; Grabowska and Michaluk, 1974) is not clear from the data presented.

Similar methodological and procedural problems undoubtedly underlie other inconclusive or even inconsistent results, such as the fact that electro-lytically produced (Baum *et al.,* 1971; Costall *et al.,* 1972) or 6-OHDA-produced (Creese and Iversen, 1975) damage to the nigrostriatal DA system differentially affects APO SB.

V. Biochemistry

As neuropsychopharmacological research allowed recognition of the role of dopaminergic brain systems in the mechanism of action of APO, biochemical research has concentrated on the effects of APO on DA biosynthesis and degradation, and on its actions on presumed DA receptor sites. The possible effects of the drug on other neurotransmitter systems have also been studied, and it appears that APO may indirectly affect these systems through links which seem to exist between different neurotransmitter systems in the brain.

A. DA TURNOVER AND DA RECEPTORS

The observation (Andén *et al.,* 1967) that APO decreases DA biosynthesis and thus interferes with DA turnover has led to four alternative explanations: (1) a transsynaptic feedback mechanism activated by APO-induced stimulation of postsynaptic DA receptors (a transsynaptic messenger possibly mediating this process), (2) stimulation of presynaptic inhibitory receptors by APO, (3) direct inhibition of tyrosine hydroxylase (TH), the rate-limiting enzyme in DA biosynthesis, and (4) inhibition of MAO, a catabolic enzyme, with subsequent inhibition of TH by the reaction end product.

In a first study on this topic, Andén *et al.* (1967) investigated the depletion of brain DA produced by the TH inhibitor H44/68. It was found that APO retards this depletion, and that this APO effect can be antagonized by haloperidol. These findings suggested that APO reduces activity in DA neurons, and the possibility was raised (Andén *et al.,* 1967) that this APO effect may be mediated by a feedback mechanism activated by the direct action of APO on DA receptors. The critical basis of this idea was the antagonism between APO and neuroleptic drugs, and subsequent studies

(Andén and Bédard, 1971; Andén et al., 1969) evidenced that APO and neuroleptic drugs compete for the same receptor sites.

Another approach was offered by the administration of the labeled catecholamine precursor tyrosine and subsequent measurement of the rate of disappearance of labeled amines from mouse brain. These experiments (Nyback et al., 1970) revealed that APO retards the disappearance rate of [^{14}C]DA, while pimozide accelerates this process; the opposite effects of APO and pimozide on the turnover rate of DA again supported the concept of DA receptor-activating and blocking actions, respectively, of both drugs.

Reduced activity in DA neurons due to APO was further substantiated by the finding (Roos, 1969) that APO decreases homovanillic acid (HVA) levels in the striatal tissue of the rat. As DA levels seemed to be unaffected by APO (Andén et al., 1967), the APO-induced reduction in HVA was believed not to be mediated by effects on DA release and instead was attributed to the activating effect of APO at DA receptor sites. Another finding supporting this view is that APO reduces the neuroleptic-induced HVA increase in mouse brain (Lahti et al., 1972).

The hypothesis that the decelerating effect of APO on striatal DA turnover is due to a neuronal feedback mechanism initiated by stimulation of postsynaptic DA receptors was later broadened by Kehr et al. (1972). These workers proposed that the above-described feedback mechanism is mediated by a transsynaptic messenger. They also postulated the existence of presynaptic DA receptors through which APO, owing to its ability to attenuate DA biosynthesis, could operate intraneuronally. This was based on the fact that APO markedly decreases the accumulation of dopa in rat forebrain after administration of a dopa decarboxylase inhibitor (Kehr et al., 1972); the effect was observed on the lesioned brain side (axotomy of the nigrostriatal fibers), as well as on the intact side. Haloperidol had the opposite effect on the intact side, but did not affect dopa accumulation on the lesioned side. When both drugs were administered to the same animals, the inhibitory effect of APO on dopa accumulation was antagonized on both sides of the brain.

The hypothesis on the existence of presynaptic receptors for which APO may possess a high affinity has gained much support from further investigations. Thus APO inhibits the firing rate of central dopaminergic neurons, probably through stimulation of presynaptic DA receptors (Aghajanian and Bunney, 1973; Bunney et al., 1973). In a study on the suppression of ethanol-induced stimulation of brain DA synthesis by DA agonists, Carlsson et al. (1974) concluded that small doses of APO preferentially activate presynaptic DA receptors.

The third alternative to explain the APO-induced decrease in DA biosynthesis is derived from the proposal (Goldstein et al., 1970) that APO affects DA turnover through direct inhibition of TH. *In vitro* experiments using brain homogenates revealed a significant inhibition only at high concentrations of the drug (10^{-4} M). However, when striatal slices were used, APO inhibited [^{14}C]DA biosynthesis at markedly lower concentrations (10^{-6}– 10^{-7} M). This prompted the suggestion (Goldstein *et al.*, 1970) that the drug accumulates in dopaminergic neurons, hence reaches an effective inhibitory concentration. *In vivo* experiments showed that APO may reduce [^{14}C]DA biosynthesis in the telencephalon and brainstem by 50%. The same investigators failed to observe a direct effect of haloperidol on TH, but Mussacchio (1970) reported increased TH as an effect of various neuroleptic drugs.

Whether the ability of APO to inhibit TH is responsible for the drug's effect on DA biosynthesis has not yet been established. This remains questionable, as another presumed (Corrodi *et al.*, 1971) dopaminergic agonist, trivastal, has no effect on TH *in vitro*, whereas the same drug, like APO, decreases DA turnover *in vivo* (Goldstein *et al.*, 1973).

Later, it was proposed (Christiansen and Squires, 1974) that APO may exert a double effect on TH; the drug may inhibit synaptosomal TH directly, as well as indirectly, by activating the postulated presynaptic inhibitory DA receptors. This seemed to be supported by experiments showing that APO effectively ($IC_{50} \simeq 6 \times 10^{-7}$ M) inhibited TH in a dispersed striatal synaptosome fraction; the effect was partly reversed by haloperidol. It was further found (Christiansen and Squires, 1976) that is *in vitro* antagonism by neuroleptic drugs parallels the potency of these drugs to antagonize APO *in vivo*. It was also noted that, at effectively antagonizing concentrations, none of the neuroleptics had a direct effect on TH; at higher concentrations these drugs also inhibited TH and, in contrast to Musacchio's (1970) finding, no activation of the enzyme was ever observed. The correlation between the *in vitro* and *in vivo* activity of neuroleptic drugs was later confirmed (Christiansen and Squires, 1976), but it was also observed that the same drugs failed to reverse the inhibition of TH produced by DA, whereas DA reuptake blockers were able to do so. These findings suggest that DA decreases TH by direct enzyme inhibition, while APO—at physiological pH—acts at least partly by an indirect mechanism, i.e., through stimulation of the postulated presynaptic DA receptors. The above-mentioned correlation between *in vitro* antagonism by neuroleptics and their *in vivo* potency further suggests that these presynaptic receptors are very similar to postsynaptic DA receptors. In several experiments on the effects of APO, DA, and haloperidol on dibutyryl cyclic adenosine monophosphate (dB-cAMP)-stimulated TH activity, Ebstein *et al.* (1974) reached a similar conclusion. APO was found to exert two distinct actions on TH; the direct action appeared to be related to the inhibitory property of the catechol moiety of the molecule, while the indirect one involved activation of the presumed presynaptic DA receptors.

In recent studies (Iversen et al., 1975), the activity of various dopaminergic agonists and antagonists was studied in a presynaptic model (i.e., synaptosomal TH) and compared to that in a postsynaptic model (i.e., DA-sensitive adenylate cyclase; see Section II, B). APO behaved as a pure agonist in the first model but had mixed agonist-antagonist effects in the second one (Iversen et al., 1975). The presynaptic model was further developed to evaluate the antagonistic effects of several antipsychotics on APO-inhibited synaptosomal TH activity; according to these studies (Iversen et al., 1976), the two models yielded different potencies for the series of neuroleptics tested, thus indicating that relatively subtle differences exist between pre- and postsynaptic receptors.

However, the exact location of the DA receptor that regulates striatal TH is still in doubt. For example, it has been hypothesized (Zivkovic et al., 1974, 1975) that, were the assumption of a presynaptic autoreceptor correct, stimulation of the autoreceptor by APO would prevent the change in the kinetic state of striatal TH induced by cerebral hemisection. APO was then found not to produce this effect, thus indicating that the altered TH kinetics are not due to the lack of occupancy of the autoreceptors by the agonist. In addition, blockage or stimulation of DA receptors affects the kinetic state of striatal TH only if the nigrostriatal pathway is intact, and it was concluded (Zivkovic et al., 1975) that postsynaptic DA receptors are involved in the regulation of the kinetic state of striatal TH.

The fourth alternative explanation of APO's effects on DA biosynthesis involves the well-documented assumption (Di Chiara et al., 1974) that APO primarily inhibits DA deamination. It was showed that, in vitro, APO competitively inhibits DA deamination in brain mitochondria ($K_i = 1.4 \times 10^{-4}$ M) and does not affect COMT activity up to a concentration of 5×10^{-4} M. In contrast with earlier data (Andén et al., 1967), APO was found (Di Chiara et al., 1974) to increase DA and to reduce HVA and dihydroxyphenyl-acetic acid (DOPAC) levels. Also, APO prevented reserpine-induced depletion of DA and a rise in HVA and DOPAC, and antagonized the increase in DOPAC after L-dopa administration. It was felt that the APO-induced decrease in HVA levels was primarily due to MAO inhibition, either through accumulation of the drug in DA neurons or by a selective APO effect on DA-sensitive MAO. The APO-induced decrease in DA biosynthesis was thought to be secondary to the blockage of DA deamination (by end-product inhibition), and it was concluded that the hypothesis of a transsynaptic feedback mechanism fails to explain the inhibition of HVA and DOPAC rise after L-dopa administration because TH is not involved in these processes. These and other considerations indeed constitute a serious challenge to the negative feedback mechanism, but do not conclusively invalidate the possibility of a stimulatory feedback mechanism for catecholamine biosynthesis secondary to receptor blockade.

B. DA-Sensitive Adenylate Cyclase

An adenylate cyclase activated by low DA concentrations has been demonstrated in mammalian superior cervical sympathetic ganglia (Kebabian and Greengard, 1971), in homogenates of different dopaminergic rat brain areas such as the caudate nucleus (Kebabian et al., 1972), in the olfactory tubercle and the nucleus accumbens (Clement-Cormier et al., 1974), and in the retina (Brown and Makman, 1972). The DA-sensitive adenylate cyclase is felt to be involved in synaptic transmission (Kebabian and Greengard, 1971) through the action of its reaction product cAMP (Greengard and Kebabian, 1974; Greengard et al., 1972). Low concentrations of APO were found (Bucher and Schorderet, 1975; Kebabian et al., 1972) to activate this enzyme, an effect that is antagonized by neuroleptic drugs. These observations suggest (Clement-Cormier et al., 1974; Forn et al., 1974; Kebabian et al., 1972) that a DA-sensitive adenylate cyclase constitutes the DA receptor in the CNS. Further studies (Iversen et al., 1975a) revealed that the DA agonists DA, APO, epinine, and 2-amino-6,7-dihydroxy-1,2,3,4-tetrahydronaphthalene are equipotent with respect to their ability to activate the enzyme; APO, however, appeared to exert mixed agonist and antagonist effects. The ability of neuroleptics to antagonize DA-induced activation of the enzyme was found (Iversen et al., 1975b) to correlate with the in vivo activity of these drugs, thus corroborating the above-mentioned suggestion.

APO also increases cAMP levels without affecting cyclic guanosine monophosphate (cGMP) levels in rats bearing unilateral electrolytic lesions of the nigrostriatal pathway (Forn et al., 1974; Stratten and Avlott, 1974) and in isolated rabbit retina (Bucher and Schorderet, 1975).

Goldstein et al. (1973) revealed the somewhat confusing finding that the cAMP analog dB-cAMP has an effect on striatal DA biosynthesis opposite to that of APO. The stimulation of TH activity elicited by dB-cAMP is thought to be of a nature distinct from the receptor-mediated elevation of DA turnover produced by neuroleptics. These investigators proposed three possible explanations of the dB-cAMP action: (1) permeability changes across the neuronal membrane, (2) direct activation of TH, and (3) an increase in the level of the TH cofactor. The last-mentioned alternative proved to be most useful with regard to the antagonism between dB-cAMP and neuroleptics on the one hand and APO on the other (Ebstein et al., 1974). Haloperidol and dB-cAMP were found to attenuate the effectiveness of APO to reduce DA biosynthesis, but the effects of both compounds were not additive, whereas APO and DA enhanced the dB-cAMP-induced activation of TH. On the basis of further experiments in which APO, dB-cAMP, and haloperidol were combined in the incubation mixture, it was concluded (Ebstein *et al.*, 1974) that "haloperidol partially reversed the enhanced stimulation of TH activity elicited by dB-cAMP in the presence of APO."

From these *in vitro* data it appears that the involvement of cAMP in the effect of APO on DA biosynthesis is highly complex, owing to numerous possible interactions. However, the extent to which these actions and interactions are operative in the *in vivo* situation remains to be elucidated.

C. *In Vitro* BINDING TO BRAIN DA RECEPTORS

The first attempt to identify DA receptors by a direct *in vitro* binding assay was made by Taylor (1974). As was done earlier for the binding of other neurotransmitters (e.g., acetylcholine, glycine), this investigator used a labeled receptor blocker ([^{14}C]fluphenazine) and tested different presumed DA receptor agonists and antagonists for their ability to displace tissue-bound radioactivity. The highest displaceable [^{14}C]fluphenazine binding was found in synaptic membranes from rat brain tissue. The specificity of the binding was supported by the correlation revealed between the potency of neuroleptics to displace labeled fluphenazine and their clinical activity. Antagonists showed much higher affinity than agonists; with a fluphenazine concentration of 1 μM, the IC_{50} value for neuroleptics was in the micromolar range, whereas that for agonists was in the order of 10^{-2} M, APO and DA being equipotent. Another model consists of the binding of labeled DA to synaptic membranes of mammalian striatal tissue (Burt *et al.*, 1975). Using [^{3}H]DA at a concentration of 5 nM, the IC_{50} values obtained for agonists were lower than those for antagonists; APO was the most potent (IC_{50} = 4 nM), and the antagonists were active in the micromolar range.

It has been claimed (Creese *et al.*, 1975) that agonist and antagonist states of the DA receptor can be differentiated. This resulted from experiments in which inhibition of binding of either [^{3}H]DA or [^{3}H]haloperidol was studied; it was found that agonists were more effective as inhibitors of agonist binding, and that antagonists were more effective as inhibitors of antagonist binding. Thus, for example, APO IC_{50} values were 6 nM for [^{3}H]DA binding and 150 nM for [^{3}H]haloperidol binding; those of DA were 22 nM and 1000 nM, respectively. APO again displayed a higher receptor affinity than the endogenous agonist; this result may explain the high *in vivo* activity of the drug. Independent work from another laboratory (Seeman *et al.*, 1974, 1975) has led to very similar conclusions.

From the above it can be inferred that APO binds to the presumed DA receptor in a way very similar to that of DA itself. However, APO's affinity for the receptor is consistently higher than that of DA.

D. Uptake and Release of Catecholamines

The findings and speculations about APO's effect on DA biosynthesis inspired Ferris *et al.* (1975) to investigate the possible effects of APO on catecholamine uptake and release in presynaptic nerve endings from rat brain. In this study, APO displayed mixed inhibition kinetics on the uptake of DA in striatal synaptosomes and on that of noradrenaline in hypothalamic homogenates. It appeared that APO was bound to the membranes, as both active (at 37°C) and passive (at 0°C) uptake were reduced. It was also shown that APO produces a dose-related DA release from striatal storage pools; no appreciable effect of APO on noradrenaline release was observed. These data suggest (Ferris *et al.*, 1975) that APO may increase the DA concentration in the synaptic cleft. However, it seems unlikely that this increased DA concentration is critically involved in APO's *in vivo* effects.

E. Other Neurotransmitters

Initial studies (Andén *et al.*, 1967) failed to reveal any effect of APO on noradrenaline turnover in rat brain after inhibition of TH. However, given a suitable time interval (at least 30 minutes) between the administration of APO and of labeled precursor ([³H]tyrosine), APO may enhance the disappearance rate of [³H]noradrenaline after inhibition of TH (Persson and Waldeck, 1970a,b). It was assumed that the change in noradrenaline turnover was due to a functional interrelationship between noradrenergic and dopaminergic neurons such that APO-induced DA receptor stimulation resulted in increased activity of noradrenaline neurons (Persson, 1970; Persson and Waldeck, 1970b).

In view of the finding (Section V,A) that APO inhibits TH it was postulated (Goldstein *et al.*, 1970) that the APO-induced increase in noradrenaline turnover after TH inhibition may be due to a potentiation of TH inhibition. However, no effect of APO on the disappearance rate of noradrenaline was detected in mice, although brain noradrenaline content was reduced by 70% (Nyback *et al.*, 1970).

Data on the possible effect of APO on serotonin turnover and metabolism are conflicting. Several investigators (e.g., Tagliamonte *et al.*, 1971) failed to observe any effect of APO on the brain level of serotonin, or on the concentration of its precursor, tryptophan, or on its most important metabolite, 5-hydroxyindoleacetic acid. Other workers (Grabowska *et al.,* 1973b) reported that APO elevates the concentration of both serotonin and its metabolite in rat brain. However, the latter effects can be reproduced only under quite specific experimental conditions (Scheel-Krüger and Hasselager, 1974). Further studies (Grabowska, 1974, 1975) favor the interpretation that APO may indirectly affect serotonergic transmission through activation by the drug of dopaminergic neurons.

APO has been reported (Stadler *et al.,* 1973) to abolish enhanced acetylcholine output into cat caudate nucleus perfusate produced by neuroleptics. This antagonism between APO and neuroleptics provided the first direct evidence that neuroleptic-induced activation of cholinergic neurons is due to DA receptor blockade.

APO increases acetylcholine levels in rat striatum (McGeer *et al.,* 1974) without affecting choline levels (Ladinsky *et al.,* 1975); this increase is more prominent in the denervated striatum than in the intact striatum (Fibiger and Grewaal, 1974). APO also reverses the depletion of acetylcholine induced by medial forebrain bundle lesions (Rommelspacher and Kuhar, 1975). The effects of APO and neuroleptics seem to be quite specific to the striatum, as these drugs do not affect acetylcholine concentrations in the diencephalon or cerebellum (Consolo *et al.,* 1975). The *in vivo* rate of acetylcholine utilization has been estimated by assessing the decline in striatal acetylcholine content after local microinjections of an acetylcholine biosynthesis blocking agent (Guyenet *et al.,* 1975). It was revealed that neuroleptics enhance striatal acetylcholine utilization; this effect was antagonized by APO, but not by 6-OHDA-induced degeneration of the nigrostriatal DA system. On the basis of these results it was hypothesized (Guyenet *et al.,* 1975) that the DA receptors presumably involved in the pharmacological interaction between neuroleptics and APO are localized on striatal acetylcholine neurons.

However, in another study (Trabucchi *et al.,* 1975), APO decreased and neuroleptics increased acetylcholine turnover rate in rat striatum without affecting the steady-state concentration of either acetylcholine or choline, and no effect of APO on cortical acetylcholine turnover was found. This led to the interpretation (Trabucchi *et al.,* 1975) that striatal DA receptor-stimulating drugs reduce the inhibitory influence of cholinergic neurons on γ-aminobutyric acid neurons, which in turn reduces the firing rate of DA neurons.

In conclusion, it seems that there is no convincing evidence to support a possible direct effect of APO on neurotransmission systems other than the dopaminergic systems, and there is even less reason to predict that any such effect is critically involved in the pharmacological actions of APO *in vivo.*

At present, a parsimonious speculation may be that APO, by virtue of its ability to increase dopaminergic activity intensively, may affect other neurotransmitter systems through interactions between dopaminergic and other neurotransmission systems, as such interactions are probably inherent to the basic functioning of the brain.

VI. Narcotic Analgesics and APO

It is known that narcotic analgesic drugs antagonize some of the pharmacological effects of APO (Sections III and IV), and evidence has accumulated to suggest (Lal, 1975; Lal et al., 1975) that narcotic analgesics may block DA receptors in the brain. However, some behavioral data (e.g., Colpaert et al., 1976b) alternatively indicate that narcotic analgesics increase central dopaminergic activity. It is therefore worthwhile to discuss some findings that seem relevant to this topic, and hence may somewhat clarify the mechanism of action of APO with respect to at least some of its pharmacological effects.

A. NARCOTIC SB

Morphine and other narcotic analgesic drugs are known to antagonize, at least in part, the SB produced by APO (Janssen et al., 1960) or by amphetamine (Van Nueten, 1962). However, narcotic analgesics may also increase behavioral activity in rats (Martin et al., 1963; Neal, 1968). This increased activity partly consists of SB and self-mutilation (Charness et al., 1975; Fog, 1970), which have also been observed following APO injection (Section IV; Baxter et al., 1974).

Fog (1970) further found that nalorphine and amphetamine may prevent the occurrence of morphine SB, and observed that the morphine antagonism of amphetamine SB, unlike that by neuroleptics, does not really constitute a restoration of normal activity. In fact, morphine may also intensify and/or prolong amphetamine and APO SB (McKenzie and Sadof, 1974; Vedernikov, 1970). The latter effect seems to disappear gradually with the progressive induction of tolerance (Vedernikov, 1970).

As the stereotypogenic effects of morphine (Ayhan and Randrup, 1972) and methadone (Ahtee, 1974) can be abolished by reserpine and α-methyltyrosine (Ayhan and Randrup, 1972), it was suggested (Ayhan and Randrup, 1973a) that this effect critically depends on catecholamine biosynthesis. Other antagonists of narcotic SB are aceperone, spiramide (Ayhan and Randrup, 1972), haloperidol (Charness et al., 1975), and naloxone (Ahtee, 1974), and noradrenergic (Ayhan and Randrup, 1972, 1973a) as well as dopaminergic brain systems (Ahtee, 1974) are thought to be critically involved.

Ayhan and Randrup (1973b) also found that amphetamine, 1-dopa, and APO, which mutually potentiate SB in rats, all antagonize morphine SB, and the SB induced by partial narcotic agonists is likewise antagonized by APO (Buckett and Shaw, 1975). A seemingly similar antagonism to APO and amphetamine SB has also been observed (Cox and Tha, 1973) with the dopaminergic drug amantadine. Although straightforward interpretations of such data are lacking (Ayhan and Randrup, 1973b), one conceivable alternative is competition at some presynaptic site.

The stereotypogenic effect of morphine develops progressively on repeated administration of the drug (Fog, 1970), and no tolerance to this effect is evident (Charness et al., 1975). Similarly, the inhibitory effects of morphine on self-stimulation disappear gradually, whereas its stimulatory effects become more and more apparent on chronic exposure to the drug (Adams et al., 1972; Lorens and Mitchell, 1973). These observations corroborate the early hypothesis (Tatum et al., 1929) that tolerance to various depressant effects of narcotic drugs develops quite readily, whereas stimulatory effects show higher resistance to this phenomenon. This implies that the progressive increase in morphine SB is due to the concomitant development of tolerance to motor suppression (Charness et al., 1975) and to catatonia (Ahtee, 1974), in the relative absence of tolerance to SB. Nevertheless, tolerance to at least some of the stimulatory effects of morphine ultimately develops (Glick and Rapaport, 1974; Holtzman, 1974), and it remains to be established to what extent morphine's stereotypogenic action is, in the long run, subject to tolerance.

B. PERCEPTION OF NOXIOUS STIMULI

Acute injection of morphine, like that of APO (Janssen et al., 1960), produces hyperexcitability (Kumar et al., 1971; Vedernikov, 1970) and increased reactivity to stimuli which otherwise fail to induce behavioral arousal (Ayhan and Randrup, 1972; Charness et al., 1975). In rats treated chronically with the drug, morphine also induces an hyperalgesic response (Kayan et al., 1973), as does APO in drug-naive animals (Tulunay et al., 1975). An acute hyperalgesic response to morphine can also be elicited by local application in the medial septum, the caudate nucleus, and the periaqueductal gray matter (Jacquet and Lajtha, 1973). Despite the fact that both compounds may thus produce hyperalgesia, APO antagonizes morphine-induced analgesia by a mechanism presumed to be distinct from direct DA receptor activation (Tulunay et al., 1975).

C. Self-Administration

As a somewhat surprising challenge to the validity of the self-administration technique in laboratory animals as an experimental model for human drug abuse (Schuster and Thompson, 1969), it was recently found that rats can self-administer APO (Baxter *et al.*, 1974), as well as haloperidol (Glick and Cox, 1975a). The suggestion (Glick and Cox, 1975a) that, in rats, a change in activity per se of central dopaminergic neurons may by itself constitute a reinforcing event, prompts the question of whether decreased or increased dopaminergic activity is involved in or associated with the reinforcing action of narcotic analgesic drugs.

The assumption that APO exerts its reinforcing action by increasing dopaminergic activity is based upon (1) the generally accepted ability of APO to activate DA receptors, and (2) the fact that the DA receptor-blocking agent, pimozide, blocks this action (Baxter *et al.*, 1974).

There is general agreement that the self-administration of narcotic analgesics can similarly be antagonized by DA receptor-blocking agents (Glick and Cox, 1975b; Hanson and Climini-Venema, 1972; Pozuelo and Kerr, 1972; Schwartz and Marchok, 1974a). However, Smith and Davis (1973) reported that haloperidol failed to block the establishment of conditioned reinforcement based on morphine injection. This finding was later contradicted by several well-designed experiments (Schwartz and Marchok, 1974b) indicating that haloperidol effectively blocks morphine reinforcement. The latter study (Schwartz and Marchok, 1974b) also showed that the time-effect course of haloperidol with respect to this blocking action is somewhat peculiar, thus accounting for the inconsistency mentioned above. Similar evidence is available to substantiate the blocking effect of haloperidol (Davis and Smith, 1975) and pimozide (Yokel and Wise, 1975) on amphetamine self-administration.

Interestingly, the self-administration of morphine is increased by low and decreased by high APO doses (Glick and Cox, 1975b). Lesions of the caudate nucleus increase the rat's sensitivity to the rewarding effect of morphine (Glick *et al.*, 1975), and it has been shown (Glick, 1974) that this effect is quantitative, rather than representing a qualitative change. It seems therefore that morphine, through an action involving the caudate nucleus, partly inhibits its own reinforcing effect (unless receptor supersensitivity is in operation). However, although morphine may increase neuronal activity in this nucleus (Stille, 1971), its site of action is likely to be located elsewhere; intrastriatal injection of morphine, unlike that of haloperidol, fails to inhibit self-stimulation (Broekkamp and Van Rossum, 1975), and the neural substrate of morphine's catatonic effect is not located in the neostriatum (Costall and Naylor, 1973d, 1974d).

D. FURTHER EXAMPLES

APO and narcotic analgesics have various other actions in common. Like APO, narcotic analgesics increase locomotor activity in mice (e.g., Davis et al., 1972; Parker, 1974; Smith et al., 1972; Rethy et al., 1971; Villarreal et al., 1973), and excellent studies on this topic (see, for example, Carroll and Sharp, 1972) have shown that various neurotransmitters, including DA, are involved in this effect. Like APO, narcotic analgesics produce aggressive behavior (Assouline, 1967; Schneider, 1968) and vomiting (Borison and Wang, 1953). APO and morphine stimulate prostaglandin biosynthesis (Collier et al., 1974), an effect that may be related to the emetic, hyperthermic, and hyperglycemic actions of both drugs.

E. RELEVANCE TO APO'S MECHANISM OF ACTION

From the above it seems that, given tolerance being developed to some otherwise masking effects, morphine and other narcotic analgesics produce several pharmacologically relevant actions (e.g., SB, hyperalgesia) which are also produced by APO in drug-naive animals. APO and morphine can be self-administered by rats, and the reinforcing action of morphine, like that of APO, is associated with increased rather than decreased dopaminergic activity in the brain. An intriguing phenomenon, however, is that, although APO and morphine produce several seemingly similar actions, they also antagonize each other with respect to at least some of the very same actions (e.g., SB, self-administration, vomiting). The presently reviewed evidence, as well as other data (Colpaert et al., 1976b), thus suggest that some of morphine's agonist characteristics are based on or associated with increased dopaminergic activity, and it seems difficult to support the position (see Lal, 1975; Lal et al., 1975) that the interference of narcotic analgesics with central dopaminergic activity consists exclusively of DA receptor blockage. This implies that an alternative explanation of the mutual antagonism between APO and morphine is to be looked for. An important possibility seems to reside in the effects of APO and morphine on DA biosynthesis. APO is known to reduce this biosynthesis in a dose-related way (Section V), and there is compelling evidence (e.g., Ahtee, 1974; Kuschinsky and Hornykiewicz, 1972; Smith et al., 1970) indicating that narcotic analgesics increase catecholamine biosynthesis. The mechanism by which the latter drugs do so is probably distinct (Iwatsubo and Clouet, 1975; Kuschinsky and Hornykiewicz, 1974) from that of neuroleptics. With respect to narcotic SB it is interesting to note that, although tolerance to the narcotic effect on catecholamine biosynthesis can readily be obtained in mice (Fukui and

256   F. C. COLPAERT, W. F. M. VAN BEVER, AND J. E. M. F. LEYSEN

Takagi, 1972; Smith *et al.*, 1972), surprisingly little tolerance is seen in rats (Ahtee, 1974; Clouet and Ratner, 1970).

Recent experiments in our laboratory (unpublished data) have shown that APO and the narcotic analgesic fentanyl (Janssen *et al.*, 1963) indeed exert an efficient mutual antagonism with respect to striatal HVA content in rats. If the mutual antagonism—at the pharmacological level—between APO and narcotic analgesics were based on their opposite actions on DA biosynthesis, this would imply that endogenous DA plays a critical role in these pharmacological effects of APO. In other words, these pharmacological effects of APO would depend on (1) a direct action at postsynaptic DA receptor sites, and (2) action at the level of the presynaptic neuron such that DA biosynthesis is reduced. This hypothesis may explain, e.g., the remarkable finding that electrolytic lesions of the substantia nigra significantly affect APO SB (Section IV).

Recent data (Connor, 1970; Klawans *et al.*, 1971; Struyker Boudier, 1975; Struyker Boudier *et al.*, 1973, 1974) evidence the existence of different DA receptors which are differentially affected by both APO and DA (Aghajanian and Bunney, 1973; Bunney *et al.*, 1973; Goldberg *et al.*, 1968). It has also been substantiated (Ferrini and Miragoli, 1972; Goldberg and Musgrave, 1971; Simon and van Maanen, 1971) that DA may selectively antagonize APO at (peripheral) DA receptors. In view of this evidence, the presumed involvement of a direct APO action, as well as of endogenous DA, in the mechanism of action of APO obviously leads to complex effects of APO at the pharmacological level and to even more complex interactions with drugs that increase DA biosynthesis (e.g., narcotic analgesics).

REFERENCES

Abrahamsson, H., Jansson, G., and Martinson, J. (1971). *Rend. R. Gastroenterol.* **3**, 114.
Abrahamsson, H., Jansson, G., and Martinson, J., (1973). *Acta Physiol. Scand.* **88**, 296–302.
Adams, W. J., Lorens, S. A., and Mitchell, C. L., (1972). *Proc. Soc. Exp. Biol. Med.* **140**, 770–771.
Aghajanian, G. K., and Bunney, B. S., (1973). In "Frontiers in Catecholamine Research" (E. Usdin and S. H. Snyder, eds.), pp. 643–648. Pergamon, Oxford.
Ahtee, L. (1974). *Eur. J. Pharmacol.* **27**, 221–230.
Amsler, C. (1923). *Arch. Exp. Pathol. Pharmakol.* **97**, 1–14.
Andén, N.-E., and Bédard, P. (1971). *J. Pharm. Pharmacol.* **23**, 460–462.
Andén, N.-E., Carlsson, A., Dahlström, A., Fuxe, K., Hillarp, N. A., and Larsson, K. (1964). *Life Sci.* **3**, 523–530.
Andén, N.-E., Rubenson, A., Fuxe, K., and Hökfelt, T. (1967). *J. Pharm. Pharmacol.* **19**, 627–629.
Andén, N.-E., Carlsson, A., and Maggendahl, J. (1969). *Annu. Rev. Pharmacol.* **9**, 119–134.

Antonaccio, M. J., and Robson, R. D. (1974). *Arch. Int. Pharmacodyn. Ther.* **212**, 89–102.

Asper, H., Baggiolini, M., Burki, H. R., Lauener, H., Ruch, W., and Stille, G. (1973). *Eur. J. Pharmacol.* **22**, 287–294.

Assouline, G. (1967). *C. R. Seances Soc. Biol. Ses. Fil.* **161**, 642–649.

Atkinson, E. R., Bullock, E. R., Granchelli, F. E., Archer, S., Rosenberg, F. J., Teiger, D. G., and Nachod, F. C. (1975). *J. Med. Chem.* **18**, 1000–1003.

Axelrod, J., and Weinshilboum, R. (1972). *N. Engl. J. Med.* **287**, 237–242.

Ayhan, I. H., and Randrup, A. (1972). *Psychopharmacologia* **27**, 203–212.

Ayhan, I. H., and Randrup, A. (1973a). *Psychopharmacologia* **29**, 317–328.

Ayhan, I. H., and Randrup, A. (1973b). *Arch. Int. Pharmacodyn. Ther.* **204**, 283–292.

Barnett, A., and Fiore, J. W. (1971). *Eur. J. Pharmacol.* **14**, 206–208.

Barnett, A., Goldstein, J., and Taber, R. I. (1972). *Arch. Int. Pharmacodyn. Ther.* **198**, 242–247.

Baum, E., Etévenon, P., Piarroux, M. C., Simon, P., and Boissier, J.-R. (1971). *J. Pharmacol.* **2**, 423–434.

Baum, E., North-Diehl, A., Piarrally, M. C., Thenint, F., and Boissier, J.-R. *J. Pharmacol.* **3**, 477–486.

Baxter, B. L., Gluckman, M. I., Stein, L., and Scerni, R. A. (1974). *Pharmacol., Biochem. Behav.* **2**, 387–391.

Berger, B., Tassin, J. P., Blanc, G., Moyne, M. A., and Thierry, A. M. (1974). *Brain Res.* **81**, 332–337.

Berney, D., Petcher, T. J., Schmutz, J., Weber, H. P., and White, T. G. *Experientia* **31**, 1327–1328.

Bevan, W., Bloom, W. L., and Lewis, G. T. (1951). *Physiol. Zool.* **24**, 231–237.

Bhargava, K. P., Gupta, P. C., and Chandra, O. (1961). *J. Pharmacol. Exp. Ther.* **134**, 329–331.

Bieger, D., Larochelle, L., and Hornykiewicz, O. (1972). *Eur. J. Pharmacol.* **18**, 128–136.

Blaschko, H. (1939). *J. Physiol. (London)* **96**, 50–55.

Bondareff, W., Routtenberg, A., Narotzky, R., and McLone, D. G. (1970). *Exp. Neurol.* **28**, 213–229.

Borenstein, P., and Bles, G. (1965). *Therapie* **20**, 975–995.

Borison, H. L. (1974). *Life Sci.* **14**, 1807–1817.

Borison, H. L., and Wang, S. C. (1953). *Pharmacol. Rev.* **5**, 193–230.

Boyd, E. M., and Boyd, C. E. (1953). *Can. J. Med. Sci.* **31**, 320–327.

Boyd, E. M., Cassell, W. A., Boyd, C. E., and Miller, J. K. (1955). *J. Pharmacol. Exp. Ther.* **113**, 299–309.

Breese, G. R., and Traylor, T. D. (1970). *J. Pharmacol. Exp. Ther.* **174**, 413–420.

Brizzee, K. R., Neal, L. M., and Williams, P. M. (1955). *Am. J. Physiol.* **180**, 659–662.

Broch, O. J., and Marsden, C. A. (1972). *Brain Res.* **38**, 425–428.

Brodal, A. (1963). *Acta Neurol Scand.* **39**, Suppl. 4, 17–38.

Broekkamp, C. L. E., and Van Rossum, J. M. (1974). *Psychopharmacologia* **34**, 71–80.

Broekkamp, C. L. E., and Van Rossum, J. M. (1975). *Arch. Int. Pharmacodyn. Ther.* **217**, 110–117.

Brown, J. H., and Makman, M. M. (1972). *Proc. Natl. Acad. Sci. U.S.A.* **69**, 539–543.

258   F. C. COLPAERT, W. F. M. VAN BEVER, AND J. E. M. F. LEYSEN

Brown, W. A., Drawbaugh, R., Gianutsos, G., Lal, H., and Brown, G. M. (1975). *Res. Commun. Chem. Pathol. Pharmacol.* 11, 671–674.
Brücke, F. I. (1935). *Naunyn-Schmiedeberg's Arch. Exp. Pathol. Pharmakol.* 179, 504–523.
Bucher, M.-B., and Schorderet, M. (1975). *Naunyn-Schmiedeberg's Arch. Pharmacol.* 288, 103–107.
Buckett, W. R., and Shaw, J. S. (1975). *Psychopharmacologia* 42, 293–297.
Bunney, B. S., Aghajanian, G. K., and Roth, R. H. (1973). *Nature (London)* 245, 123–125.
Bunney, W. E., and Davis, J. M. (1965). *Arch. Gen. Psychiatry* 13, 483–494.
Burkman, A. M. (1960). *J. Am. Pharm. Assoc.* 49, 558–559.
Burkman, A. M. (1973). *Neuropharmacology* 12, 83–85.
Burt, D. R., Enna, S. J., Creese, I., and Snyder, S. H. (1975). *Proc. Natl. Acad. Sci. U.S.A.* 72, 4655–4659.
Butcher, L. L. (1968). *Eur. J. Pharmacol.* 3, 163–166.
Butcher, L. L., and Andén, N.-E. (1969). *Eur. J. Pharmacol.* 6, 255–264.
Butcher, L. L., Butcher, S. G., and Larsson, K. (1969). *Eur. J. Pharmacol.* 7, 283–288.
Cannon, J. G., Hensiak, J. H., and Burkman, A. M. (1963). *J. Pharm. Sci.* 52, 1112–1113.
Cannon, J. G., Smith, R. V., Modini, A., Sod, P. J., Borgman, R. J., and Aleem, M. A. (1972a). *J. Med. Chem.* 15, 273–282.
Cannon, J. G., Kim, J. C., Aleem, H. A., and Long, J. P. (1972b). *J. Med. Chem.* 15, 348–350.
Cannon, J. G., Boryman, R. G., and Aleem, M. A. (1973). *J. Med. Chem.* 16, 219–224.
Cannon, J. G., Smith, R. V., and Aleem, M. A. (1975a). *J. Med. Chem.* 18, 108–110.
Cannon, J. G., Khonje, P. R., and Long, J. P. (1975b). *J. Med. Chem.* 18, 110–112.
Cannon, W. B. (1898). *Am. J. Physiol.* 1, 359–382.
Carlsson, A., Engel, J., Strömbau, U., Svensson, T. H., and Waldeck, B. (1974). *Naunyn-Schmiedeberg's Arch. Pharmacol.* 283, 117–128.
Carlsson, S. G. (1972). *Physiol. Behav.* 9, 127–130.
Carroll, B. J., and Sharp, P. T. (1972). *Br. J. Pharmacol.* 46, 124–139.
Castaigne, P., Laplane, D., and Dordain, G. (1971). *Res. Commun. Chem. Pathol. Pharmacol.* 2, 154–158.
Charness, M. E., Amit, Z., and Taylor, M. (1975). *Behav. Biol.* 13, 71–80.
Christensen, N. J., Neubauer, B., Brandsborg, O., Mathias, C. J., and Frankel, H. L. (1975). *Lancet* 1, 1084–1085.
Christiansen, J., and Squires, R. F. (1974). *J. Pharm. Pharmacol.* 26, 367–369.
Christiansen, J., and Squires, R. F. (1976). In press.
Clement-Cormier, Y. C., Kebabian, J. W., Petzold, G. L., and Greengard, P. (1974). *Proc. Natl. Acad. Sci. U.S.A.* 71, 1113–1117.
Clouet, D. H., and Ratner, M. (1970). *Science* 168, 854–855.
Collier, H. O. J., McDonald-Gibson, W. G., and Saeed, S. H. (1974). *Nature (London)* 252, 56–58.
Colpaert, F. C., Niemegeers, C. J. E., Kuyps, J. J. M. D., and Janssen, P. A. J. (1975). *Eur. J. Pharmacol.* 32, 383–386.
Colpaert, F. C., Niemegeers, C. J. E., and Janssen, P. A. J. (1976a). Submitted for publication.

Colpaert, F. C., Niemegeers, C. J. E., and Janssen, P. A. J. (1976b). *Neuropharmacology* **15** (in press).

Conner, J. D. (1968). *Science* **160**, 899–900.

Connor, J. D. (1970). *J. Physiol. (London)* **208**, 691–703.

Consolo, S., Ladinsky, H., and Bianchi, S. (1975). *Eur. J. Pharmacol.* **33**, 345–351.

Cools, A. R. (1971). *Arch. Int. Pharmacodyn. Ther.* **194**, 259–269.

Cools, A. R. (1973). Ph.D. Dissertation, University of Nijmegen, The Netherlands.

Corrodi, H., and Hardegger, E. (1955). *Helv. Chim. Acta* **38**, 2038–2043.

Corrodi, M., Fuxe, K., and Ungerstedt, U. (1971). *J. Pharm. Pharmacol.* **23**, 989–991.

Costall, B., and Naylor, R. J. (1972). *Life Sci.* **11**, 1135–1146.

Costall, B., and Naylor, R. J. (1973a). *Eur. J. Pharmacol.* **21**, 350–361.

Costall, B., and Naylor, R. J. (1973b). *Eur. J. Pharmacol.* **24**, 8–24.

Costall, B., and Naylor, R. J. (1973c). *Naunyn-Schmiedeberg's Arch. Pharmacol.* **278**, 117–133.

Costall, B., and Naylor, R. J. (1973d). *Arzneim.-Forsch.* **23**, 674–683.

Costall, B., and Naylor, R. J. (1974a). *J. Pharm. Pharmacol.* **26**, 30–33.

Costall, B., and Naylor, R. J. (1974b). *Naunyn-Schmiedeberg's Arch. Pharmacol.* **285**, 71–81.

Costall, B., and Naylor, R. J. (1974c). *Naunyn-Schmiedeberg's Arch. Pharmacol.* **285**, 83–88.

Costall, B., and Naylor, R. J. (1974d). *Psychopharmacologia* **34**, 233–241.

Costall, B., and Naylor, R. J. (1975). *Eur. J. Pharmacol.* **32**, 87–92.

Costall, B., Naylor, R. J., and Olley, J. E. (1971). *Neuropharmacology* **10**, 581–594.

Costall, B., Naylor, R. J., and Olley, J. E. (1972). *Eur. J. Pharmacol.* **18**, 95–106.

Costall, B., Naylor, R. J., and Pinder, R. M. (1974). *J. Pharm. Pharmacol.* **26**, 753–762.

Costall, B., Naylor, R. J., and Neumeyer, J. L. (1975). *Eur. J. Pharmacol.* **31**, 1–16.

Costentin, J., Protais, P., and Schwartz, J. C. (1975). *Nature (London)* **257**, 405–407.

Cotzias, G. C., Van Woert, M. H., and Schiffer, L. M. (1967). *N. Engl. J. Med.* **276**, 374–379.

Cotzias, G. C., Papavisiliou, P. S., Fehling, C., Kaufman, B., and Mena, J. (1970). *N. Engl. J. Med.* **282**, 31–33.

Cox, B., and Tha, S. J. (1973). *Eur. J. Pharmacol.* **24**, 96–100.

Creese, I., and Iversen, S. D. (1972). *Nature (London) New Biol.* **228**, 247–248.

Creese, I., and Iversen, S. D. (1973). *Brain Res.* **55**, 369–382.

Creese, I., and Iversen, S. D. (1975). *Brain Res.* **83**, 419–436.

Creese, I., Burt, D. R., and Snyder, S. H. (1975). *Life Sci.* **17**, 993–1002.

Dahlström, A., and Fuxe, K. (1964). *Acta Physiol. Scand., Suppl.* **232**, 1–55.

Davies, J. A., Jackson, B., and Redfern, P. H. (1973). *Neuropharmacology* **12**, 735–740.

Davies, J. A., Jackson, B., and Redfern, P. H. (1974). *Neuropharmacology* **13**, 199–204.

Davis, W. M., and Smith, S. G. (1975). *J. Pharm. Pharmacol.* **27**, 540–542.

Davis, W. M., Babbini, M., and Khalsa, J. H. (1972). *Res. Commun. Chem. Pathol. Pharmacol.* **4**, 267–279.

Dengler, H., and Reichel, G. (1958). *Naunyn-Schmiedeberg's Arch. Exp. Pathol. Pharmakol.* **234**, 275–281.

Dent, J. Y. (1955). "Anxiety and Its Treatment," Vol. III. Skeffington, London.

De Oliveira, L., and Graeff, F. G. (1972). *Eur. J. Pharmacol.* **18**, 159–165.

Dhawan, B. N., and Saxena, P. N. (1960). *Br. J. Pharmacol.* **15**, 285–289.

Dhawan, B. N., Saxena, P. N., and Gupta, G. P. (1961). *Br. J. Pharmacol.* **16**, 137–145.

Di Chiara, G., Balakleevsky, A., Porceddu, M. L., Tagliamonte, A., and Gessa, G. L. (1974). *J. Neurochem.* **23**, 1105–1108.

Dismukes, R. K., and Rake, A. V. (1972). *Psychopharmacologia* **23**, 17–25.

Divac, I. (1972). *Psychopharmacologia* **27**, 171–178.

Dresse, A., and Niemegeers, C. (1961). *C.R. Seances Soc. Biol. Ses. Fil.* **155**, 1713–1715.

Ebstein, B., Roberge, C., Tabachnick, J., and Goldstein, M. (1974). *J. Pharm. Pharmacol.* **26**, 975–977.

Emele, J., Shanaman, J., and Warren, M. (1961). *Fed. Proc. Fed. Am. Soc. Exp. Biol.* **20**, 328.

Enero, S., and Langer, P. (1975). *Naunyn-Schmiedeberg's Arch. Pharmacol.* **289**, 179–203.

Ernst, A. M. (1962). *Acta Physiol. Pharmacol. Neerl.* **11**, 48–53.

Ernst, A. M. (1965). *Psychopharmacologia* **7**, 391–399.

Ernst, A. M. (1967). *Psychopharmacologia* **10**, 316–323.

Ernst, A. M. (1969). *Acta Physiol. Pharmacol. Neerl.* **15**, 141–154.

Ernst, A. M., and Smelik, E. (1966). *Experientia* **22**, 837–838.

Everitt, B. J., Fuxe, K., and Hökfelt, T. (1974). *Eur. J. Pharmacol.* **29**, 187–191.

Fadhel, N. (1967). *Diss. Abstr.* **28**, 1632B.

Faull, R. I., and Laverty, R. (1969). *Exp. Neurol.* **23**, 332–340.

Fekete, M., Kurti, A. M., and Pribusz, I. (1970). *J. Pharm. Pharmacol.* **22**, 377–379.

Ferrini, R., and Miragoli, G. (1972). *Pharm. Res. Commun.* **4**, 347–352.

Ferris, R. M., Tang, F. L., and Russell, A. V. (1975). *Biochem. Pharmacol.* **24**, 1523–1527.

Fibiger, H. C., and Grewaal, D. S. (1974). *Life Sci.* **15**, 57–63.

Finch, L., and Haeusler, G. (1973). *Eur. J. Pharmacol.* **21**, 264–270.

Fog, R. (1970). *Psychopharmacologia* **16**, 305–312.

Fog, R., and Pakkenberg, H. (1971). *Acta Neurol. Scand.* **47**, 475–484.

Fog, R., Randrup, A., and Pakkenberg, H. (1970). *Psychopharmacologia* **18**, 346–356.

Forn, G., Krueger, B. K., and Greengard, P. (1974). *Science* **186**, 1118–1120.

Frigyesi, T. L., and Purpura, D. F. (1967). *Brain Res.* **6**, 440–456.

Frommel, E. (1965). *Arch. Int. Pharmacodyn. Ther.* **154**, 231–234.

Frommel, E., Ledebur, I. V., and Seydoux, J. (1965). *Arch. Int. Pharmacodyn. Ther.* **154**, 227–230.

Fukui, K., and Takagi, H. (1972). *Br. J. Pharmacol.* **44**, 45–51.

Fuxe, K., and Sjöqvist, F. (1972). *J. Pharm. Pharmacol.* **24**, 702–705.

Fuxe, K., Agnati, L. F., Hökfelt, T., Jonsson, G., Lidbrink, P., Ljungdahl, A., Lofstrom, A., and Ungerstedt, U. (1975). *J. Pharmacol.* **6**, 117–129.

Garcia, J., Ervin, F. R., and Koelling, R. A. (1966). *Psychon. Sci.* **5**, 121.

Gianutsos, G., Hynes, M. D., and Lal, H. (1975). *Biochem. Pharmacol.* **24**, 581–582.

Giesecke, J. (1973). *Acta Crystallogr., Sect. B* **29**, 1785–1791.

Ginos, J. Z., Cotzias, G. C., Tolosa, E., Tang, L. C., and Lo Monte, A. (1975). *J. Med. Chem.* **18**, 1194–1200.

Glick, S. D. (1974). *Arch. Int. Pharmacodyn. Ther.* **212**, 214–220.

Glick, S. D., and Cox, R. S. (1975a). *Life Sci.* **16**, 1041–1046.

Glick, S. D., and Cox, R. D. (1975b). *Res. Commun. Chem. Pathol. Pharmacol.* **12**, 17–24.

Glick, S. D., and Marsanico, R. G. (1974). *Br. J. Pharmacol.* **51**, 353–357.

Glick, S. D., and Rapaport, G. (1974). *Res. Commun. Chem. Pathol. Pharmacol.* 9, 647–652.

Glick, S. D., Cox, R. S., and Crane, A. M. (1975). *Psychopharmacologia* 41, 219–224.

Goetz, C., and Klawans, H. L. (1974). *Acta Pharmacol. Toxicol.* 34, 119–130.

Goldberg, L. I. (1972). *Pharmacol. Rev.* 24, 1–29.

Goldberg, L. I. (1975). *Biochem. Pharmacol.* 24, 651–653.

Goldberg, L. I., and Musgrave, G. (1971). *Pharmacologist* 13, 227.

Goldberg, L. I., Sonneville, P. F., and McNay, J. L. (1968). *J. Pharmacol. Exp. Ther.* 163, 188–197.

Goldstein, M., Anagnoste, B., Battista, A. F., Owen, W. S., and Nakatani, S. (1969). *J. Neurochem.* 16, 645–653.

Goldstein, M., Freedman, L., and Backstrom, T. (1970). *J. Pharm. Pharmacol.* 22, 715–717.

Goldstein, M., Anagnoste, B., and Shirron, C. (1973). *J. Pharm. Pharmacol.* 25, 348–351.

Grabowska, M. (1974). *Psychopharmacologia* 39, 315–322.

Grabowska, M. (1975). *Pharmacol., Biochem. Behav.* 3, 589–591.

Grabowska, M., and Michaluk, J. (1974). *Pharmacol., Biochem. Behav.* 2, 263–266.

Grabowska, M., Michaluk, J., and Antkiewicz, L. (1973a). *Eur. J. Pharmacol.* 23, 82–89.

Grabowska, M., Antkiewcz, L., Maj, J., and Michaluk, J. (1973b). *Pol. J. Pharmacol. Pharm.* 25, 29–39.

Greengard, P., and Kebabian, J. W. (1974). *Fed. Proc., Fed. Am. Soc. Exp. Biol.* 33, 1059–1067.

Greengard, P., McAfee, D. A., and Kebabian, J. W. (1972). *Adv. Cyclic Nucleotide Res.* 1, 373–390.

Gudelsky, G. A., Thornburg, J. E., and Moore, K. E. (1975). *Life Sci.* 16, 1331–1338.

Guyenet, P. G., Agid, Y., Javoy, F., Beaujouan, J. C., Rossier, J., and Glouriski, J. (1975). *Brain Res.* 84, 227–244.

Håkanson, R. (1970). *Acta Physiol. Scand., Suppl.* 340, 1–134.

Håkanson, R., and Owman, C. (1967). *Life Sci.* 6, 759–766.

Håkanson, R., Owman, C. H., Sjöberg, N.-O., and Sporrong, B. (1970). *Histochemie* 21, 189–220.

Hamburger-Bar, R., and Rigter, H. (1975). *Eur. J. Pharmacol.* 32, 357–360.

Hanson, H. M., and Climini-Venema, C. A. (1972). *Fed. Proc., Fed. Am. Soc. Exp. Biol.* 31, 503.

Harnack, E. (1874). *Arch. Exp. Pathol. Pharmakol.* 2, 254–306.

Hensiak, J. H., Cannon, J. G., and Burkman, A. M. (1965). *J. Med. Chem.* 8, 557–559.

Hess, S. M., Connamacher, R. H., Ozaki, M., and Udenfriend, S. (1961). *J. Pharmacol. Exp. Ther.* 134, 129–138.

Hill, H. F., and Horita, A. (1972). *J. Pharm. Pharmacol.* 24, 490–491.

Hökfelt, T., and Fuxe, K. (1972). *Neuroendocrinology* 9, 100–122.

Hökfelt, T., Fuxe, K., Johansson, O., and Ljungdahl, A. (1974a). *Eur. J. Pharmacol.* 25, 108–112.

Hökfelt, T., Ljungdahl, K., Fuxe, K., and Johansson, O. (1974b). *Science* 184, 177–179.

Holtzman, S. G. (1974). *Psychopharmacologia* 39, 23–37.

Horn, A. S. (1974). *J. Pharm. Pharmacol.* 26, 735–737.

Hornykiewicz, O. (1966). *Pharmacol. Rev.* **18**, 925–964.

Hornykiewicz, O. (1972). *In* "The Structure and Function of Nervous Tissue" (G. H. Bourne, ed.), Vol. 6, pp. 367–415. Academic Press, New York.

Hornykiewicz, O. (1973). *Br. Med. Bull.* **29**, 172–178.

Horowski, R., Neumann, F., and Graf, K.-J. (1975). *J. Pharm. Pharmacol.* **27**, 532–534.

Hull, C. D., Buchwald, N. A., and Ling, G. (1967). *Brain Res.* **6**, 22–35.

Isaacs, B., and MacArthur, J. G. (1954). *Lancet* **2**, 570–572.

Iversen, L. L., Horn, A. S., and Miller, R. J. (1975). *In* "Pre- and Postsynaptic Receptors" (E. Usdin and W. E. Bunney, eds.), pp. 207–240. Dekker, New York.

Iversen, L. L., Rogawski, M. J., and Miller, R. J. (1976). *Mol. Pharmacol.* **12**, 251–262.

Iversen, S. D. (1971). *Brain Res.* **31**, 295–311.

Iwatsubo, K., and Clouet, D. H. (1975). *Biochem. Pharmacol.* **24**, 1499–1503.

Jacobs, B. L. (1974). *Eur. J. Pharmacol.* **27**, 363–366.

Jacoby, H. I., and Brodie, D. A. (1967). *Gastroenterology* **52**, 676–684.

Jacquet, Y. F., and Lajtha, A. (1973). *Science* **182**, 490–492.

Jalfre, M., and Haefely, W. (1971). *In* "6-Hydroxydopamine and Catecholamine Neurons" (T. Malinfors and H. Thoenen, eds.), pp. 333–346. North-Holland Publ., Amsterdam.

Janssen, P. A. J. (1967). *Int. J. Neuropsychiat.* **3**, 10–18.

Janssen, P. A. J., and Niemegeers, C. J. E. (1959). *Arzneim.-Forsch.* **9**, 765–767.

Janssen, P. A. J., Niemegeers, C. J. E., and Jageneau, A. H. M. (1960). *Arzneim.-Forsch.* **10**, 1003–1005.

Janssen, P. A. J., Niemegeers, C. J. E., and Verbruggen, F. (1962). *Psychopharmacologia* **3**, 114–123.

Janssen, P. A. J., Niemegeers, C. J. E., and Dony, J. G. H. (1963). *Arzneim.-Forsch.* **13**, 502–507.

Janssen, P. A. J., Niemegeers, C. J. E., and Schellekens, K. H. L. (1965a). *Arzneim.-Forsch.* **15**, 104–117.

Janssen, P. A. J., Niemegeers, C. J. E., and Schellekens, K. H. L. (1965b). *Arzeim.-Forsch.* **15**, 1196–1206.

Janssen, P. A. J., Niemegeers, C. J. E., Schellekens, K. H. L., and Lenaerts, F. M. (1967). *Arzneim.-Forsch.* **17**, 841–854.

Janssen, P. A. J., Niemegeers, C. J. E., Schellekens, K. H. L., Dresse, A., Lenaerts, F. M., Pinchard, A., Schaper, W. K. A., Van Nueten, J. M., and Verbruggen, F. J. (1968). *Arzneim.-Forsch.* **18**, 261–287.

Janssen, P. A. J., Niemegeers, C. J. E., Schellekens, K. H. L., Lenaerts, F. M., Verbruggen, F. J., Van Nueten, J. M., and Schaper, W. K. A. (1970). *Eur. J. Pharmacol.* **11**, 139–154.

Janssen, P. A. J., Niemegeers, C. J. E., Schellekens, K. H. L., Lenaerts, F. M., and Wauquier, A. (1975). *Arzneim.-Forsch.* **25**, 1287–1294.

Jansson, G., and Martinson, J. (1966). *Acta Physiol. Scand.* **68**, 184–192.

Justin-Besançon, L. (1964). *Sem. Hop.* **40**, 2337–2338.

Kadzielawa, K. (1974). *Arch. Int. Pharmacodyn. Ther.* **209**, 214–226.

Kamberi, J. A., Mical, R. S., and Porter, J. C. (1970). *Experientia* **26**, 1150–1151.

Kaul, P. N., and Conway, M. W. (1971). *J. Pharm. Sci.* **60**, 93–95.

Kaul, P. N., Brochmann-Hanssen, E., and Way, E. L. (1961a). *J. Pharm. Sci.* **50**, 244–247.

Kaul, P. N., Brochmann-Hansen, E., and Way, E. L. (1961b). *J. Pharm. Sci.* **50**, 248–251.

Kaul, P. N., Brochmann-Hanssen, E., and Way, E. L. (1961c). *J. Pharm. Sci.* **50**, 840–842.

Kayan, S., Woods, L. A., and Mitchell, C. L. (1973). *J. Pharmacol. Exp. Ther.* **177**, 509–513.

Kebabian, G. W., and Greengard, P. (1971). *Science* **174**, 1346–1349.

Kebabian, G. W., Petzold, G. L., and Greengard, P. (1972). *Proc. Natl. Acad. Sci. U.S.A.* **69**, 2145–2149.

Kehr, W., Carlsson, A., Lindqvist, M., Magnusson, T., and Atack, C. (1972). *J. Pharm. Pharmacol.* **24**, 744–747.

Kelly, P. H., Seviour, P. W., and Iversen, S. D. (1975). *Brain Res.* **94**, 507–522.

Kety, S. S. (1970). *In* "The Neurosciences: Second Study Program" (F. O. Schmitt, ed.), pp. 324–336. Rockefeller Univ. Press, New York.

Kjellberg, B., and Randrup, A. (1974). *Arch. Int. Pharmacodyn. Ther.* **210**, 61–66.

Klawans, H. L. (1968). *Dis. Nerv. Syst.* **29**, 805–812.

Klawans, H. L., Ilahi, M. M., and Ringel, S. P. (1971). *Confin. Neurol.* **33**, 297–304.

Kloch, M. V., Cannon, J. G., and Burkman, A. M. (1968). *J. Med. Chem.* **11**, 977–981.

Konzett, H., and Strieder, N. (1969). *Z. Kreislaufforsch.* **58**, 210–214.

Koster, R. (1957). *J. Pharmacol. Exp. Ther.* **119**, 406–417.

Kostrzewa, R. M., and Jacobowitz, D. M. (1974). *Pharmacol. Rev.* **26**, 199–288.

Kruk, Z. L. (1972). *Life Sci.* **11**, 845–850.

Kruk, Z. L., and Brittain, R. T. (1972). *J. Pharm. Pharmacol.* **24**, 835–837.

Kulkarni, S. K., and Dandiya, P. C. (1975). *Pharmakopsychiatrie* **1**, 45–50.

Kumar, R., Mitchell, E., and Stolerman, I. P. (1971). *Br. J. Pharmacol.* **42**, 473–484.

Kuschinsky, K., and Hornykiewicz, O. (1972). *Eur. J. Pharmacol.* **19**, 119–122.

Kuschinsky, K., and Hornykiewicz, O. (1974). *Eur. J. Pharmacol.* **26**, 41–50.

Ladinsky, H., Consolo, S., Bianchi, S., Samanin, R., and Gheszi, D. (1975). *Brain Res.* **84**, 221–226.

Lahti, R. A., McAllister, B., and Wozniak, J. (1972). *Life Sci.* **11**, 605–613.

Lal, H. (1975). *Life Sci.* **17**, 483–496.

Lal, H., O'Brien, J., and Puri, S. K. (1971). *Psychopharmacologia* **22**, 217–223.

Lal, H., Gianutsos, G., and Puri, S. K. (1975). *Life Sci.* **17**, 29–34.

Lal, S., and Sourkes, T. L. (1973). *Arch. Int. Pharmacodyn. Ther.* **202**, 171–182.

Lal, S., Sourkes, T. L., Missala, K., and Belendiuk, G. (1972a). *Eur. J. Pharmacol.* **20**, 71–79.

Lal, S., de La Vega, C. E., Sourkes, T. L., and Friesen, H. G. (1972b). *Lancet* **2**, 661.

Lal, S., de la Vega, C. E., Garelis, E., and Sourkes, T. I. (1973). *Psychiatr., Neurol., Neurochir.* **76**, 113–117.

Lapin, I. P., and Samsonova, M. L. (1968). *Farmakol. Toksikol. (Moscow)* **31**, 563–567.

Lecomte, J., and Dresse, A. (1962). *Arch. Int. Pharmacodyn. Ther.* **139**, 604–610.

Liebmann, J. M., and Butcher, L. L. (1973). *Naunyn-Schmiedeberg's Arch. Pharmacol.* **277**, 305–318.

Liebmann, J. M., and Butcher, L. L. (1974). *Naunyn-Schmiedeberg's Arch. Pharmacol.* **284**, 167–194.

Lindvall, O., and Björklund, A. (1974). *Acta Physiol. Scand. Suppl.* **412**, 1–48.

264   F. C. COLPAERT, W. F. M. VAN BEVER, AND J. E. M. F. LEYSEN

Lindvall, O., Björklund, A., Moore, R. Y., and Steveni, U. (1974). *Brain Res.* **81**, 325–331.
Lindzey, G., Winston, H., and Manosevitz, M. (1961). *Nature (London)* **191**, 474–476.
Long, J. P., Heintz, S., Cannon, J. G., and Kim, J. (1975). *J. Pharmacol. Exp. Ther.* **192**, 336–342.
Lorens, S. A., and Mitchell, C. L. (1973). *Psychopharmacologia* **32**, 271–277.
McDermed, J. D., McKenzie, G. M., and Philips, A. P. (1975). *J. Med. Chem.* **18**, 362–367.
McGeer, P. L., Grewaal, D. S., and McGeer, E. G. (1974). *Brain Res.* **80**, 211–217.
McKenzie, G. M. (1971a). *Brain Res.* **34**, 323–330.
McKenzie, G. M. (1971b). *Pharmacologist* **13**, 279.
McKenzie, G. M. (1972). *Psychopharmacologia* **23**, 212–219.
McKenzie, G. M., and Sadof, M. (1974). *J. Pharm. Pharmacol.* **26**, 280–282.
McKenzie, G. M., and Soroko, F. E. (1972). *J. Pharm. Pharmacol.* **24**, 696–701.
McKenzie, G. M., and White, H. L. (1973). *Biochem. Pharmacol.* **22**, 2329–2336.
McLennan, H. (1965). *Experientia* **21**, 725.
Macleod, R. M., and Lehmeyer, J. E. (1974). *Endocrinology* **94**, 1077–1085.
Maj, J., Grabowska, M., and Gajda, L. (1972). *Eur. J. Pharmacol.* **17**, 208–214.
Malmnäs, C. O. (1973). *Acta Physiol. Scand., Suppl.* **395**, 96–116.
Martin, W. R., Wikler, A., Eades, C. G., and Pescor, F. T. (1963). *Psychopharmacologia* **4**, 247–260.
Martinson, J. (1965). *Acta Physiol. Scand.* **65**, Suppl. 255, 1–24.
Masur, J., and Benedito, M. A. C. (1974a). *Behav. Biol.* **10**, 527–531.
Masur, J., and Benedito, M. A. C. (1974b). *Behav. Biol.* **10**, 533–540.
Masur, J., Maroni, J. B., and Benedito, M. A. C. (1975). *Behav. Biol.* **14**, 21–30.
Matthiessen, A., and Wright, C. R. A. (1870). *Anal. Chem., Suppl.* **7**, 170–176.
Mayer, E. L. (1871). *Chem. Ber.* **4**, 121–129.
Meites, J., and Clemens, A. (1972). *Vitam. Horm. (N.Y.)* **30**, 165–221.
Missala, K., Lal, S., and Sourkes, T. L. (1973). *Eur. J. Pharmacol.* **22**, 54–58.
Mitchell, L. (1950). *Science* **112**, 154.
Muacevic, G., Stötzer, H., and Wick, H. (1965). *Arzneim.-Forsch.* **15**, 613–618.
Munkvad, I., and Randrup, A. (1966). *Acta Psychiatr. Scand.* **42**, Suppl. 191, 178–187.
Musacchio, M. (1970). *Symp. Brain Chem. Ment. Dis., 1970* p. 192.
Nahorski, S. R. (1975). *Psychopharmacologia* **42**, 159–162.
Naylor, R. J., and Olley, J. E. (1972). *Neuropharmacology* **11**, 91–99.
Neal, M. J. (1968). *J. Pharm. Pharmacol.* **20**, 950–953.
Neumeyer, J. L., Neustadt, B. R., Oh, K. H., Weinhardt, K. K., Boyce, C. B., Rosenberg, F. J., and Teiger, D. G. (1973). *J. Med. Chem.* **16**, 1223–1228.
Neumeyer, J. L., Granchelli, F. E., Fuxe, K., Ungerstedt, U., and Corrodi, H. (1974). *J. Med. Chem.* **17**, 1090–1095.
Niemegeers, C. J. E. (1960). Dr. Sc. Dissertation, Paris.
Niemegeers, C. J. E. (1971). *Pharmacology* **6**, 353–364.
Nilsson, K. O. (1975). *Acta Endocrinol. (Copenhagen)* **80**, 230–236.
Nilsson, K. O., Wide, L., and Hökfelt, B. (1975). *Acta Endocrinol. (Copenhagen)* **80**, 220–229.
Nybäck, H., Schubert, J., and Sedvall, G. (1970). *J. Pharm. Pharmacol.* **22**, 622–624.
Nymark, M. (1972). *Psychopharmacologia* **26**, 361–368.
Parker, R. B. (1974). *Psychopharmacologia* **38**, 15–23.

Patil, P. N., Burkman, A. M., Yamauchi, D., and Hetey, S. (1973). *J. Pharm. Pharmacol.* **25**, 221–228.
Patni, S. K., and Dandiya, P. C. (1974). *Life Sci.* **14**, 737–745.
Pedersen, V. (1967). *Acta Pharmacol. Toxicol.* **25**, Suppl. 4, 63.
Pedersen, V. (1968). *Br. J. Pharmacol.* **34**, 219–220.
Peng, M. T. (1963). *J. Pharmacol. Exp. Ther.* **139**, 345–349.
Peng, M. T., and Wang, S. C. (1962). *Proc. Soc. Exp. Biol. Med.* **110**, 211–215.
Persson, T. (1970). *Acta Pharmacol. Toxicol.* **28**, 49–56.
Persson, T., and Waldeck, B. (1970a). *Acta Physiol. Scand.* **78**, 142–144.
Persson, T., and Waldeck, B. (1970b). *Eur. J. Pharmacol.* **11**, 315–320.
Portig, P. J., and Vogt, M. (1968). *J. Physiol. (London)* **197**, 20–21.
Portig, P. J., and Vogt, M. (1969). *J. Physiol. (London)* **204**, 687–715.
Pozuelo, J., and Kerr, F. W. L. (1972). *Mayo Clin. Proc.* **47**, 621–628.
Pschorr, R. (1907). *Chem. Ber.* **40**, 1984–1993.
Pschorr, R., Jaeckel, B., and Fecht, H. (1902). *Chem. Ber.* **35**, 4377–4383.
Puech, A. J., Simon, P., Chermat, R., and Boissier, J. R. (1974). *J. Pharmacol.* **5**, 241–254.
Puri, S. K., and Lal, H. (1973). *Psychopharmacologia* **32**, 113–120.
Quock, R. M., and Horita, A. (1974). *Science* **183**, 539–540.
Quock, R. M., Carino, M. A., and Horita, A. (1975). *Life Sci.* **16**, 525–532.
Ramsbottom, N., and Hunt, J. N. (1970). *Gut* **11**, 989–993.
Randrup, A., and Munkvad, I. (1965). *Psychopharmacologia* **7**, 416–422.
Randrup, A., and Munkvad, I. (1967). *Psychopharmacologia* **11**, 300–310.
Rekker, R. F., Engel, D. J. C., and Nys, G. G. (1972). *J. Pharm. Pharmacol.* **24**, 589–591.
Rethy, C. R., Smith, C. B., and Villarreal, J. E. (1971). *J. Pharmacol. Exp. Ther.* **176**, 472–479.
Rommelspacher, H., and Kuhar, M. J. (1975). *Life Sci.* **16**, 65–70.
Roos, B. E. (1969). *J. Pharm. Pharmacol.* **21**, 263–264.
Roszell, D. K., and Horita, A. (1975). *J. Psychiatr. Res.* **12**, 117–123.
Rotrosen, J., Wallach, M. B., Angrist, B. N., and Gershon, S. (1972a). *Psychopharmacologia* **26**, 185–194.
Rotrosen, J., Angrist, B. M., Wallach, M. B., and Gershon, S. (1972b). *Eur. J. Pharmacol.* **20**, 133–135.
Routtenberg, A. (1972). *Behav. Biol.* **7**, 601–641.
Saari, W. S., and King, S. (1973). *J. Med. Chem.* **16**, 171–172.
Saari, W. S., King, S., Lotti, V. J., and Scriabine, A. (1974). *J. Med. Chem.* **17**, 1086–1090.
Sahakian, B. J., and Robbins, T. W. (1975). *Neuropharmacology* **14**, 251–257.
Sahakian, B. J., Robbins, T. W., Morgan, M. J., and Iversen, S. D. (1975). *Brain Res.* **84**, 195–205.
Sayers, A. C., Bürki, H. R., Ruch, W., and Asper, H. (1975). *Psychopharmacologia* **41**, 97–104.
Scheel-Krüger, J. (1970). *Acta Pharmacol. Toxicol.* **28**, 1–16.
Scheel-Krüger, J., and Hasselager, E. (1974). *Psychopharmacologia* **36**, 189–202.
Scheel-Krüger, J., and Randrup, A. (1976). *Life Sci.* **6**, 1389–1398.
Schelkunov, E. L., and Stabrovsky, E. M. (1971). *Farmakol. Toksikol. (Moscow)* **34**, 653–657.
Schneider, C. (1968). *Nature (London)* **220**, 586–587.

266   F. C. COLPAERT, W. F. M. VAN BEVER, AND J. E. M. F. LEYSEN

Schoenfeld, R. I., Neumeyer, J. L., Dafeldecker, W., and Roffler-Tarlov, S. (1975). Eur. J. Pharmacol. 30, 63–68.
Schuster, S. R., and Thompson, T. (1969). Ann. Rev. Pharmacol. 9, 483–502.
Schwab, R. S., Amadoz, L. V., and Lettvin, J. Y. (1951). Trans. Am. Neurol. Assoc. 76, 251–253.
Schwartz, A. S., and Marchok, P. L. (1974a). Nature (London) 248, 257–258.
Schwartz, A. S., and Marchok, P. L. (1974b). Rep. 6th Annu. Sc. Meet. Comm. Problems Drug Dependence, 1974.
Seeman, P., Wong, M., and Lee, T. (1974). Fed. Proc. Fed. Am. Soc. Exp. Biol. 33, 246.
Seeman, P., Chau-Wong, M., Tedesco, J., and Way, K. (1975). Proc. Natl. Acad. Sci. U.S.A. 72, 4376–4380.
Senault, B. (1968). J. Physiol. (London) 60, Suppl. 2, 543–544.
Senault, B. (1970). Psychopharmacologia 18, 271–287.
Senault, B. (1971). Psychopharmacologia 20, 389–394.
Setler, P. E., Pendleton, R. G., and Finlay, E. (1975). J. Pharmacol. Exp. Ther. 192, 702–712.
Share, N. N., Chai, C. Y., and Wang, S. C. (1965). J. Pharmacol. Exp. Ther. 147, 416–421.
Shemano, I., Wendel, H., and Ross, S. D. (1961). J. Pharmacol. Exp. Ther. 132, 258–263.
Shintomi, K., and Yamamura, M. (1975). Eur. J. Pharmacol. 31, 273–280.
Simon, A., and van Maanen, E. F. (1971). Fed. Proc., Fed Am. Soc. Exp. Biol. 30, 624.
Simpson, B. A., and Iversen, S. D. (1971). Nature (London) 230, 30–32.
Singer, G., and Montgomery, R. B. (1973). Pharmacol., Biochem. Behav. 1, 211–221.
Small, L., Faris, B. F., and Mallonee, J. E. (1940). J. Org. Chem. 5, 334–349.
Smelik, P. G., and Ernst, A. M. (1966). Life Sci. 5, 1485–1488.
Smith, C. B., Villarreal, J. E., Bednarczyk, J. H., and Sheldon, M. I. (1970). Science 170, 1106–1108.
Smith, C. B., Sheldon, M. I., Bednarczyk, J. H., and Villarreal, J. E. (1972). J. Pharmacol. Exp. Ther. 180, 547–557.
Smith, S. G., and Davis, W. M. (1973). Psychol. Rec. 23, 215–221.
Soroko, F. E., and McKenzie, G. M. (1970). Pharmacologist 12, 253.
Sourkes, T. L. (1954). Arch. Biochem. 51, 444–456.
Sourkes, T. L., and Poirier, L. S. (1968). Adv. Pharmacol. 6, 35–46.
Spector, S., Sjoerdsma, A., and Undenfriend, S. (1965). J. Pharmacol. Exp. Ther. 147, 86–95.
Srimal, R. C., and Dhawan, B. N. (1970). Psychopharmacologia 18, 99–107.
Stadler, H., Lloyd, K. G., Gadea-Ciria, M., and Bartholini, G. (1973). Brain Res. 55, 476–480.
Stille, G. (1971). Arzneim.-Forsch. 21, 650–654.
St.-Laurent, J., Leclerc, R. R., and Mitchell, M. L. (1973). Pharmacol., Biochem. Behav. 1, 581–588.
Stratten, W. P., and Avlott, M. V. (1974). Fed. Proc., Fed. Am. Soc. Exp. Biol. 50, 1595.
Struppler, A., and von Uexküll, T. (1953). Z. Klin. Med. 152, 46–57.
Struyker Boudier, H. A. J. (1975). Ph.D. Dissertation, University of Nijmegen, The Netherlands.

Struyker Boudier, H. A. J., Gielen, W., and Van Rossum, J. M. (1973). *In* "Frontiers in Catecholamine Research" (E. Usdin and S. H. Snyder, eds.), pp. 673–674. Pergamon, Oxford.

Struyker Boudier, H. A. J., Gielen, W., Cools, A. R., and Van Rossum, J. M. (1974). *Arch. Int. Pharmacodyn. Ther.* 209, 324–331.

Tagliamonte, A., Tagliamonte, P., Perz-Cruet, J., Stern, S., and Gessa, G. L. (1971). *J. Pharmacol. Exp. Ther.* 177, 475–480.

Tagliamonte, A., Fratta, W., and Gessa, G. L. (1974). *Experientia* 30, 381–382.

Tarsy, D., and Baldessarini, R. J. (1973). *Nature (London), New Biol.* 245, 262–263.

Tarsy, D., and Baldessarini, R. J. (1974). *Neuropharmacology* 13, 927–940.

Tatum, A. L., Seevers, M. H., and Collins, K. H. (1929). *J. Pharmacol. Exp. Ther.* 36, 447–475.

Taylor, K. M. (1974). *Nature (London)* 252, 238–241.

Taylor, K. M., and Snyder, S. H. (1971). *Brain Res.* 28, 295–309.

Terada, C. W., and Masur, J. (1973). *Eur. J. Pharmacol.* 24, 375–380.

Tesařová, O. (1972). *Pharmakopsychiatr. Neuro-Psychopharmakol.* 5, 13–19.

Ther, L., and Schramm, H. (1962). *Arch. Int. Pharmacodyn. Ther.* 138, 302–319.

Thierry, A. M., Stinus. L., Blanc, G., and Glowinski, J. (1973). *Brain Res.* 50, 230–234.

Thierry, A. M., Hirsch, J. C., Tassin, J. P., Blanc, G., and Glowinski, J. (1974). *Brain Res.* 79, 77–88.

Thomas, J. (1970). *Fed. Proc., Fed. Am. Soc. Exp. Biol.* 29, 1488.

Thorner, M. O. (1975). *Lancet* 1, 662–664.

Tolosa, E. S., and Sparber, S. B. (1974). *Life Sci.* 15, 1371–1380.

Trabucchi, M., Cheney, D. L., Racagni, G., and Costa, E. (1975). *Brain Res.* 85, 130–134.

Tseng, L.-F., and Loh, H. H. (1974). *J. Pharmacol. Exp. Ther.* 189, 717–724.

Tulunay, F. C., Sparber, S. B., and Takemori, A. E. (1975). *Eur. J. Pharmacol.* 33, 65–70.

Ungerstedt, U. (1971a). *Acta Physiol. Scand., Suppl.* 367, 1–68.

Ungerstedt, (1971b). *Acta Physiol. Scand., Suppl.* 367, 69–93.

Ungerstedt, U. (1971c). *Acta Physiol. Scand., Suppl.* 367, 95–122.

Uretsky, N. J., and Iversen, L. L. (1970). *J. Neurochem.* 17, 269–278.

Van Nueten, J. M. (1962). Dr. Sc. Dissertation, Paris.

Van Rossum, J. M. (1966). *Arch. Int. Pharmacodyn. Ther.* 160, 492–494.

Van Rossum, J. M. (1970). *In* "The Neuroleptics" (D. P. Bobon, P. A. J. Janssen, and J. Bobon, eds.), pp. 65–67. Karger, Basel.

Vedernikov, V. P. (1970). *Psychopharmacologia* 17, 283–288.

Vernier, V. G. (1952). *Fed. Proc., Fed. Am. Soc. Exp. Biol.* 11, 399.

Vernier, V. G., and Unna, K. R. (1951). *J. Pharmacol. Exp. Ther.* 103, 365.

Villarreal, J. E., Guzman, M., and Smith, C. B. (1973). *J. Pharmacol. Exp. Ther.* 187, 1–7.

Vogt, M. (1969). *Br. J. Pharmacol.* 37, 325–337.

von Uexküll, T. (1953). *Verh. Dtsch. Ges. Inn. Med.* 59, 104–107.

Vonvoigtlander, P. F., Losey, E. G., and Triezenberg, H. J. (1975). *J. Pharmacol. Exp. Ther.* 193, 88–94.

Votava, L., and Dyntarova, H. (1968). *Act. Nerv. Super.* 10, 303–304.

Wang, S. C., and Borison, H. L. (1950). *Arch. Neurol. Psychiatry* 63, 928–941.

Wang, S. C., and Borison, H. L. (1952). *Gastroenterology* 22, 1–11.

Wauquier, A., and Niemegeers, C. J. E. (1973). *Psychopharmacologia* **30**, 163–172.
Weiner, W. J., Goetz, C., and Klawans, H. L. (1975). *Acta Pharmacol. Toxicol.* **36**, 155–160.
Weinstock, M., and Speiser, Z. (1974). *Eur. J. Pharmacol.* **25**, 29–35.
Weissman, A. (1966). *Arch. Int. Pharmacodyn. Ther.* **160**, 330–332.
Weissman, A. (1975). *Eur. J. Pharmacol.* **33**, 267–275.
Weissman, A., Koe, B. K., and Tenen, S. S. (1966). *J. Pharmacol. Exp. Ther.* **151**, 339–352.
White, H. L., and McKenzie, G. M. (1971). *Pharmacologist* **13**, 313.
Willems, J. L. (1973). *Naunyn-Schmiedeberg's Arch. Pharmacol.* **279**, 115–126.
Willems, J. L., and Bogaert, M. G. (1975). *Naunyn-Schmiedeberg's Arch. Pharmacol.* **286**, 413–428.
Willner, J., Samach, M., Angrist, B., Wallach, M., and Gershon, S. (1970). *Commun. Behav. Biol.* **5**, 135–141.
Wolfarth, S. (1974). *Pharmacol., Biochem. Behav.* **2**, 181–186.
Yarbrough, G. G. (1975). *Eur. J. Pharmacol.* **31**, 367–369.
Yokel, R. A., and Wise, R. A. (1975). *Science* **187**, 547–549.
Ziegler, B., and Schneider, E. (1974). *Arzneim.-Forsch.* **24**, 1117–1119.
Zivkovic, B., Guidotti, A., and Costa, E. (1974). *Mol. Pharmacol.* **10**, 727–735.
Zivkovic, B., Guidotti, A., and Costa, E. (1975). *Brain Res.* **92**, 516–521.

THYMOLEPTIC AND NEUROLEPTIC DRUG PLASMA LEVELS IN PSYCHIATRY: CURRENT STATUS

By Thomas B. Cooper, George M. Simpson, and J. Hillary Lee

Rockland Research Institute, Orangeburg, New York

I. Introduction

Since the introduction of neuroleptic drugs in the middle 1950s, and tricyclic antidepressant drugs in the late 1950s and early 1960s, considerable investigation and refinement of the mode of administration of these drugs have been made (e.g., efficacy of once-a-day medication and of long-acting medication). In terms of the quantity of drug to be administered to each individual patient, however, the clinician to date has essentially been forced to treat the variety of mental illnesses with drugs at his disposal simply by starting the patient on what is regarded as a reasonable dose of medication and then, if a clinical response is not obtained, increasing the amount of medication given until either the patient shows clinical improvement or troublesome side effects, or the amount of medication given exceeds a sometimes arbitrary upper limit. Thus a patient who does not respond is then moved to another medication or to some other treatment. In the case of neuroleptic drugs it is a common practice to "titrate" the patient until extra-pyramidal side effects are observed and then to reduce the medication slightly, and hopefully the patient will improve at the new level.

In some branches of medicine the value of plasma levels of a drug required to optimize patient treatment or avoid toxicity has been well documented (e.g., digoxin, digitoxin phenylhydantoin salicylate, lidocaine, hormone therapy). In psychiatry, however, with one exception (i.e., lithium), the techniques available for quantitating plasma drug levels until recently have been totally inadequate in that they lacked the sensitivity and/or specificity for accurate measurement of the very low levels of drugs found in the plasma of patients receiving psychotropic drugs (ca. 10^{-7}–10^{-12} gm/ml).

A major breakthrough occurred in 1967 when Hammer and Brodie published an article describing a technique which involved the acetylation of a secondary amine [desmethylimipramine (DMI)] with radioactive labeled acetic anhydride (^{3}H). This technique demonstrated the sensitivity to measure, in relatively small plasma samples (3 ml) levels of drug in the nanogram-per-milliliter range (10^{-9} gm). Then Curry (1968) introduced a quantitative method for the neuroleptic, chlorpromazine, involving gas-liquid chromatography (GLC) coupled to a highly sensitive and selective electron-capture detector, again with sensitivity in the 10^{-9}-gm range. Ryhage (1968) and Hammar et al. (1968) identified chlorpromazine and its metabolites using GLC–mass fragmentography which has subsequently been demonstrated in some instances to be sensitive to 10^{-12} gm/ml. These three techniques published within such a short time of each other have resulted in a major reevaluation of the various approaches to rational drug therapy and experimentation in psychiatry.

Use of these techniques, and modifications of them developed for the specific properties of various drug molecules, allows the following issues to be examined:

1. Whether or not the patient is taking the medication.

2. The possibility that the plasma level or the whole-blood level of a drug and/or its metabolites in the steady state can be correlated with clinical efficacy and/or side effects.

3. Evaluation of drug interactions.

4. Evaluation of biochemical changes (e.g., neurotransmitters and their metabolites) in relation to plasma drug levels.

5. Investigation, in controlled experiments, of the effects of psycho-pharmaceuticals not by fixed-dosage schedule but by controlling blood levels

within a predetermined range. (Clearly of value in animal experiments as well as for humans.)

6. Whether a drug is inducing enzymes and thus accelerating its own metabolism.

7. The kinetics of single-dose administration of a drug and the appearance of metabolites.

8. The kinetics of multidose administration of a drug.

9. Use of the single-dose pharmacokinetic approach to determine whether or not the steady-state plasma level can be predicted for individual patients.

10. Checking the bioavailability of the same drug (e.g., generic versus tradename product).

II. Lithium (The Ideal Prototype)

The role of lithium in the treatment of mania is well established (Cade, 1949; Schou, 1968), but some controversy exists regarding its efficacy in depression (Mendels, 1973).

Lithium is the ideal drug to demonstrate the value of blood level determination in clinical psychiatry for the following reasons. (1) It is very easily measured in plasma or other body fluids and has no metabolites. (2) There is clear evidence of a therapeutic range for lithium; thus patients who are above a certain plasma level manifest signs of toxicity (Warwick, 1966; Gershon, 1970; Schou et al., 1971; Prien et al., 1971; Brown, 1973). The relationship therefore is curvilinear, and dosage is actually controlled by means of the plasma lithium level. (3) Techniques have been described to predict the individual lithium dosage requirements of patients. (4) The red blood cell concentration and/or red blood cell to plasma ratio of lithium has been suggested to be an indicator of the brain level of the drug and an indicator of pending toxicity. (5) The same ratio has also been claimed to be the basis of a technique for delineating a subgroup of depressed patients who may show a clinical response to lithium therapy.

A. METHODOLOGY

Chemical analysis of blood samples (whole blood, plasma, serum, or red blood cells involves the use of either atomic emission or atomic absorption instrumentation. Atomic emission techniques have been described by Fournis and Chazot (1971), Brown and Legg (1970), Sideman (1970), Combs (1971), and Klaus (1971), and atomic absorption techniques by Amdisen (1968), Brown and Legg (1970), Frazer et al. (1972), Malenfant (1970), Pybus and Bowers (1970), and Wittrig et al. (1970). The two techniques have been compared by Pybus and Bowers (1970), Blijenberg and Leijnse (1968), and Levy and Katz (1970). Robertson *et al.* (1973) and Horn-castle (1973) showed that lithium flame emission photometry may actually be more sensitive than atomic absorption spectrophotometry. It is our opinion that either technique used by competent personnel is equally acceptable. The limits of sensitivity are of little importance, because the therapeutic levels of lithium are such that either system measures concentrations many times higher than its lower limit of sensitivity. Two micro-techniques, one using flame photometry (Villeneuve *et al.*, 1971) requiring 0.2 ml of serum, and one using atomic absorption requiring 50 μl of plasma (Cooper *et al.*, 1974), have been described.

Previous criticism of atomic absorption systems focused on the initial cost factor, but this no longer applies because systems are now available that are competitive in price with comparable flame instrumentation.

B. Prediction of Individual Patient Dosage Requirements

Schou *et al.* (1970) described a method for the prediction of individual dosage requirements using the renal clearance of lithium. The renal clearance can be determined from a single oral dose of lithium by means of a timed urine sample and blood samples at the beginning and end of the urine collection. The elimination phase of the kinetic curve ($t_o + 7$ hours) is used for this test. The equation used by Schou was:

Maintenance dosage (meq/liter) = average lithium concentration (meq/liter) $\times$ renal lithium clearance (ml/minute) $\times$ 1.44

This gave the average lithium level during a medication period but not the steady-state level. These investigators suggested that this level is approximately 30% higher than the steady-state level. Sedval *et al.* (1970), using 10 healthy normal volunteers, demonstrated a high negative correlation ($r = -0.87$) between the steady-state blood level and the product of lithium clearance and body weight (Fig. 1) and suggested that this may be indicative of clearance of lithium by routes other than the kidney. However, both techniques can be used effectively to determine individual patient drug requirements.

Bergner *et al.* (1973) described a pharmacokinetic approach to the analysis of data collected from the administration of a single 600-mg dose of lithium carbonate. These workers showed that they could predict with acceptable clinical accuracy the individual dosage requirement of each patient. This experimental approach, however, required a minimum of eight blood samples collected over a 24-hour period, plus the use of a large

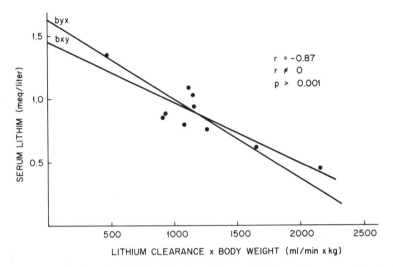

Fig. 1. Correlation of product of body weight and lithium clearance with steady-state plasma lithium level. [Reproduced with permission of Editors of *European Journal of Clinical Pharmacology* Vol. 2, p. 231 (1970).]

computer. In a second report (Cooper *et al.*, 1973), the same group demonstrated that each patient's dosage requirement could be ascertained from a single blood sample collected 24 hours after a single 600-mg oral dose of lithium carbonate, without the use of the computer, simply by referring to a table. This procedure was based on the observation that a very high correlation ($r = 0.97$) was obtained when the 24-hour blood level was compared to the steady-state level reached after a fixed-dosage regimen (Fig. 2). Since this work was first published, the observation has been confirmed in more than 100 patients, and this method is in routine use in the lithium clinic at the Rockland Research Institute (Cooper and Simpson, 1976).

The reproducibility of the prediction is shown in Table I. The convenience of the technique is best seen in an outpatient situation in which each patient is given 600 mg of lithium carbonate by the clinician, or given the medication to take at a later time. The patient is then requested to attend the laboratory or the clinician's office 24 hours after ingesting the medication, and a single blood sample is taken at that time. The plasma lithium level is determined from the sample and reported to the clinician. The result is checked with Table II, and the clinician can then start the patient on a dosage schedule that will result in a plasma lithium level between 0.6 and 1.2 meq/liter. Recently, Seifert *et al.* (1975) confirmed the clinical usefulness of this technique in 58 patients, but modified the procedure because they used a delayed-release preparation. Obviously, the differ-

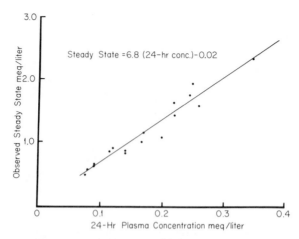

Fig. 2. Correlation of 24-hour and steady-state serum lithium levels ($r = .97$, $n = 17$) where patients received 600 mg t.i.d. [*American Journal of Psychiatry* Vol. 130, pp. 601–603 (1973). Copyright 1973, the American Psychiatric Association. Reprinted by permission.]

ences in the kinetics of standard and delayed-release forms of a medication must be considered.

Schou (1969) reported that renal clearance of lithium was decreased in older patients. In a recent study of the effects of lithium on late-onset, drug-related dyskinesias, in which the single blood sample prediction technique was used (Cooper and Simpson, 1976), the predicted dosages were found to be accurate in all cases ($n = 10$). Of interest was the observation that these older patients (mean 72 years, range 57–82 years) required 600 mg/day, with two exceptions (one requiring 300 mg/day and the other 1200 mg/day), to achieve the therapeutic range, confirming Schou's observation and the general clinical experience that older patients seem to require less lithium.

C. Intracellular Studies

Maggs (1968) examined the concentration of lithium in the red blood cell and observed that patients on treatment who maintained a low RBC/plasma lithium ratio tended to "run a fluctuating clinical course with further episodes of mania and occasionally depression." Frazer *et al.* (1973) administered lithium to rats (acute and chronic experiments) and reported that erythrocyte levels of lithium provided better predictions of brain levels than plasma. Elizur *et al.* (1972) examined the relationship between erythrocyte and plasma levels of lithium in psychiatric patients and in hospitalized

TABLE I

LITHIUM LEVELS 24 HOURS AFTER A 600-mg DOSE
OF LITHIUM CARBONATE[a]

Patient number	8/22/74	9/6/74	9/12/74
1	0.18	0.19	0.16
2	0.23	0.25	0.21
3	0.24	0.24	0.21
4	0.29	0.30	0.30
5	0.23	0.25	0.24
6	0.21	0.20	0.19
7	0.25	0.27	
8	0.31	0.31	0.27
9	0.20	0.17	0.18
10	0.22	0.22	0.21
11	0.21	0.23	0.21
12	0.19	0.19	0.16
13	0.26	0.27	0.28
14	0.18	0.17	0.18

[a] Three separate loading doses were given to each patient. [*American Journal of Psychiatry* Vol. 133, pp. 440–443 (1976). Copyright 1976, the American Psychiatric Association. Reprinted by permission.]

TABLE II

DOSAGE REQUIRED TO ACHIEVE A SERUM
LEVEL OF 0.6–1.2 meq/liter[a,b]

24-Hour serum level after single loading dose	Dosage required
Less than 0.05	1200 mg t.i.d.
0.05–0.09	900 mg t.i.d.
0.10–0.14	600 mg t.i.d.
0.15–0.19	300 mg q.i.d.
0.20–0.23	300 mg t.i.d.
0.24–0.30	300 mg b.i.d.
More than 0.30	300 mg b.i.d.[c]

[a] *American Journal of Psychiatry* Vol. 130, pp. 601–603 (1973). Copyright 1973, the American Psychiatric Association. Reprinted by permission.

[b] The regimen selected minimizes fluctuation in the plasma level while maintaining a schedule the patient can adhere to. Variation in this regimen can be made at the choice of the clinician, but the total daily dose must remain the same. All steady-state values are collected just before the next medication is to be taken.

[c] Use extreme caution.

nonpsychiatric subjects. These investigators' findings indicated that both mania and depression are associated with lower erythrocyte lithium concentrations than noted in the controls or in manic depressive patients in their interphase. Soucek *et al.* (1974) reported essentially similar findings with, however, much higher RBC/plasma ratios. Lytkkens *et al.* (1973) reported a statistically significant higher RBC/plasma lithium ratio in manic females compared to manic males and control subjects. Mendels and Frazer (1973, 1974) suggested that there may be an abnormality in the cell membrane systems that regulate the movement of electrolytes across the plasma membrane in a subgroup of depressed patients, and these patients appeared to be responsive to lithium. There is both *in vitro* and *in vivo* evidence that the distribution of lithium between plasma and the red blood cell is under genetic control (Dorus *et al.*, 1974, 1975; Schless *et al.*, 1975). Thus it appears that the RBC lithium concentration indicates a subgroup of patients with endogenous depression who will respond to lithium and who cannot be categorized in any other way. A recent article by Kupfer *et al.* (1975) discussed an experiment in which members of a group of unipolar depressives were separated according to their response or lack of response to tricyclic antidepressants, and the personality traits and clinical characteristics of each subgroup compared to those of bipolar patients. The conclusion of these investigators again attests to the lack of homogeneity of unipolar depression, and it may be that the subgroup described by Kupfer *et al.* (1975) is the same one that has the cell membrane abnormality postulated by Mendels and Frazer (1973, 1974). Hokin-Neaverson *et al.* (1974) have described a deficiency of erythrocyte sodium pump activity in manic-depressive patients, and Naylor *et al.* (1973) demonstrated increased $Na^+–K^+$-ATPase activity, after clinical recovery in a group of "psychotic" depressive patients, and that lithium treatment increased this activity in manic-depressive patients (Naylor *et al.*, 1974; Naylor and Dick, 1974).

If Mendels and Frazer's work can be confirmed, it will be of major importance in that a biological marker, easily detected, will enable clinicians to select lithium responders from among depressed patients, and will also allow the research investigator to study a less heterogeneous group of depressed patients. The reduction in heterogeneity obviously applies to both the responding and nonresponding groups.

The picture, however, is not as clear-cut as stated above. Rybakowski *et al.* (1974a) were unable to demonstrate differences in the RBC/plasma lithium ratio between groups of manic-depressive and control patients, nor were they able to differentiate lithium responders from nonresponders in a group of depressed patients, using this ratio. Zakowska-Dabrowska and Rybakowski (1973) did demonstrate a positive correlation between this ratio and the intensity of EEG changes.

In another study by Rybakowski *et al.* (1974b), the same ratio was investigated in patients in remission who were on lithium prophylactic therapy. Again the findings contradicted the findings of Elizur *et al.* (1972) and Lyttkens *et al.* (1973), in that the ratios in the patients in remission were not different from those in comparable patients in the acute psychotic state, nor were there any differences between males and females in the different diagnostic groups. These workers also investigated the variability of the RBC/plasma lithium ratio and found it to be quite variable; they expresed this variability as the relative standard deviation (standard deviation as percent of the mean) and, if the work of Mendels and Frazer (1973) is examined, it is apparent that their data show essentially the same range of variability. Findings similar to those of Rybakowski have recently been presented by Carroll (1975) but with a much larger number of subjects (94) and diagnostic categories. There was no significant difference between 36 bipolar and 25 unipolar patients with respect to the RBC/plasma lithium ratio. Ratios in males ($n = 40$) were significantly lower than in females ($n = 54$), but the schizophrenic group was the only diagnostic category in which this difference was significant. Fourteen patients (with neuroses and personality disorders) had significantly lower ratios when compared to all other categories. In 20 depressed patients treated with lithium, 7 of

TABLE III

RBC/Plasma Lithium Ratio $\times$ 100[a]

Source	Pooled data	Bipolar			Pooled data	Unipolar	
		Normo-thymic	Manic	Depres-sive		Depres-sive	Remis-sion
Elizur *et al.* (1972)	27.7 (35)	30.5 (16)			28.4 (12)		28.1 (9)
		27.3 (16)[b]	18.9 (16)				
		14.8 (3)[b]		7.7 (3)			
						40 (3)	29.3 (3)
Lyttkens *et al.* (1973)	45.4 (37)						
Mendels and Frazer (1973)					47.6 (13)		
Rybakowsky *et al.* (1974b)	54 (28)	54 (28)			55 (9)		55 (9)
Soucek *et al.* (1974)	43.3 (52)	47 (36)	34 (8)		45.3 (23)		44.6 (12)
		48.2 (6)		48.9 (6)		50.7 (4)	46 (11)
Carroll (1975)	49.7 (36)				53 (25)		

[a] Figure in parentheses indicates number of patients in a group.

[b] Where data are on the same patients in different phases, the mean is calculated from the interphase data.

8 bipolar and 4 of 12 unipolar patients responded. There was no significant difference between responders and nonresponders in the unipolar group in the RBC/plasma lithium ratio. These data are listed in Table III.

As stated at the beginning of this section, lithium, because of its simplicity, has been selected as the ideal drug for demonstrating the possible importance of blood levels in psychiatry, both at the research and clinical practice level. The preceding section demonstrates many of the values at the clinical level, and also the valuable hypotheses that can be tested to attempt to delineate the basic mechanism of action of this most important cation. However, even with this "simple" drug there are contradictory data. Therefore one can anticipate the difficulties in investigating drugs with complex metabolic pathways and centrally active metabolites, to be discussed in the following sections.

III. Tricyclic Antidepressants

A. CHEMICAL ANALYSIS

Early methods for the quantitation of these drugs using spectrofluorimetric procedures were insensitive, and the separation techniques were such that many of the metabolites were included in the analysis (Hermann et al., 1959; Hermann and Pulver, 1960). Moody et al. (1967) described a spectrofluorimetric procedure for the determination of imipramine and DMI capable of measuring steady-state plasma levels. Perel et al. (1974) modified this procedure to increase the sensitivity.

Hammer and Brodie (1967) used a procedure involving in vitro acteylation of the secondary amine (DMI) with tritium-labeled acetic anhydride. Quantitation was achieved by relating the radioactivity count to a standard curve obtained by acetylating known amounts of DMI. The method was modified for the quantitation of nortriptyline by Sjöqvist et al. (1969), Burrows (1972), and Frederickson-Overø (1972), and has been used extensively in the investigation of nortriptyline plasma levels and clinical correlates.

Harris et al. (1970) have described a method for the quantitation of imipramine and DMI, using a combination of the Hammer–Brodie (1967) technique plus methylation of the tertiary amine (imipramine) to form a quaternary ammonium compound. ^{3}H or ^{14}C counts are then related to their respective standard curves as described above.

Several gas chromatographic methods have been described for tricyclic secondary amines, the majority of which use the sensitive and selective electron-capture detector (Sisenwine et al., 1969; Borga and Garle, 1972; Ervik et al., 1970; Walle and Ehrsson, 1971). It is worth noting that the sensitivity of the latter technique is in the picograms-per-milliliter range (10^{-12} gm).

Braithwaite and Widdop (1971) measured both amitriptyline and nortriptyline (after derivatizing) using GLC with a flame ionization detector. The technique is sensitive enough to measure steady-state plasma levels. Hucker and Stauffer (1974) claimed some difficulties with this method and described a technique which did not require a derivative of nortriptyline be formed. Jorgensen (1975), using a heated nitrogen detector, found increased sensitivity, so that he was able to measure amitriptyline and nortriptyline derivatized after single loading doses of 50 mg. Nagy and Treiber (1973) have described a thin-layer chromatographic (TLC) method with a lower limit of sensitivity of 5 ng/ml (5-ml sample). T. B. Cooper et al. (1975a,c) have reported a technique using a nitrogen detector which quantitated 5 ng/ml (3 ml plasma extracted) of imipramine, DMI, amitriptyline, and nortriptyline without requiring derivation. Gas chromatography linked with mass fragmentography has been used to identify various metabolites of these compounds (Hammar et al., 1971) and to quantitate nortriptyline (Borga and Garle, 1972) and imipramine (Frigerio et al., 1972).

B. CLINICAL STUDIES INVOLVING PLASMA LEVEL DETERMINATIONS

Patients treated with identical doses of tricyclic antidepressants show great interindividual differences in their steady-state plasma concentrations (Fig. 3) and in the ratio between the tertiary amine and its secondary amine metabolite when given the tertiary compound (Moody et al., 1967; Hammer and Sjöqvist, 1967; Hammer et al., 1969; Sjöqvist et al., 1969; Braithwaite et al., 1972). Much of the variation is genetically determined (Alexanderson et al., 1969). However, within patients, the steady-state plasma level is directly proportional to the administered dose (Hammer and Sjöqvist, 1967; Sjöqvist et al., 1969).

1. Clinical Response and Plasma Levels

As early as 1962, in a group of psychotic depressives, Haydu et al. observed that, of eight patients on 150 mg of imipramine per day, four responded well to imipramine therapy, while the other four proved refractory. The responders had statistically significant lower levels of imipramine 7 hours after a single dose. Thus patients who had high levels were claimed not to respond to the medication. Yates et al. (1963) noted that the clinical response to DMI was poor in two patients with high plasma levels when compared to four cases with lower levels. (As noted in Section III, A, the methods used by the above workers were not specific.) Zeidenberg et al.

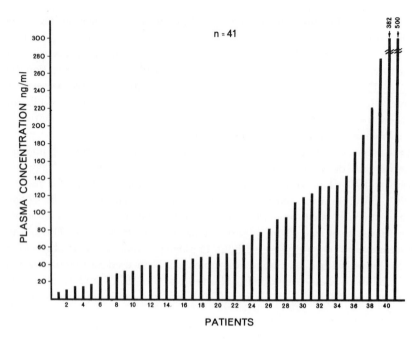

Fig. 3. Variation observed in steady-state plasma level of DMI when patients received 50 mg t.i.d.

(1971) showed that six out of seven severely depressed patients improved rapidly on very high doses of imipramine. Clinical improvement correlated well with drug blood levels, but blood levels varied greatly from patient to patient and were characteristic of individual patients rather than of dose. One patient showed marked deterioration when her plasma levels of the drug decreased, and striking improvement when they increased (the increase was achieved by administering methylphenidate concomitantly). Walter (1971) found a significant correlation ($r = 0.73$) between the therapeutic response to imipramine and the plasma concentration of the drug in 16 patients. This investigation used the method of Moody *et al.* (1967) and reported values ranging from 2.5 to 71 ng/ml. In a study of 15 patients, Braithwaite *et al.* (1972) demonstrated a positive linear correlation between the plasma concentration of amitriptyline plus nortriptyline and clinical response ($r = 0.86$).

Asberg *et al.* (1971) treated 29 patients with nortriptyline and did not find a linear correlation but a curvilinear one; that is, patients at each end of the plasma drug level spectrum did not improve, whereas the majority of the patients in the middle range did. The best range was found to be 50–140 ng/ml. A series of exact probabilities was calculated on the distributions obtained when progressively higher plasma levels were used as cutoff points. Kragh-Sorensen et al. (1973) confirmed this finding ($n = 30$), though with a slightly different range (50–175 ng/ml). It is interesting to note that six of eight nonresponders with plasma levels outside the therapeutic range were considered well and discharged from the hospital within a week of adjustment (most often a reduction) of dosage. Kragh-Sorensen reported confirmation of the previous work and that of others in a triple-blind study in which one group of patients was adjusted to a high plasma drug level of >180 ng/ml and another group to a plasma level of <150 ng/ml. At the end of 4 weeks of continuous nortriptyline treatment, the high-plasma level patients were randomly allocated to two subgroups, one continuing on the same dosage and the other on a decreased dosage. This regimen was continued for two more weeks. The conclusion of this study was in agreement with previous studies, thus giving strong evidence for the assumption that high plasma concentrations of nortriptyline lead to a decreased therapeutic effect in patients suffering from endogenous depression. These workers claim that the best therapeutic results were obtained at a plasma level ranging from 50 to 150 ng/ml nortriptyline (a slight modification of their previous range).

The original Asberg study has been criticized because the patients were on medication only for a 2-week period, they received other medication, and the medication dosage varied from patient to patient. The statistical procedure used has also been criticized (Lader, 1974). Asberg herself (1973) points out that the prerequisites for proper hypotheses testing were not fulfilled, since the hypothesis tested was derived from inspection of the data.

In contrast, Burrows et al. (1972, 1974a) were unable to show any correlation between the plasma levels of nortriptyline and clinical efficacy when looking at their patients as a group. However, when individual patients who were in a steady state on nortriptyline were given identical capsules of different potency, either decreasing their medication or increasing it, these investigators claim that a clear worsening of the depression occurred as the oral dose and plasma level fell, and an improvement as the original dosage was reinstituted (cf. Zeidenberg et al., 1971; Cooper and Simpson, 1973). The original study of Burrows et al. (1972) has been criticized on two grounds (Asberg, 1973; Kragh-Sorensen, 1974): (1) patient selection, and (2) chemical methodology. In terms of patient selection, the more seriously depressed patients were treated with electroconvulsive therapy (ECT) and in the remaining patients (who were less ill) no distinction was made between endogenous and other types of depression. The criticism of the methodology is that the fluctuations in the steady-state levels of individual patients were very high, which was not the experience of other workers in the field. Kragh-Sorensen (1974) correctly points out that the correlation between plasma level and receptor site concentration depends heavily on the assumption of a true steady state; if the patients were not in a steady state (as the data seem to suggest), the assumption of equilibrium between plasma and receptor site is less tenable. However, the patients used were patients who commonly received antidepressants, and a good proportion of them were in a steady state. In addition, the consistent changes in clinical status with changes in blood levels (intraindividual changes) are exceedingly convincing (Fig. 4).

In further studies Burrows et al. (1974b) tested hypotheses that high levels of nortriptyline (140 ng/ml) can lead to greater clinical improvement than plasma levels of less than 50 ng/ml. With the use of a sequential skew restricted design, 20 paired patients were entered into the study, and the analysis at the end point indicated that it was highly unlikely that, if the experiment had been continued, a significant difference between the treatment regimens would have been detected.

Gram et al. (1975) reported that 24 patients, carefully screened and diagnosed as endogenous depressives, were given imipramine (150–225 mg on a t.i.d. regimen) after a 7-day placebo period. Of 12 patients who responded to the treatment, 11 had plasma concentrations of imipramine and DMI greater than or equal to 45 ng/ml and 75 ng/ml, respectively. The 12 patients who did not respond satisfactorily all had concentrations of imipramine and/or DMI below these limits. It is very interesting to note that these workers suggest that it is necessary to have both the parent compound and the metabolite above their respective lower limits to exert an effect. They go on to suggest that, in cases in which imipramine levels are adequate but DMI levels are low, DMI can be administered concomitantly. Where demethylation is rapid, parenteral administration of imipramine may be indicated to eliminate the "first-pass" effect. Gram and Christiansen (1975) demonstrated that this first-pass effect for amitriptyline can result in up to 30–70% demethylation.

These data agree in some respects with the data of Braithwaite et al. (1972), in that there was no upper threshold above which the therapeutic effect diminished. However, as Gram et al. (1975) point out, the data of Braithwaite did not show that the parent compound and metabolite both had to be above minimum levels. In other words, Braithwaite's data indicated that amitriptyline and nortriptyline can be substituted for each other, whereas imipramine and DMI cannot. Olivier-Martin et al. (1975) found a significant correlation in endogenous depressives between the degree of clinical improvement, DMI level, and imipramine and DMI levels, but not imipramine level alone. Neurotic depressives ($n = 6$) did not improve.

In several clinical studies higher dosages have been shown to produce more improvement than lower dosages. Blashki et al. (1971) demonstrated that 150 mg/day of amitriptyline produced significantly better results than

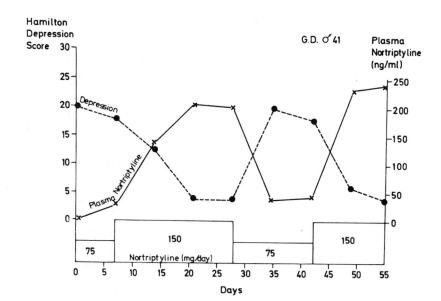

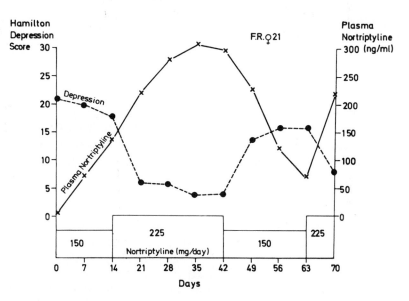

FIG. 4. Relationship between clinical response and plasma nortriptyline level in a male and a female patient receiving varying dosages of nortriptyline in identical capsules. [Reproduced with permission of Editors of *Symposia Medica Hoechst* 8, pp. 173–179 (1974).]

75 mg/day. Simpson *et al.* (1976b) showed similar findings for 300 mg of imipramine versus 150 mg in a double-blind controlled study.

Muscettola *et al.* (1972) described a marked improvement in patients suffering from Parkinson's disease ($n = 13$), who were treated with DMI. The patients in the study had not benefited from previous therapies, and these investigators claimed a significant correlation ($r = 0.89$) between DMI plasma levels and a clinical rating score. Several of these patients were receiving anti-Parkinson drugs together with DMI. When comparing these groups, i.e., DMI alone and DMI plus anti-Parkinson medication, the mean values were not significantly different even though the DMI group received 75 mg/day, while the other group received only 50 mg/day. These workers suggested that this may indicate some interaction between the drugs.

Angst and Rothweiler (1974), in the study of 20 patients treated at two different dosage levels of maprotiline, were unable to demonstrate significant differences in clinical effect in the two treatment groups. However, a trend toward increased effectiveness of the higher dosage was apparent. Two patients (one from each group) were found to have excessively high blood levels and, if these two patients are excluded from the analysis, statistically significant correlations between blood levels and clinical effects and between blood levels and neurological side effects can be demonstrated. These workers speculate that patients with excessively high maprotiline levels may be rather resistant to therapy, perhaps suggesting a curvilinear relationship between plasma levels.

Basic Problems in Clinical Studies. When tricyclic drugs containing a tertiary amine, e.g., imipramine, amitriptyline, are given, the investigator must consider the active demethylated metabolites together with, or as well as, the parent compound. The ratio of parent compound to metabolite varies greatly among individuals (Table IV). However, studies with monomethylated antidepressants (e.g., nortriptyline, DMI) are less complicated in that they do not involve psychoactive major metabolites.

The diagnosis and classification of depression has been and continues to be the subject of much controversy in psychiatry (Kendell, 1968). Problems of patient diagnosis and selection are particularly pertinent at the plasma level–clinical efficacy interface. Simpson *et al.* (1976a) point out that it seems unlikely that hospitalized patients, who represent ca. 5% of the total population of depressives, are typical of the total population. It is quite possible that investigators are dealing with an atypical "hard-core" group of patients who probably would have a poorer response rate to any type of treatment. A further and major problem in experimental design is spontaneous remission. Actual figures are difficult to obtain, but it is a general impression that a significant number of patients recover during the first week of hospitalization whether treated or not. Thus in studies without

TABLE IV
VARIATION IN METABOLISM OF AMITRIPTYLINE AND IMIPRAMINE IN 20 PATIENTS
(10 IN EACH GROUP) AS EVIDENCED BY RATIOS OF DEMETHYLATED
METABOLITE TO PARENT COMPOUND[a]

Amitriptyline (ng/ml)	Nortriptyline (ng/ml)	AMI/NT ratio	Imipramine (ng/ml)	DMI (ng/ml)	IMI/DMI ratio
68	242	0.28	43	95	0.45
70	144	0.49	38	62	0.61
61	123	0.50	82	132	0.62
39	66	0.59	16	21	0.76
87	98	0.89	46	43	1.07
162	163	0.99	70	50	1.40
83	82	1.01	106	56	1.89
153	69	2.22	112	29	3.86
135	40	3.38	131	31	4.23
95	22	4.32	293	45	6.51

[a] Each patient received 150 mg/day. AMI, Amitriptyline; NT, nortriptyline; IMI, imipramine; DMI, desmethylimipramine. (Unpublished data, collaborative study with Dr. A. Nies and Dr. D. Robinson, Dept. Pharmacology, University of Vermont, Burlington.)

at least a 1-week drug-free period, there is still a significant group which responds for non-drug-related reasons and which therefore introduces considerable additional variance in the overall design.

Kuhn (1957) stated, in his initial studies with imipramine, that the therapeutic effects were better in "vital," i.e., endogenous (psychotic) depression as compared with reactive (neurotic) depression. Glassman et al. (1975) observed in their blood level studies that depressed patients with delusions were markedly unresponsive to tricyclic drug therapy, a finding recently confirmed by Simpson et al. (1976b). They suggest that, if such patients are included in a study, they will tend to obscure a potential relationship between plasma levels of the drug and therapeutic outcome. These factors clearly indicate the need in future studies for clearly defined patient selection criteria to provide representative and reasonably homogeneous groups of depressives.

More recently, two major biochemical hypotheses of depression have been proposed, which may enable the investigator to select more homogeneous groups. Thus recent research on the biochemical correlates of depression has focused on two neurotransmitters: noradrenaline and serotonin. Noradrenaline (Schildkraut, 1965) and serotonin hypotheses (Lapin and Oxenkrug, 1969) have been advanced and have been reviewed by Schildkraut (1973).

Imipraminelike drugs inhibit uptake of transmitters into noradrenergic neurons, and this has been suggested to be their mode of action as antidepressants (Carlsson, 1965). These same drugs, however, are poor inhibitors of serotonin uptake. Carlsson et al. (1969) demonstrated that chlorimipramine is the most potent inhibitor of serotonin among the tricyclic antidepressants but has little if any effect on noradrenergic neurons. The demethylated metabolite, however, is a potent inhibitor of noradrenaline uptake (Hamberger and Tuck, 1974). Braithwaite (1974) reported the following potencies for the reuptake of norepinephrine and serotonin: for norepinephrine, DMI > imipramine, amitryptyline > chlorimipramine; for serotonin, chlorimipramine > amitriptyline, imipramine > DMI.

Maas et al. (1972) reported that depressed patients in whom the pretreatment level of urinary 3-methoxy-4-hydroxyphenylglycol (MHPG) was low responded well to treatment with DMI or imipramine (MHPG is a major metabolite of brain norepinephrine and ca. 30–50% of the MHPG found in the urine is thought to be from the brain). This study was replicated, and again these investigators found a significant inverse correlation between low predrug MHPG and response to imipramine. Beckmann and Goodwin (1975) reported that depressed patients who showed a good response to imipramine had low pretreatment MHPG levels, whereas patients with higher pretreatment levels showed a favorable response to treatment with amitriptyline.

If these original studies are confirmed, the additional complications of using selective inhibitors such as DMI may make it more difficult to separate and determine correlations between clinical outcome and depression. Thus, given that the monoamine hypotheses are correct, a patient with a serotonergic-type depression cannot be expected to respond when treated with DMI, even with adequate plasma levels. Drugs that give rise to metabolites with an effect opposite that of the parent compound may be the drugs of choice, e.g., the dual action on serotonin and norepinephrine when chlorimipramine is metabolized to desmethylchlorimipramine.

It should be noted that iprindole, a tricyclic compound which compares favorably with imipramine in antidepressant activity, has been shown to have no effect on the peripheral uptake of amines (Fann et al., 1972), suggesting that the problem may be even more complex than the biogenic amine hypotheses indicate.

Protein binding of tricyclics is extensive, and Borga et al. (1969) have claimed that only about 5% of the total amount of the drug is "free." These data have been challenged by Glassman et al. (1973), who questioned the determination of the binding measurement at room temperature rather than at body temperature. Glassman et al. (1973) claimed that plasma binding of imipramine was not constant from one patient to another and that the percent bound at body temperature was ca. 85%, not 95% as found by Borga et al. (1969). Glassman and his co-workers claim that their findings indicate there can be more than a fourfold difference (5.4–23%) in the amount of free drug available to different patients. These investigators suggest that differences in this magnitude may explain in part the discrepancies seen in studies that attempt to correlate plasma levels and clinical outcome. These data have in turn been questioned by Vesell (1974), who suggested that much of the variance demonstrated may be due to competitive binding by bilirubin. Alexanderson and Borga (1972) agreed that individual differences exist in protein binding but claim that they are very small in comparison to the overall variability in drug plasma level. Until studies are made in which both total and free levels are determined in a clinical efficacy protocol, the problem will remain unresolved.

2. Side Effects and Plasma Levels

Asberg (1973) correlated drug-related side effects to plasma nortriptyline levels and found a significant correlation in patients ($r = 0.5$) and in healthy volunteers ($p < 0.05$). Braithwaite (1974), Burrows (1972), and Gram et al. (1975) were unable to correlate plasma levels with side effects.

Asberg (1973) reported three potentially dangerous reactions which seemed to be associated with high plasma levels. There were two "sudden falls," with plasma levels of 428 and 340 ng/ml, in a patient and a volunteer, respectively. One patient had a bundle branch block with a plasma level of 235 ng/ml (Freyschuss et al., 1970). Kantor et al. (1975) have also reported a bundle branch block which was reversible and reproducible and which correlated with plasma imipramine levels. Winsberg et al. (1975) reported on drug-induced electrocardiograph changes in seven hyperactive children. All seven showed abnormalities during treatment, but these changes did not correlate with plasma imipramine levels.

Winsberg et al. (1974) studied plasma levels of imipramine and DMI in children receiving 5 mg/kg dosages of imipramine and estimated the amount of circulating free drug. These workers demonstrated blood levels of the order of 150 ng/ml as early as 30 minutes after a single 50-mg oral dose and found that children have more free drug circulating than adults. Thus their findings showed that, within the concentration range studied, binding was constant and characteristic for each patient, and therefore the amount of free drug available increased with increasing dosage. They therefore urge that once-a-day administration of imipramine for behavior disorders, where large doses are involved, should be discouraged.

C. DRUG INTERACTIONS

The fairly common practice of administering combinations of drugs to depressed patients (e.g., hypnotics and sedatives in addition to antidepressants) may have profound effects on the plasma level of the anti-depressant drug. The interactions of barbiturates with tricyclic antidepressants were elegantly demonstrated by Sjöqvist et al. (1968). This effect, i.e., the lowering of the plasma level of the drug of interest, is caused by stimulation (enzyme induction) of the hepatic microsomal enzyme system by the barbiturate drug (Conney, 1967, 1969; Prescott, 1971). This has particular pertinence for clinical practice, where barbiturates are often used as hypnotics. Because they lower tricyclic antidepressant plasma levels, they may interfere with the clinical efficacy of the latter. Burrow and Davies (1971) demonstrated a similar interaction between amylobarbitone and nortriptyline plasma levels.

Gram and Fredericson-Overø (1972) found that the administration of perphenazine to patients already receiving tricyclic antidepressant drugs resulted in an increase in the plasma level of the antidepressants. In studies with animals (Gram et al., 1974) the metabolism of ^{14}C-labeled imipramine and nortriptyline was studied after intraperitoneal administration of single doses of the drug. Results indicated that perphenazine inhibits the hydroxylation and/or glucuronide formation of imipramine, whereas demethylation, N-oxidation, and dealkylation seemed unaffected. These workers also stated that perphenazine and chlorpromazine appear to have equal potency in this effect.

Olivier-Martin et al. (1975) demonstrated that the administration of levopromazine together with imipramine to patients ($n = 6$) produced markedly increased DMI levels as compared to the administration of imipramine alone ($n = 18$). Moody et al. (1967) described a patient who, while receiving 75 mg of imipramine per day together with 150 mg of chlorpromazine, showed increased imipramine and DMI plasma levels.

Silverman and Braithwaite (1973) investigated the effect of several benzodiazepines (nitrazepam, diazepam, oxazepam, and chlordiazepoxide) on steady-state plasma levels of amitriptyline and nortriptyline and found no interaction. Gram et al. (1974) tested diazepam and chlordiazepoxide using ^{14}C-labeled nortriptyline and again found no significant pharmacokinetic interaction.

Zeidenberg et al. (1971) described a patient who showed clear clinical improvement when given methylphenidate in addition to imipramine. Wharton et al. (1971) investigated the effects of methylphenidate given to patients who were already in a steady state with respect to imipramine and observed a marked increase in both imipramine and DMI plasma levels. Five of seven patients so treated showed "prompt and striking" clinical recovery. Cooper and Simpson (1973) confirmed this observation in a difficult, treatment-resistant patient who despite high levels of imipramine and DMI showed no clinical improvement. After the addition of methylphenidate, the plasma level of imipramine and DMI increased, and clinical improvement was marked; the patient regressed when the methylphenidate was withdrawn (Fig. 5). Perel and Black (1970) demonstrated that this effect is caused by competitive inhibition of hydroxylation in the microsomal enzyme system.

Prange *et al.* (1969) have claimed a synergistic effect of triiodothyronine, thyroxine, and imipramine. The findings seem to indicate that the onset of clinically quantifiable recovery is accelerated if these hormones are administered together with imipramine. In a careful study, Wheatley (1972) confirmed the observation using amitriptyline, and this form of therapy is used by many clinicians who add thyroxine to patients' drug regimens when they have patients not responding to treatment. This effect, however, is not the result of an increased plasma level of the drug or its active metabolites (Simpson and Cooper, unpublished data).

It is clear that in studies involving tricyclic antidepressants, in which the patient needs additional medication, only drugs that have been tested and shown not to have any pharmacokinetic interaction should be used. That this has been a problem is demonstrated in the differences between Asberg's first study (Asberg *et al.*, 1971) and her second study in collaboration with Kragh-Sorensen *et al.* (1973). In the second study, the patients had significantly higher steady-state plasma levels ($141 \pm$ S.D., 42.8 ng/ml) than the patients in the first study ($92 \pm$ S.D., 33.1 ng/ml). Methodological errors were ruled out, since the method used in the second sample yielded slightly lower values, and the investigators have suggested that the use of barbiturates in the first study is the only logical explanation (Asberg, 1973).

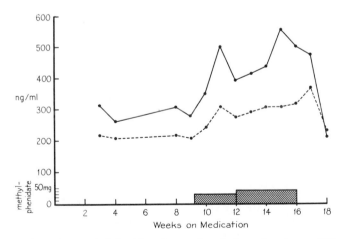

FIG. 5. Imipramine–methylphenidate interaction. Imipramine dosage 300 mg/day. Plasma levels: (———) IMI, (– – – –) DMI.

Many other drug interactions with tricyclic antidepressants have been documented, and for a detailed listing the publication by Hansten (1973) is recommended. The interactions discussed above are of clinical and theoretical importance in psychiatry and would not have been so readily interpreted had good analytical tools not been available.

D. PREDICTION OF PLASMA LEVELS OF DRUGS

Alexanderson (1972, 1973) clearly demonstrated the ability to predict steady-state plasma levels of nortriptyline and DMI from single-dose plasma level data (Table V). The area under the curve of the beta slope was calculated by collecting five blood samples for nortriptyline analysis beginning 20 hours after a single dose was given. Blood samples were then collected during the next 4–5 days without the patient being given additional medication. The ability to predict the steady-state level accurately has been confirmed by Alexanderson (1972) in a study of twins (monozygous and dizygous), in which he found that estimates of the pharmacokinetic parameters used in predicting the steady-state plasma levels in nortriptyline gave an accurate prediction of the steady-state data collected on the same subjects 2 years previously (thus demonstrating the stability of the parameters over time). The importance of the stability of these parameters over time cannot be overstated. Nortriptyline appears to be the only antidepressant for which we have reasonable though not unquestioned evidence of a therapeutic window (i.e., a lower and an upper threshold), and it would clearly be advantageous to determine individual patient dosage requirements for this medica-

TABLE V
COMPARISON OF OBSERVED STEADY-STATE VALUES
AND VALUES PREDICTED FROM SINGLE-DOSE
PLASMA CLEARANCE DATA[a]

Observed steady-state nortriptyline (ng/ml)[b]	Predicted steady-state nortriptyline (ng/ml)
110 ± 4.9	116
60.5 ± 1.3	53
51.7 ± 3.1	46
92.3 ± 3.0	78
76.7 ± 3.4	75
113.8 ± 5.8	119

[a] Reproduced with permission of Editors of *European Journal of Clinical Pharmacology* Vol. 4, pp. 82–91 (1972).
[b] Mean ± S.E.

tion. Thus patients could be brought rapidly to their optimal dosage based on a kinetic procedure and would achieve the therapeutic window within a reasonably short time. In addition, the physician would not be faced with a clinical decision of whether to increase or decrease the medication simply on an intuitive basis. The requirement of 4–5 days without medication to determine these parameters is not unreasonable when one considers the significant number of spontaneous remissions occurring during the first week of hospitalization. Again, this would benefit patients capable of rapid or slow biotransformation of the drug, in that rapid metabolizers could be built up to high levels efficiently, whereas slow metabolizers could be started on a lower dosage schedule than normally used. Asberg (1973) emphasized this point, stating that dosage adjustments based on clinical response have to be delayed until the response can be assessed with reasonable accuracy (usually several weeks). Dosage adjustment decisions based on plasma level analyses can be formed as soon as a steady-state level is reached (usually 1 week) but, with a predictive technique such as that described above, patients' requirements would be known within a week without the necessity for multiple adjustments.

Even without a clear therapeutic window or lower threshold, such techniques are of value in that they indicate which patients require much more or much less than the standard dose of medication.

E. Summary

The preceding data demonstrate that the availability of chemical methods with sufficient sensitivity has allowed the elucidation of many perplexing problems and testing of hypotheses, which were not possible by other means.

Studies on pharmacokinetics, first-pass effects, drug interactions, dosage predictions, etc., have been well executed, and the results are convincing.

The investigation into the relationship between plasma levels of a drug and clinical efficacy, however, have not been as well executed, nor are these data as convincing. The data of Braithwaite et al. (1972) for amitriptyline involved only 15 patients and the correlation ($r = 0.86$) was high, but it clearly must be confirmed in case it was fortuitous. To date, neither the original investigators nor other groups have done this.

The recent article by Gram et al. (1975) indicates that it may be necessary to have certain minimum levels of both imipramine and DMI in the plasma to achieve a therapeutic effect, but again the number of patients was small ($n = 24$), only 12 of whom were judged improved.

The Scandinavian workers appear to have demonstrated a therapeutic window for nortriptyline (Asberg et al., 1971; Kragh-Sorensen et al., 1975). Yet in a large number of patients and in several studies, Burrows et al.

(1974a,b) did not find a therapeutic range. Their work has been criticized because the patients were not in a steady state, the technique they used is difficult, and their patient population included neurotic depressives. However, the data from these investigators on specific patients relating improvement to blood levels is convincing evidence that, in their hands, the chemical technique is acceptable. In terms of the diagnosis criticism, Burrows *et al.* (1974a) state that the patients they studied are those that normally would be given tricyclic medication. Therefore one is left with the possibility that the Scandinavian workers used a diagnostic classification which enabled them to select a subpopulation that responds to tricyclic medication and in which the plasma level of the drug is correlated with clinical efficacy. This seems quite possible to us, because it is well documented that the reliability of most psychiatric diagnoses is quite low (Sandifer *et al.*, 1964), but that this reliability is improved if the psychiatrists involved are trained at or work at the same center (Kendell, 1973). The admirable way in which the Scandinavians work in collaboration with each other make the latter point particularly pertinent.

Thus it may be that for a specific subgroup of depressed patients a therapeutic window or at least a lower threshold for tricyclic antidepressants exists, but until more data are obtained such procedures remain of research interest rather than practical clinical tools.

IV. Neuroleptics

A. CHEMICAL METHODS

The methodology for the analysis of chlorpromazine has been critically reviewed by Usdin (1971). Representative techniques include direct scanning of thin-layer chromatographic plates (Turano and Turner, 1972; Chan and Gershon, 1973), thin-layer chromatography of dansylated derivatives with spectrofluorescent quantitation (Kaul *et al.*, 1970), radioactive derivative formation (Efron *et al.*, 1971), GLC–microcoulometric detection (Johnson and Burchfield, 1965), GLC–electron-capture detection (Curry, 1968), and GLC–mass fragmentography (Hammar *et al.*, 1968). Radioimmunoassay is also being investigated by Shostak (1973) and Spector (1974). Turner *et al.* (1976) have reported on an attempt to establish accuracy and precision in making specific metabolite determinations in a multicenter collaborative study in which the apparent inability to quantitate a variety of metabolites is most disturbing.

Thioridazine methods involve fluorescence techniques (Ragland *et al.*, 1965; Martin, 1966; Mellinger and Keeler, 1964; Pacha, 1969). Zingales

(1969) used TLC to determine thioridazine and chlorpromazine in red blood cells. One GLC method has been published (Curry and Mould, 1969), and a modification of this technique is referred to in Dinovo *et al.* (1974). Less extensively investigated neuroleptic drugs include: butaperazine, using fluorescence (Simpson *et al.*, 1973; Bruce *et al.*, 1974; Manier *et al.*, 1974); perphenazine and fluphenazine, using GLC–electron capture (Larsen and Naestoft, 1973; Hansen and Larsen, 1974); penfluridol, using GLC–electron capture (S. F. Cooper *et al.*, 1975; Airoldi *et al.*, 1974); thiothixene, using fluorescence (Mjorndal and Oreland, 1971) and GLC–mass fragmentography (Hobbs *et al.*, 1974); and butyrophenones (trifluperidol and halperidol), using GLC–electron capture (Zingales, 1971; Marcucci *et al.*, 1971a,b). An exquisitely sensitive technique for reserpine, utilizing TLC and fluorimetric scanning, has recently been described (Tripp *et al.*, 1975). Methods exist for other neuroleptics, but they have not been used to any extent in psychiatry to date.

B. CLINICAL STUDIES

Neuroleptics have not been studied in such detail as tricyclic antidepressants, with the notable exception of chlorpromazine and to a lesser extent three other drugs (thioridazine, butaperazine, and thiothixene). At two NIMH workshops, chlorpromazine and the clinical efficacy plasma level interface have been thoroughly investigated, and yet with few exceptions, all of which are yet to be confirmed, little of substance has been resolved. It was only recently that the 7-hydroxychlorpromazine metabolite was shown to cross the blood–brain barrier (Brookes *et al.*, 1970; Maickel *et al.*, 1971; Manian *et al.*, 1971), a possibility that many pharmacologists did not even consider. Huang and Ruskin (1964), using fluorimetric procedures, found levels 1–2 hours after administration of 200 mg of chlorpromazine to be 0–0.2 μg/ml and 0.3–1.9 μg/ml for chlorpromazine and chlorpromazine sulfoxide, respectively. These investigators found large variations among individuals and recorded the presence in serum of phenolic metabolites in excess of the nonphenolic compounds. No attempt was made to separate these individual metabolites. Wechsler *et al.* (1967) attempted separation of the individual metabolites by TLC but did not quantitate the data. With the introduction of the GLC–electron capture technique by Curry (1968), in contrast to the previously mentioned work, very different levels were found. These workers describe quantitation of chlorpromazine, chlorpromazine sulfoxide, and mono- and didemethylated chlorpromazine. Values were in the nanogram-per-milliliter range, as contrasted to the microgram-per-milliliter range reported by earlier workers. March *et al.* (1972), using a colorimetric procedure, demonstrated essentially the same large interpatient variability in nonphenolic chlorpromazine metabolites but did not separate these metabolites further. An example of the variability found in chronic schizophrenic populations who have been on a fixed regimen of medication for many months is seen in data we obtained in a study several years ago, which are presented in graphic form in Fig. 6. Some workers have claimed that the steady-state plasma chlorpromazine level varies considerably from day to day and, indeed, Curry (1970) has claimed 50% differences within a few minutes.

Curry et al. (1971) demonstrated in a isolated guinea pig ileum loop that only one-sixth of the dosage of chlorpromazine was absorbed unchanged, the remainder being metabolized in the gut wall before entering the portal circulation.

Curry et al. (1970) investigated factors affecting chlorpromazine levels in psychiatric patients, using intravenous, intramuscular, and oral dosage forms (liquid, tablets, and slow-release). These data were consistent with the route of administration, and large differences were demonstrated in the plasma level of the drug in individual patients receiving the same dosage, but for individual patients the plasma level appeared to be dose-related. In two bioequivalency studies in which steady-state plasma levels of chlor-promazine were measured on three consecutive days, this degree of varia-

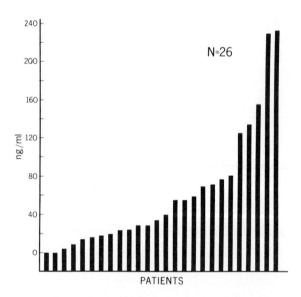

Fig. 6. Variation observed in steady-state plasma levels of chlorpromazine when patient received 200 mg b.i.d. [Reproduced with permission from "Pharmacokinetics of Psychoactive Drugs: Blood Levels and Clinical Response" (L. A. Gottschalk and S. Merlis, eds.). Spectrum Publ., New York. 1976.]

TABLE VI
STEADY-STATE PLASMA CHLORPROMAZINE LEVELS[a]

Patient number	Dose (mg/day)	Day 1	Day 2	Day 3
1	900	45	51	41
2	600	11	21	17
3	450	29	26	29
4	600	28	43	35
5	600	43	40	44
6	375	152	139	164
7	1200	140	139	100
8	900	109	87	79
9	650	28	11	22
10	650	100	114	126

[a] Samples collected from patients in a steady state on three consecutive days. All patients were on a t.i.d. regimen. All blood samples were collected immediately prior to morning dose. Values are given in nanograms per milliliter.

bility was not observed (Table VI). It is emphasized, however, that, when considerable variations are observed, in our experience this was always proven to be the result of improper supervision of administration of the medication. In this respect, for these studies one is tempted to insist on the use of liquid medication and that medication be administered only by staff capable of totally accurate dispensing and of checking that patients in fact swallow the medication.

1. Clinical Response and Plasma Levels

a. Chlorpromazine. Curry (1970) reported that a patient who had elevated levels of chlorpromazine (ca. 700 ng/ml) and who was aggressive and assaultive, improved markedly when her dosage was reduced and her plasma levels were ca. 300 ng/ml. Sakalis et al. (1972) gave chlorpromazine in a liquid form on a t.i.d. basis for 5–6 weeks and investigated a series of physiological parameters which they attempted to relate to drug plasma levels. They found that peripheral autonomic measures correlated with drug plasma levels, but changes in central measures were inconsistent. The drug plasma level and clinical improvement were weakly correlated and only during the first 2 weeks of a 6-week study. Physiological measures that changed significantly included blood pressure, pulse, pupil size, salivary excretion, palmar skin conductance, EEG, and evoked response. These investigators also demonstrated that the plasma levels of their patients steadily declined throughout the study, and suggest that this was due to enzyme induction by the drug itself. Loga et al. (1975) confirmed these findings in two studies in acutely ill psychotic patients receiving a fixed dosage of chlorpromazine (300 mg/day).

Mackay *et al.* (1974), in a large study (86 chronic schizophrenics), measured plasma concentrations of chlorpromazine, 7-hydroxychlorpromazine, and chlorpromazine sulfoxide. In general, the metabolites measured were of magnitude similar to that of the chlorpromazine concentration. These investigators again demonstrated the wide variability in the plasma level of the unchanged drug and metabolites among patients receiving similar daily doses, but of great interest was the observation that patients who were well controlled had higher concentrations of the biologically active 7-hydroxy metabolite, whereas patients who were poorly controlled had high levels of the inactive sulfoxide. The sulfoxide level was significant between groups ($p < 0.05$), and the average ratio of 7-hydroxychlorpromazine to the sulfoxide was significantly greater ($p < 0.01$) in well-controlled patients. The number of patients involved in this aspect of the study, however, was much smaller (a total of 12 patients), and presumably this ratio could not be determined in many of the patients. Inspection of the data indicates that many of the patients had extremely low drug plasma concentrations. Sakalis *et al.* (1973) provide some support for this observation; in a study of eight schizophrenic patients responders ($n = 4$) showed a relatively higher 7-hydroxychlorpromazine level, whereas nonresponders ($n = 4$) showed high sulfoxide levels.

Rivera-Calimlim *et al.* (1973) reported on plasma chlorpromazine levels in psychiatric patients monitored over a 6-week period and collected blood samples 2, 3, and 4 hours after a standard dose of chlorpromazine. Their study suggested that schizophrenic patients with negligible plasma levels (less than 30 ng/ml) are not likely to improve clinically. Most patients who showed clinical improvement achieved higher plasma levels (30–300 ng/ml). Patients showing toxicity, manifested in the form of tremors and convulsions, were shown to have high plasma levels (750–1000 ng/ml). Rivera-Calimlim *et al.* (1976), in a second study, claimed that the number of patients showing some degree of clinical improvement increased with increasing plasma levels up to the 100–300 ng/ml range. Above 300 ng/ml, few patients seemed to improve. These workers claim that patients on a single-dose regimen had "more consistent levels" compared to patients on a multiple-dose regimen (however, this experiment was not controlled by a cross-over design). This finding contradicts some of our work with butaperazine demonstrating that steady-state levels of the drug are lower the less frequently the medication is given (Bergner *et al.*, 1973; T. B. Cooper *et al.*, 1975b), especially when one considers that the plasma half-life of chlorpromazine is relatively short. This observation, however, is less critical in a situation in which a drug has a long half-life (e.g., amitriptyline).

Braithwaite *et al.* (1974), however, have recently demonstrated a trend (though not significant) to lower values of amitriptyline when patients were changed from a three-times-a-day regimen to a once-a-day regimen.

b. Butaperazine. Simpson *et al.* (1973) described two trials in which single loading doses of butaperazine were administered with different forms of butaperazine (tablet, concentrate, syrup, capsule, and intramuscular), and in the second trial they demonstrated clear differences between bioavailability when the intramuscular form was compared to the tablet or the concentrate. The peak levels for the intramuscular form occurred later than the peak levels obtained with oral doses of the medication. These workers state that there was a tendency for responders to have slightly higher steady-state levels than nonresponders, though the number of patients involved in this study was small.

Davis *et al.* (1974) demonstrated in a total of 19 schizophrenic patients that several pharmacokinetic parameters are highly correlated with steady-state blood levels. They report a linear relationship between dosage and plasma level and show that the curves obtained for acute and chronic administration are similar in shape. They analyze the initial curve with respect to steady-state blood level achieved with various dosages and report a very high correlation ($r = 0.9$) between the butaperazine peak, the area under the curve, and the half-life following acute administration of 20 and 40 mg of butaperazine. Peak height area under the curve and steady-state butaperazine levels were all highly correlated. These investigators also conclude from this study that chronic administration of butaperazine does not lead to marked changes in butaperazine metabolism. They also claim there is considerably less interpatient variation in butaperazine serum levels than in chlorpromazine levels.

T. B. Cooper *et al.* (1975b) demonstrated that there is a significant difference in the steady-state blood level of butaperazine depending on the frequency of administration, i.e., the more frequently the medication is given the higher the steady-state level. These workers also describe a patient who they claim showed clear evidence of enzyme induction with butaperazine. This patient was given a 40-mg single oral dose, and blood samples were collected for pharmacokinetic analysis during the next 24 hours. The patient was then given butaperazine for several weeks and showed a good clinical response with measurable blood levels. The clinical condition of the patient thereafter deteriorated, even though the medication was increased to 100 mg/day (butaperazine in the plasma was not measurable at this time). At this point an additional single loading dose kinetic was obtained, and the results of this experiment are shown in Fig. 7. It is emphasized that extreme care was taken to ensure that the patient took the

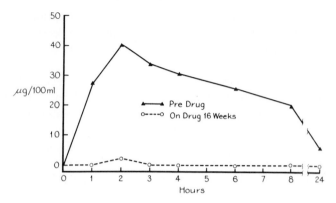

FIG. 7. Kinetic data obtained when patient was given a 40-mg single oral dose before receiving the drug and after 16 weeks of continuous medication. [Reproduced with permission of Editors of *Archives of General Psychiatry* Vol. 32, p. 903 (1975).]

medication, to the point that the patient was given the medication dissolved in a liquid and a technician stayed in the same room throughout the first 8 hours of blood collection.

c. Thioridazine. Buyze et al. (1973), in a study of chronic schizophrenic patients, found that the plasma level of the drug was dose-related ($n = 42$). In 53 patients receiving other medication concomitantly, this relationship did not hold, and the suggestion was made that this was evidence for drug interaction. This same study again demonstrates the large interindividual variability occurring when patients are given a fixed dosage. In a comparison of two forms of medication (standard and long-acting) the data indicated greater variability (a threefold change) during a cycle with the standard form than with the long-acting form. Of interest in this study was the observation that the variability of the drug plasma level while the patient was receiving the standard medication would have been obscured if a fluorimetric procedure rather than a GLC technique had been used, because the sum of the parent compound plus the various metabolites did not show this threefold change. A correlation of the parent compound and/or metabolites with respect to clinical efficacy was not found. Viukari and Salmimies (1973) compared standard and slow-release tablets and a suspension from different manufacturers, using blood level data. Standard preparations given two or three times daily showed comparable plasma levels, as did slow-release preparations given once per day. The suspension, however, gave lower plasma levels, which the investigators ascribe to a considerable loss due to the medication adhering to the dispensing cup.

Martensson and Roos (1973), in a study of 46 patients receiving less than 5 mg of thioridazine/kg body weight, demonstrated that plasma levels were significantly correlated with dosage and the age of the patient. The sex of the patient did not appear to have any effect on the data. In a study of 10 healthy volunteers the same investigators found no effect of weight or sex on the pharmacokinetics of the drug. Klein *et al.* (1975) made similar observations in 18 schizophrenic patients, but in addition claimed a curvilinear relationship between drug plasma level and remission of symptoms. Their data confirm the work of Buyze *et al.* (1973) (i.e., the plasma concentrations of the drug declined though the dosage was kept constant), which they suggest indicates the autoinduction of enzymes. DeJonghe *et al.* (1973) studied the blood level of thioridazine in a group of patients suffering from depression. They were unable to demonstrate a significant correlation between either dose or drug blood level and therapeutic range. Dinovo *et al.* (1974) and Gruenke *et al.* (1975) have reported the isolation and identification of a major metabolite of thioridazine and mesoridazine not previously described, and this work again emphasizes the importance of the requirement for specific methodology in this area.

d. Thiothixene. Mjorndal and Oreland (1971), using a fluorometric procedure, describe kinetic curves derived from five normal subjects given 20 mg of thiothixene. The method used was not specific in that approximately 40% of the demethylated metabolite was also measured as thiothixene. Hobbs *et al.* (1974) suggest that other metabolites may also interfere, because in a comparison of the fluorimetric method with a GLC–mass fragmentography procedure, using a deuterated thiothixene as an internal standard, the more specific GLC procedure gave results approximately 50% lower. These investigators noted in 20 chronic schizophrenic patients "titrated" to control symptoms that despite the widely different dosage schedules required (15–60 mg/day) the plasma levels fell within a narrow range (10–22.5 ng/ml), and suggest that in fact the individual dosage schedules were being adjusted to this therapeutic window.

e. Other Neuroleptics. Perphenazine quantitation in human blood has proven difficult to date, and little has been accomplished. Hansen and Larsen (1974) described a pilot study of perphenazine in three different formulations. These investigators noted that an acute dystonic reaction seen in one patient was related to a peak plasma level. The slow-release form of perphenazine tested showed a marked peak approximately 10–12 hours after injection. The plasma curve continued thereafter to remain at a constant lower level. S. F. Cooper *et al.* (1975) describe similar findings for penfluridol. This is probably indicative of free drug rather than the esterified long-acting form, but may have other pertinent interpretations.

C. Drug Interactions

Rivera-Calimlim *et al.* (1973) demonstrated a decrease in the steady-state plasma level of chlorpromazine when patients were given an anti-Parkinson medication (trihexyphenidyl) concomitantly. These workers suggested that this observation may be due to the anticholinergic effect of the drug on gastric motility and that this delay favors metabolism in the intestine wall. This finding was confirmed by Rivera-Calimlim *et al.* (1976). Loga *et al.* (1975) investigated the interaction of orphenadrine (an anti-Parkinson agent) and phenobarbitone with chlorpromazine. These investigators demonstrate that chlorpromazine levels fell with the addition of orphenadrine, but that these changes were relatively small; they suggested that orphenadrine acts by means of its anticholinergic effect rather than through a decrease in plasma chlorpromazine level.

El-Yousef and Manier (1974a) examined the effect of anti-Parkinson agents on the plasma level of butaperazine. Five patients were maintained on a b.i.d. fixed-dosage regimen for 5 weeks. One week was allowed to achieve a steady state. During the next 2-week period patients were given butaperazine alone, and at the start of the fourth week benztropine mesylate was administered. Blood samples were drawn 12 hours after the evening dose throughout the trial. Analysis of these data indicated that at least for the duration of the study there was no interaction between the anti-Parkinson medication and the butaperazine. El-Yousef and Manier (1974b) carried out a similar protocol in which they tested the effects of conjugated estrogens on plasma butaperazine levels in postmenopausal female subjects. Significantly higher butaperazine levels were found following a single loading dose, and with maintenance doses of butaperazine when conjugated estrogens were administered concomitantly, than when only butaperazine was administered. They discuss these findings in terms of possible changes in absorption or inhibition of microsomal enzyme activity, but state that a clear-cut relationship of estrogen and changes in plasma levels to clinical efficacy and side effects was not demonstrated.

D. Drug Plasma Levels and Prolactin Response

Single doses of chlorpromazine produce a rise in plasma prolactin levels in human subjects (Kleinberg *et al.*, 1971; Friesen *et al.*, 1972; Sachar, 1975). Sachar (1975) has suggested that, if prolactin response correlates with drug blood levels, prolactin level measures may replace drug blood measures, producing a physiological index of the actual degree of brain dopaminergic antagonism achieved in individual patients. Sachar (1975) also demonstrated the dose dependence of the prolactin response and that a patient who has a strong prolactin response to one drug also shows a similar response to other medication. Kolakowska *et al.* (1975) demonstrated a correlation between the plasma levels of prolactin and chlorpromazine in 14 subjects ($r = 0.60$). Plasma levels were measured 2 hours after the morning dose. A similar correlation was found ($r = 0.69$) with steady-state plasma levels. Correlations between prolactin levels and extrapyramidal side effects were examined in 12 patients. The results of this analysis are shown in Fig. 8. These investigators state that none of the patients with prolactin levels below 35 ng/ml showed extrapyramidal symptoms, while all patients with higher levels developed mild or moderate parkinsonism. Mean levels of chlorpromazine were also higher in patients with extrapyramidal side effects than in subjects free from these symptoms. These workers suggest that the therapeutic effect of chlorpromazine was not related to prolactin levels. However, the steady-state plasma chlorpromazine levels in this study were in many instances extremely low (high levels, 37 ± 27 ng/ml; low levels, 11 ± 7 ng/ml).

These reports are exciting, even though the number of subjects studied is small. Clearly a physiological measure such as prolactin release, if indicative of central nervous system activity of the drug and thus proof of penetration of the blood–brain barrier, may be a measure of considerable importance. Despite the essentially unproved status of the clinical efficacy–blood plasma level interface, if laboratories are needed to evaluate numerous drugs with a variety of fairly sophisticated techniques, this will be self-limiting. If, however, a few physiological measures can be found that correlate with improvement and/or side effects for particular groups of drugs, perhaps a laboratory will only be required to carry out three or four such assays as a routine. This clearly would be more feasible, and for this reason alone the hypothesis is attractive. However, the case is far from proven, and prolactin

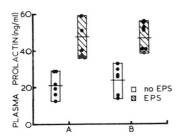

FIG. 8. Prolactin level and extrapyramidal side effects in 12 patients: A, individual means of morning plasma prolactin; B, individual means of plasma prolactin 2 hours after morning dose of chlorpromazine. [Reproduced with permission of Editors of *Psychological Medicine* Vol. 5, p. 214 (1975).]

level determinations require very much more technical expertise than many GLC techniques in use at this time.

E. SUMMARY

These neuroleptic data are disappointing in that considerable effort has been expended on chlorpromazine metabolism and clinical efficacy and yet Rivera-Calimlim *et al.* (1973, 1975) are the only group to claim a therapeutic range. Other investigators have demonstrated, though with very small numbers of patients, interesting differences in the metabolite profile of responders and nonresponders, and this clearly is an area that requires more detailed investigation. The clinical value of such metabolite profiles (does one change the medication or attempt to alter the metabolism?) are still to be determined. Similar statements apply to the other neuroleptics studied; indeed, these data appear to follow a depressingly similar pattern. In medical centers where such research is being done, the physician can use these facilities with benefit to detect drug defaulters and nonresponders who metabolize a drug rapidly, but the cost of setting up routine laboratory procedures for such a small group of patients is a luxury which in our opinion is not justified at this time. The imminent introduction of radio-immunoassay procedures may change this observation during the next few years, even if clinical efficacy and side effect relationships with plasma levels remain elusive.

V. Conclusion

There is no doubt that the investigation of plasma and whole-blood levels of drugs has been of considerable value to further understanding of the pharmacology and pharmacokinetics of psychotropic drugs. In as much as the clinical psychiatrist has gained insight into possible pitfalls in the use of these drugs (alone and in combination), these investigations have been of clinical value.

The clinical psychiatrist has gained some additional insight into treatment problems (e.g., drug interactions), but the exciting prospect of individually tailored medication schedules to optimize patient treatment has proven elusive.

Despite the considerable effort expended, the paucity of data attests to the difficulty in obtaining suitable patients for clinical efficacy studies and the practical (and ethical) problems encountered in maintaining patients in such studies for the duration of the experimental design.

However, it is essential that in future studies investigators

1. Clearly define the diagnostic criteria used to select patients for each study.
2. Ensure that, whenever appropriate, some initial period of placebo medication is part of the experimental design to reduce the variance introduced by early spontaneous remission or placebo response.
3. Utilize improvement rating scales which are accepted and have been cross-validated.
4. Ensure that medication is given at reasonably equal time intervals and that blood samples are collected immediately prior to the next dose of medication to ensure data that will be comparable across studies.
5. Take special care to check that the patient does indeed ingest the medication (not a trivial task).
6. Avoid as much as possible the concomitant administration of other medication, and if for ethical reasons this is not possible use only medications that do not interact with the drug of interest.

We strongly urge that such well-designed experiments be carried out and that sufficiently large sample sizes be studied. If such criteria are met, the promise of positive findings seems high, and meaningful practical clinical findings will ensue.

ACKNOWLEDGMENTS

The expert technical assistance of Mr. D. Allen, Mrs. R. Lonow, Mrs. A. Meister, and Mrs. B. Katof is gratefully acknowledged. Mrs. S. Marsico is especially thanked for her secreterial assistance in the preparation of the manuscript.

This work was supported in part by grants MH 08240 and GRS 05651.

REFERENCES

Airoldi, L., Marcucci, F., Mussini, E., and Garattini, S. (1974). *Eur. J. Pharmacol.* 25, 291.
Alexanderson, B. (1972). *Eur. J. Clin. Pharmacol.* 4, 82.
Alexanderson, B. (1973). *Eur. J. Clin. Pharmacol.* 6, 44.
Alexanderson, B., and Borga, O. (1972). *Eur. J. Clin. Pharmacol.* 4, 196.
Alexanderson, B., Evans, D. A., and Sjöqvist, F. (1969). *Br. Med. J.* 4, 764.
Amdisen, A. (1968). *Scand. J. Clin. Lab. Invest.* 20, 104.
Angst, J., and Rothweiler, R. (1974). *In* "Classification and Prediction of Outcome of Depression" (J. Angst, ed.), Symp. Med. Hoechst No. 8, pp. 237–244. Schattauer, Stuttgart.
Asberg, M. (1973). M.D. Dissertation, Karolinska Institutet, Stockholm, Sweden.
Asberg, M., Cronholm, B., Sjöqvist, F., and Tuck, D. (1971). *Br. Med. J.* 3, 331.
Beckmann, H., and Goodwin, F. K. (1975). *Arch. Gen. Psychiatry* 32, 17.
Bergner, P.-E. E., Berniker, K., Cooper, T. B., Gradijan, J. R., and Simpson, G. M. (1973). *Br. J. Pharmacol.* 49, 328.

Bertilsson, L., Asberg, M., and Thoren, P. (1974). *Eur. J. Clin. Pharmacol.* **7**, 365.
Blashki, T. G., Mowbray, R., and Davies, B. (1971). *Br. Med. J.* **1**, 133.
Blijenberg, B. G., and Leijnse, B. (1968). *Clin. Chim. Acta* **19**, 97.
Borga, O., and Garle, M. (1972). *J. Chromatogr.* **68**, 77.
Borga, O., Azarnoff, D. L., Forshell, G. M., and Sjöqvist, F. (1969). *Biochem. Pharmacol.* **18**, 2135.
Braithwaite, R. A. (1974). Presented at *World Psychiatr. Assoc. Workshop Biol. Deficit Affective Disorders.*
Braithwaite, R. A., and Widdop, B. (1971). *Clin. Chim. Acta* **35**, 461.
Braithwaite, R. A., Goulding, R., Theano, G., Bailey, J., and Coppen, A. (1972). *Lancet* **1**, 1297.
Braithwaite, R. A., Nakra, B. R. S., and Grand, R. (1974). *Psychol. Med.* **4**, 338.
Brookes, L. G., Holmes, M. A., Serra, M. T., and Forrest, I. S. (1970). *Proc. West. Pharmacol. Soc.* **13**, 127.
Brown, P. B., and Legg, E. R. (1970). *Ann. Clin. Biochem.* **7**, 13.
Brown, W. T. (1973). *Can. Med. Assoc. J.* **108**, 742.
Bruce, R. B., Turnball, L. B., Newman, J. H., Kinzie, J. M., Morris, P. H., and Pinchbeck, F. M. (1974). *Xenobiotica* **4**, 197.
Burrows, G. D. (1972). M.D. Thesis, University of Melbourne, Melbourne, Australia.
Burrows, G. D., and Davies, B. (1971). *Br. Med. J.* **4**, 113.
Burrows, G. D., Davies, B., and Scoggins, B. A. (1972). *Lancet* **2**, 619.
Burrows, G. D., Scoggins, B. A., and Davies, B. (1974a). In "Classification and Prediction of Outcome of Depression" (J. Angst, ed.), Symp. Med. Hoechst No. 8, pp. 173–179. Schattauer, Stuttgart.
Burrows, G. D., Turece, K., Davies, B., Mowbray, R., and Scoggins, B. (1974b). *Aust. N. Z. J. Psychiatry* **8**, 21.
Buyze, G., Egberts, P. F. C., Muunsze, R. G., and Poslavska, A. (1973). *Psychiatr., Neurol., Neurochir.* **76**, 229.
Cade, J. F. J. (1949). *Med. J. Aust.* **36**, 349.
Carlsson, A. (1966). *Handb. Exp. Pharmakol.* **19**, 529–592.
Carlsson, A., Corrodi, H., Fuxe, K., and Hokfelt, T. (1969). *Eur. J. Pharmacol.* **5**, 357.
Carroll, B. J. (1975). Personal communication.
Chan, T. L., and Gershon, S. (1973). *Mikrochim. Acta* **4**, 435.
Conney, A. H. (1967). *Pharmacol. Rev.* **19**, 317.
Conney, A. H. (1969). *N. Engl. J. Med.* **280**, 653.
Coombs, H. I. (1971). *Br. J. Psychiatry* **118**, 225.
Cooper, S. F., Albert, J. M., and Dugal, R. (1975). *Int. Pharmacopsychiatry* **10**, 78.
Cooper, T. B., and Simpson, G. M. (1973). *Am. J. Psychiatry* **130**, 721.
Cooper, T. B., and Simpson, G. M. (1976). *Am. J. Psychiatry* **133**, 440.
Cooper, T. B., Bergner, P.-E. E., and Simpson, G. M. (1973). *Am. J. Psychiatry* **130**, 601.
Cooper, T. B., Simpson, G. M., and Allen, D. (1974). *At. Absorp. Newsl.* **13**, 119.
Cooper, T. B., Allen, D., and Simpson, G. M. (1975a). *Psychopharmacol. Comm.* **1**, 445.
Cooper, T. B., Simpson, G. M., Haher, E. J., and Bergner, P.-E. E. (1975b). *Arch. Gen. Psychiatry* **32**, 903.
Cooper, T. B., Allen, D., and Simpson, G. M. (1976). *Psychopharmacol. Comm.* (in press).
Curry, S. H. (1968). *Anal. Chem.* **40**, 1251.
Curry, S. H. (1970). *J. Pharm. Pharmacol.* **22**, 753.

Curry, S. H., and Mould, G. P. (1969). *J. Pharm. Pharmacol.* 21, 674.
Curry, S. H., Davis, J. M., Janowska, D. S., and Marshall, J. H. L. (1970). *Arch. Gen. Psychiatry* 22, 209.
Curry, S. H., D'Mello, A., and Mould, G. P. (1971). *Br. J. Pharmacol.* 42, 403.
Davis, J. M., Janowska, D. S., Sekerti, H. J., Manier, D., and El-Yousef, M. K. (1974). *In* "Phenothiazines and Structurally Related Drugs" (I. S. Forrest, C. J. Carr, and E. Usdin, eds.), pp. 433–443. Raven, New York.
DeJonghe, F. E., Van Der Helm, H. J., Schalken, H. F., and Thiel, J. H. (1973). *Acta Psychiatr. Scand.* 49, 535.
Dinovo, E. C., Gottschalk, L. A., Nobel, E. P., and Biener, R. (1974). *Res. Commun. Chem. Pathol. Pharmacol.* 7, 489.
Dorus, E., Pandey, G. M., Frazer, A., and Mendels, J. (1974). *Arch. Gen. Psychiatry* 31, 463.
Dorus, E., Pandey, G. M., Davis, J., and Dekirmenjian, H. (1975). *Am. Psychiatr. Assoc. Meet., 1975, Sci. Proc. Summary Form* p. 167.
Efron, D. H., Harris, S. R., Manian, A. A., and Gaudette, L. E. (1971). *Psychopharmacologia* 19, 207.
Elizur, A., Shopsin, B., Gershon, S., and Ehlenberger, A. (1972). *Clin. Pharmacol. Ther.* 13, 947.
El-Yousef, M. K., and Manier, D. H. (1974a). *Am. J. Psychiatry* 131, 471.
El-Yousef, M. K., and Manier, D. H. (1974b). *Psychopharmacologia* 39, 39.
Ervik, M., Walle, T., and Ehrsson, H. (1970). *Acta Pharm. Seuc.* 7, 625.
Fann, W. E., Davis, J., Janowska, D., Kaufmann, J. S., Griffith, J. D., and Oates, J. A. (1972). *Arch. Gen. Psychiatry* 26, 158.
Fournis, Y., and Chazot, G. (1971). *Pathol. Biol.* 19, 787.
Frazer, A., Secunda, S. K., and Mendels, J. (1972). *Clin. Chim. Acta* 36, 499.
Frazer, A., Mendels, J., Secunda, S. K., Cochrane, C. M., and Bianchi, C. P. (1973). *J. Psychiatr. Res.* 10, 1.
Frederickson-Overø, K. F. (1972). *Acta Pharmacol. Toxicol.* 3, 433.
Freyschuss, U., Sjöqvist, F., and Tuck, D. (1970). *Pharmacol. Clin.* 2, 72.
Friesen, H. G., Guyda, H., Hwang, P., Tyson, J. E., and Barbeau, A. (1972). *J. Clin. Invest.* 51, 706.
Frigerio, A., Belvedere, G., De Nadai, F., Fanelli, R., Pantarotto, C., Riva, E., and Morselli, P. L. (1972). *J. Chromatogr.* 74, 201.
Gershon, S. (1970). *Clin. Pharmacol. Ther.* 11, 168.
Glassman, A. H., Hurwic, M. J., and Perel, J. M. (1973). *Am. J. Psychiatry* 130, 1367.
Glassman, A. H., Kantor, S. J., and Shostak, M. (1975). *Am. J. Psychiatry* 132, 716.
Gram, L. F., and Christiansen, J. (1975). *Clin. Pharmacol. Ther.* 17, 555.
Gram, L. F., and Frederickson-Overø, K. (1972). *Br. Med. J.* 1, 463.
Gram, L. F., Frederickson-Overø, K., and Kirk, L. (1974). *Am. J. Psychiatry* 131, 863.
Gram, L. F., Reisby, N., Ibsen, I., Nagy, A., Dencher, S., Beck, P., Peterson, G., and Christiansen, J. (1975). *Clin. Pharmacol. Ther.* 19, 318.
Gruenke, L. D., Craig, J. C., Dinova, E. C., Gottschalk, L. A., Noble, E. P., and Biener, R. (1975). *Res. Commun. Chem. Pathol. Pharmacol.* 10, 221.
Hamberger, B., and Tuck, J. R. (1974). Cited in Bertilsson *et al.* (1974).
Hammar, C.-G., Holmstedt, B., and Ryhage, R. (1968). *Anal. Biochem.* 25, 533.
Hammar, C.-G., Alexanderson, B. Holmstedt, B., and Sjöqvist, F. (1971). *Clin. Pharmacol. Ther.* 12, 496.

Hammer, W. M., and Brodie, B. (1967). *J. Pharmacol. Exp. Ther.* **157,** 503.

Hammer, W. M., and Sjöqvist, F. (1967). *Life Sci.* **6,** 1895.

Hammer, W. M., Martens, S., and Sjöqvist, F. (1969). *Clin. Pharmacol. Ther.* **10,** 44.

Hansen, E. E., and Larsen, N.-E. (1974). *Psychopharmacologia* **37,** 31.

Hansten, P. D. (1973). "Drug Interaction." Lea & Febiger, Philadelphia, Pennsylvania.

Harris, S. R., Gaudette, L. E., Efron, D. H., and Manian, A. A. (1970). *Life Sci.* **9,** 781.

Haydu, G. G., Dhrymiotis, A., and Quinn, G. P. (1962). *Am. J. Psychiatry* **119,** 574.

Hermann, B., and Pulver, R. (1960). *Arch. Int. Pharmacodyn. Ther.* **126,** 454.

Hermann, B., Schindler, W., and Pulver, R. (1959). *Med. Exp.* **1,** 381.

Hobbs, D. C., Welch, W. M., Short, M. J., Moody, W. A., and Van Der Velde, C. D. (1974). *Clin. Pharmacol. Ther.* **16,** 473.

Hokin-Neaverson, M., Spiegel, D. A., and Lewis, W. C. (1974). *Life Sci.* **15,** 1739.

Horncastle, D. C. (1973). *Med., Sci. Law* **13,** 3.

Huang, C. L., and Ruskin, B. H. (1964). *J. Nerv. Ment. Dis.* **139,** 381.

Hucker, H. B., and Stauffer, S. C. (1974). *J. Pharm. Sci.* **63,** 296.

Johnson, D. E., and Burchfield, H. P. (1965). *In* "Lectures on Gas Chromatography: Vol. 2. Agricultural and Biological Application" (L. R. Mattick and H. A. Szymanski, eds.), Vol. 2, p. 109. Plenum, New York.

Jorgensen, A. (1975). *Acta Pharmacol. Toxicol.* **36,** 79.

Kantor, S. J., Bigger, J. T., Glassman, A. H., Macken, M. D., and Perel, J. M. (1975). *J. Am. Med. Assoc.* **231,** 1364.

Kaul, P. N., Conway, M. W., Clark, M. L., and Huffine, J. (1970). *J. Pharm. Sci.* **59,** 1745.

Kendell, R. E. (1968). "The Classification of Depressive Illnesses." Oxford Univ. Press, London and New York.

Kendell, R. E. (1973). *Br. J. Psychiatry* **122,** 437.

Klaus, R. (1971). *Z. Klin. Chem. Klin. Biochem.* **9,** 107.

Klein, H. E., Chaldra, O., and Matussek, N. (1975). *Pharmakopsychiatr. Neuro-Psychopharmakol.* **8,** 122.

Kleinberg, D. L., Noel, L. G., and Frantz, A. G. (1971). *J. Clin. Endocrinol. Metab.* **33,** 873.

Kolakowska, T., Wiles, D. H., McNeilly, A. S., and Gelder, M. G. (1975). *Psychol. Med.* **5,** 214.

Kragh-Sorensen P. (1974). *In* "Classification and Prediction of Outcome of Depression" (J. Angst, ed.), Symp. Med. Hoechst No. 8, p. 197. Schattauer, Stuttgart.

Kragh-Sorensen, P., Hansen, C. E., and Asberg, M. (1973). *Acta Psychiatr. Scand.* **49,** 444.

Kragh-Sorensen, P., Bastrup, P. C., Hansen, C. E., and Hvidberg, E. F. (1975). *Am. Psychiatr. Assoc. Meet., 1975, Sci. Proc. Summary Form* p. 169.

Kuhn, R. (1957). *Schweiz. Med. Wochenschr.* **87,** 1135.

Kupfer, D. J., Picker, D., Himmelhock, J. M., and Detre, T. P. (1975). *Arch. Gen. Psychiatry* **32,** 866.

Lader, M. (1974). *Br. J. Pharmacol.* **1,** 281.

Lapin, I. P., and Oxenkrug, G. F. (1969). *Lancet* 1, 132.

Larsen, N.-E., and Naestoft, J. (1973). *Med. Lab. Technol.* 30, 129.

Levy, A. L., and Katz, E. M. (1970). *Clin. Chem.* 16, 840.

Loga, S., Curry, S., and Lader, M. (1975). *Br. J. Clin. Pharmacol.* 2, 197.

Lyttkens, L., Soderberg, U., and Wetterberg, L. (1973). *Lancet* 1, 40.

Maas, J. A., Fawcett, J. A., and Dekirmenjian, H. (1972). *Arch. Gen. Psychiatry* 26, 252.

Mackay, A. V. P., Healey, A. F., and Baker, J. (1974). *Br. J. Clin. Pharmacol.* 1, 425.

Maggs, R. (1968). *Proc. World Congr. Psychiatry, 4th, 1966* (J. J. López Ibor, ed.), p. 2211. Excerpta Med. Found., Amsterdam.

Maickel, R. P., Potter, W. Z., and Manian, A. A. (1971). *Fed. Proc., Fed. Am. Soc. Exp. Biol.* 30, 336.

Malenfant, A. L. (1970). *Am. Lab.* 2, 9.

Manian, A. A., Efron, D. H., and Harris, S. R. (1971). *Life Sci.* 10, 679.

Manier, D. H., Sekerke, H. J., Dingell, J. V., and El-Yousef, M. K. (1974). *Clin. Chim. Acta* 57, 225.

March, J. E., Donato, D., Turano, P., and Turner, W. J. (1972). *J. Med.* 3, 146.

Marcucci, F., Airoldi, L., Mussini, E., and Garattini, S. (1971a). *J. Chromatogr.* 59, 174.

Marcucci, F., Mussini, E., Airoldi, L., Fanelli, R., Frigerio, A., DeNadai, F., Bizzi, A., Rizzo, M., Morselli P. L., and Garattini, S. (1971b). *Clin. Chim. Acta* 34, 321.

Martensson, E., and Roos, B. E. (1973). *Eur. J. Clin. Pharmacol.* 6, 181.

Martin, E. A. (1966). *Can. J. Chem.* 44, 1783.

Mellinger, T. J., and Keeler, C. E. (1964). *Anal. Chem.* 36, 1840.

Mendels, J. (1973). *In* "Lithium: Its Role in Psychiatric Research Treatment" (S. Gershon and B. Shopsin, eds.), p. 253. Plenum, New York.

Mendels, J., and Frazer, A. (1973). *J. Psychiatr. Res.* 10, 9.

Mendels, J., and Frazer, A. (1974). *Am. J. Psychiatry* 121, 1240.

Mjorndal, T., and Oreland, L. (1971). *Acta Pharmacol. Toxicol.* 29, 295.

Moody, J. P., Tait, A. C., and Todrick, A. (1967). *Br. J. Psychiatry* 113, 183.

Muscettola, G. B., Giovannucci, M., Montanini, R., Morselli, P. L., and Garattini, S. (1972). *Rev. Eur. Etud. Clin. Biol.* 17, 375.

Nagy, A., and Treiber, L. (1973). *J. Pharm. Pharmacol.* 25, 599.

Naylor, G. J., and Dick, D. A. T. (1974). *Lancet* 1, 97.

Naylor, G. J., Dick, D. A. T., Dick, E. G., Le Poidevin, D., and Whyte, S. F. (1973). *Psychol. Med.* 3, 502.

Naylor, G. J., Dick, D. A. T., Dick, E. G., and Moody, J. P. (1974). *Psychopharmacologia* 37, 81.

Olivier-Martin, R., Marzin, D., Buschenschutz, E., Pichot, P., and Boissier, J. (1975). *Psychopharmacologia* 41, 187.

Pacha, W. L. (1969). *Experientia* 25, 103.

Perel, J. M., and Black, M. (1970). *Fed. Proc., Fed. Am. Soc. Exp. Biol.* 29, 345.

Perel, J. M., O'Brien, L., Black, G. D., Bellward, G. D., and Dayton, P. G. (1974). *In* "Phenothiazines and Structurally Related Drugs" (I. S. Forrest, C. J. Carr, and E. Usdin, eds.), p. 201. Raven, New York.

Prange, A. J., Jr., Wilson, I. C., Rabon, A. M., and Lipton, M. A. (1969). *Present Status Psychotropic Drugs, Proc. Int. Congr. Coll. Int. Neuro-Psychopharmacol., 6th, 1968* Excerpta Med. Found., Int. Congr. Ser. No. 180, p. 532.

Prescott, L. F. (1971). *Scott. Med. J.* **16**, 121.
Prien, R. F., Caffey, E. M., and Klett, D. J. (1972). *Arch. Gen. Psychiatry* **26**, 146.
Pybus, J., and Bowers, G. N., Jr. (1970). *Clin. Chem.* **16**, 139.
Ragland, J. B., Kinross-Wright, V. J., and Ragland, R. (1965). *Anal. Biochem.* **12**, 60.
Rivera-Calimlim, L., Casteneda, L., and Lasagna, L. (1973). *Clin. Pharmacol. Ther.* **14**, 978.
Rivera-Calimlim, L., Nasrallah, J., Strauss, J., and Lasagna, L. (1976). *Am. J. Psychiatry* **133**, 646.
Robertson, R., Fritze, K., and Grof, P. (1973). *Clin. Chim. Acta* **45**, 25.
Rybakowski, J., Chlopacka, M., Kapelski, Z., Hernacha, B., Szajnerman, Z., and Kasprzak, K. (1974a). *Int. Pharmacopsychiatry* **9**, 166.
Rybakowski, J., Chlopacka, M., Lisowska, J., and Czerwinski, A. (1974b). *Psychiatr. Pol.* **2**, 129.
Ryhage, R., and Swedish Medical Research Council. (1968). *Anal. Biochem.* **25**, 532.
Sachar, E. (1976). "Neuro-Regulators and Psychiatric Disorders" (E. Usdin, D. Hamburg, and J. Barcus, eds.). Oxford Univ. Press, London and New York (in press).
Sakalis, G., Curry, S. H., Mould, G. P., and Lader, M. H. (1972). *Clin. Pharmacol. Ther.* **13**, 931.
Sakalis, G., Chan, T. L., Gershon, G., and Park, S. (1973). *Psychopharmacologia* **32**, 279.
Sandifer, M. G., Pettus, C., and Quade, D. (1964). *J. Nerv. Ment. Dis.* **139**, 350.
Schildkraut, J. J. (1965). *Am. J. Psychiatry* **122**, 509.
Schildkraut, J. J. (1973). *Annu. Rev. Pharmacol.* **13**, 427.
Schless, A., Frazer, A., Mendels, J., Pandey, G., and Theodorides, V. (1975). *Arch. Gen. Psychiatry* **32**, 337.
Schou, M. (1968). *J. Psychiatr. Res.* **6**, 67.
Schou, M. (1969). *Present Status Psychotropic Drugs, Proc. Int. Congr. Coll. Int. Neuro-Psychopharmacol., 6th, 1968* Excerpta Med. Found. Int. Congr. Ser. No. 180, pp. 120–122.
Schou, M., Baastrup, P. C., Grof, P., Weis, P., and Angst, J. (1970). *Br. J. Psychiatry* **116**, 615.
Schou, M., Amdisen, A., and Baastrup, P. C. (1971). *Br. J. Hosp. Med.* **6**, 53.
Sedval, G., Petterson, U., and Fyrov, B. (1970). *Pharmacol. Clin.* **2**, 231.
Seifert, R., Bremkamp, H., and Junge, C. (1975). *Psychopharmacologia* **43**, 285.
Shostak, M. (1973). *Psychopharmacol. Bull.* **9**, 24.
Sideman, L. (1970). *Clin. Chem.* **16**, 618.
Silverman, G., and Braithwaite, R. A. (1973). *Br. Med. J.* **3**, 18.
Simpson, G. M., Lament, R., Cooper, T. B., Lee, J. H., and Bruce, R. B. (1973). *J. Clin. Pharmacol.* **13**, 288.
Simpson, G. M., Cooper, T. B., and Lee, J. H. (1976a). In "Depression: Behavioral, Biochemical, Diagnostic and Treatment Concepts" (D. M. Gallant and G. M. Simpson, eds.), p. 109. Spectrum Publ., New York.
Simpson, G. M., Lee, J. H., Cuculic, Z., and Kellner, R. (1976b). *Arch. Gen. Psychiatry* (in press).
Sisenwine, S. F., Knowles, J. A., and Ruelins, H. W. (1969). *Anal. Lett.* **2**, 315.
Sjöqvist, F., Hammer, W., Idestrom, C.-M., Lind, M., Tuck, D., and Åsberg, M., (1968). *Proc. Eur. Soc. Study Drug Toxic.* **9**, 246.
Sjöqvist, F., Hammer, W., Borga, O., and Azarnoff, D. (1969). *Present Status*

Psychotropic Drugs, Proc. Int. Congr. Coll. Int. Neuro-Psychopharamacol., 6th, 1968 Excerpta Med. Found. Int. Congr. Ser. No. 180, p. 128.

Soucek, K., Zvolsky, P., Krulik, R., Filip, V., Vinarova, E., and Dostal, T. (1974). *Act. Nerv. Super.* **16**, 193.

Spector, S. (1974). *Adv. Biochem. Psychopharmacol.* **9**, 363.

Tripp, S. L., Williams, E., Wagner, W. E., Jr., and Lukas, G. (1975). *Life Sci.* **16**, 116.

Turano, P., and Turner, W. J. (1972). *J. Chromatogr.* **64**, 347.

Turner, W. J., Turano, P., and Badzinski, S. (1976). *In* "Pharmacokinetics of Psychoactive Drugs: Blood Levels and Clinical Response" (L. A. Gottschalk and S. M. Merlis, eds.), p. 33. Spectrum Publ., New York.

Usdin, E. (1971). *Crit. Rev. Clin. Lab. Sci.* **2**, 347.

Vesell, E. (1974). *Clin. Pharmacol. Exp.* **16**, 212.

Villeneuve, A., Dery, R., and Genest, P. H. (1971). *Clin. Biochem.* **4**, 194.

Viukari, N. M., and Salmimies, P. (1973). *Lancet* **2**, 1271.

Walle, T., and Ehrsson, J. (1971). *Acta Pharm. Suec.* **8**, 27.

Walter, C. J. S. (1971). *Proc. R. Soc. Med.* **64**, 282.

Warwick, L. H. (1966). *Dis. Nerv. Syst.* **27**, 527.

Wechsler, M. B., Warton, R. N., Tanato, E., and Malitz, S. (1967). *J. Psychiatr. Res.* **5**, 327.

Wharton, R. N., Perel, J. M., Dayton, P. G., and Malitz, S. (1971). *Am. J. Psychiatry* **127**, 55.

Wheatley, D. (1972). *Arch. Gen. Psychiatry* **26**, 229.

Winsberg, B. G., Perel, J. M., Hurwic, M. J., and Klutch, A. (1974). *In* "The Phenothiazines and Structurally Related Drugs" (I. S. Forrest, C. J. Carr, and E. Usdin, eds.), p. 425. Raven, New York.

Winsberg, B. G., Goldstein, S., Yepes, L., and Perel, J. M. (1975). *Am. J. Psychiatry* **132**, 542.

Wittrig, J., Anthony, E. J., and Lucarno, H. E. (1970). *Dis. Nerv. Syst.* **31**, 408.

Yates, C. M., Todrick, A., and Tait, A. C. (1963). *J. Pharm. Pharmacol.* **15**, 432.

Zakowska-Dabrowska, T., and Rybakowski, J. (1973). *Acta Psychiatr. Scand.* **49**, 457.

Zeidenberg, P., Perel, P., Kanzler, M., Wharton, R. N., and Malitz, S. (1971). *Am. J. Psychiatry* **127**, 1321.

Zingales, I. A. (1969). *J. Chromatogr.* **44**, 547.

Zingales, I. A. (1971). *J. Chromatogr.* **54**, 15.

SUBJECT INDEX

A

Acetaldehyde, from ethanol metabolism, oxidation of, 127
N-Acetylation, of microamines in invertebrates, 192
Acetylcholine, in brain ethanol effects on, 147
Active transport, ethanol effects on, 140–143
Adenylate cyclase
  apomorphine activation of, 248–249
  in brain, ethanol effects on, 139
Addiction, neurotransmitter role in, 155
Adrenaline
  determination of, 180
  structure of, 175
Aggression, apomorphine effects on, 241
Alcohol, see Ethanol
Alcohol dehydrogenase (ADH)
  ethanol metabolism by
    in brain, 125–126
    in liver, 128–129
Alcoholic mothers, offspring abnormalities in, 156–160
Aldehyde dehydrogenase, in acetaldehyde oxidation, 127
Aldehyde reductase, in acetaldehyde oxidation, 128
Amino acids, effect on alcohol metabolism, 166–167
γ-Aminobutyric acid, see GABA
4-Aminobutyrate 2-oxoglutarate aminotransferase, ethanol effects on, 150
Amnesia
  frontal lobe type, 11–14
  hippocampal lesions and, 1–49
  temporal lobe type, 10–11
Annelids, octopamine function in, 210–211
Apomorphine, 225–268
  adenylate cyclase activation by, 248–249

biochemistry of, 244–252
chemistry of, 226–231
clinical data of, 226
effects on
  aggression, 241
  blood pressure, 233
  convulsions, 234
  dopamine turnover and receptors, 244–248
  EEG, 234
  hormone release, 233–234
  locomotor activity, 240–241
  metabolism, 234
  neurotransmitter release, 250–252
  sexual behavior, 242
as emetic, 231–232
hyperthermic response to, 232–233
in vitro binding to brain dopamine receptors, 249–250
mechanism of action of, 254
modification of, 227–231
narcotic analgesics and, 252–256
neuropsychopharmacology of, 235–244
in perception of noxious stimuli, 253
pharmacology of, 231–234
self-administration of, 254
stereotyped behavior from, 235–240
Arthropods, octopamine function in, 205–207

B

Biogenic amines. (See also Microamines)
  ethanol effects on urinary excretion of, 151–152
Blood pressure, apomorphine effects on, 233
Brain
  ethanol effects on, 130–136
    carbon dioxide metabolism, 132–133
    energy metabolism, 136–139
    oxidative metabolism, 130–132
    oxygen metabolism, 131–132
    redox changes, 135–136
    TCA cycle in, 134–135

311

CONTENTS OF PREVIOUS VOLUMES

317

A 6
B 7
C 8
D 9
E 0
F 1
G 2
H 3
I 4
J 5